N. Talal H. M. Moutsopoulos
S. S. Kassan (Eds.)

Sjögren's Syndrome

Clinical and Immunological Aspects

With 51 Figures and 63 Tables

Springer-Verlag Berlin Heidelberg New York
London Paris Tokyo

Norman Talal, M. D.
The University of Texas Health Science Center at San Antonio
7703 Floyd Curl Drive
San Antonio, TX 78284-7874, USA

Haralampos M. Moutsopoulos, M. D., F. A. C. P.
Department of Internal Medicine
School of Medicine
453 32 Ioannina, Greece

Stuart S. Kassan, M. D., F. A. C. P.
Rehabilitation Center, Lutheran Medical Center,
7760 West 38th Avenue 290
Wheat Ridge, CO 80033, USA

ISBN 978-3-642-50120-3 ISBN 978-3-642-50118-0 (eBook)
DOI 10.1007/978-3-642-50118-0

Library of Congress Cataloging-in-Publication Data
Sjögren's syndrome. Bibliography: p. Includes index. 1. Sjogren's syndrome. 2. Sjogren's syndrome - Immunological aspects. I. Talal, Norman.
II. Moutsopoulos, Haralampos M. III. Kassan, Stuart S.
RC647.5.S5S56 1987 616.4 87-4860
ISBN 978-3-642-50120-3

Softcover reprint of the hardcover 1st edition 1987

2127/3145-5 4 3 2 1 0

Dedication

This book is dedicated to the memory of Henrik Sjögren who died in September 1986 from pneumonia after being confined to a nursing home for several years because of a stroke. He will long be remembered for his enthusiasm, his love of teaching and his important contributions to clinical medicine.

Preface

I have been a student of Sjögren's syndrome for virtually all of my professional life. My education in this disease began in 1962 when I arrived at the National Institutes of Health to begin a Clinical Associateship with Dr. Joseph J. Bunim. Bunim introduced me to a patient with Sjögren's syndrome of 8 years duration who had developed malignant lymphoma 6 months previously. He told me that there were other such patients. I obtained serum samples from these patients and studied them by the then new technique of immunoelectrophoresis. We observed that an initial hypergammaglobulinemia could progressively decline to hypogammaglobulinemia with loss of autoantibodies. One patient in this initial series had macroglobulinemia. We published this report and suggested that the autoimmunity predisposed to the malignant transformation. Thus began my love affair with this disease.

In those days many rheumatologists considered Sjögren's syndrome simply a variant of rheumatoid arthritis. It's curious that two decades ago there was little confusion between Sjögren's syndrome and systemic lupus erythematosus, whereas today there is great confusion. There is still a great need for internationally agreed upon diagnostic criteria, which merely illustrates once again the difficulty of accurate diagnosis in our profession.

The multidisciplinary aspects of Sjögren's syndrome require authorities in several areas of medicine. The various chapter contributors are experts in their field and have often put aside other responsibilities to complete their contributions and not delay publication. To them I express my sincere gratitude.

It is a personal pleasure to see that several of my former students have made important contributions to this text. One in particular, Dr. H. M. Moutsopoulos, along with Dr. S. Kassen, was instrumental in providing the initial spark that launched this publication. A special note of appreciation goes to Dr. Anders Bjelle who hosted an extraordinatory meeting on Sjögren's syndrome 10 years ago in Umea, Sweden, when it was my particular delight to meet Professor Henrik Sjögren (Figure). I'm also deeply grateful to the Sjögren's Syndrome Foundation for contributing a chapter from the patient's perspective. It is, after all, for our patients that we strive in this en-

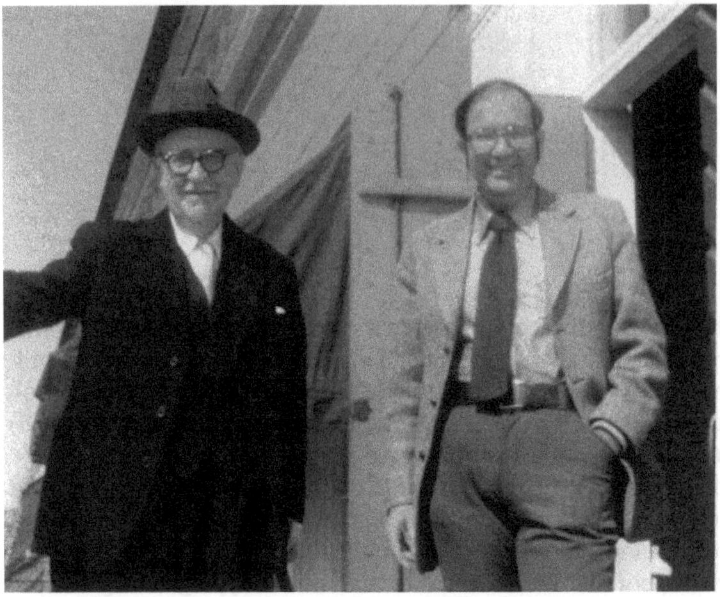

deavor to better understand the cause and find the cure for this disabling autoimmune disorder.

I hope the reader will find this book useful in that it not only reviews the historical past but also points to the future which I believe will see great accomplishments thanks to contemporary developments in molecular biology, medical technology, and immunopharmacology. We hope and trust that continued advancements can be made and that one day a final chapter can be written which will represent a successful conclusion to this enigmatic illness.

Norman Talal
San Antonio, Texas

Table of Contents

I. Introduction

II. Clinical Spectrum

A. Glandular Findings

B. Extraglandular Findings

III. Laboratory Abnormalities

IV. Treatment of Sjögren's Syndrome

List of Contributors

ALEXANDER, Elaine, M. D., Ph. D.
Good Samaritan Hospital, 5601 Loch Raven Blvd., Baltimore, MD 21239, U. S. A.

AUFDEMORTE, Thomas B., D. D. S.
Department of Pathology, The University of Texas, Health Science Center at San Antonio, 7703 Floyd Curl Drive, San Antonio, TX 78284, U. S. A.

BAUM, Bruce J., M. D., Ph. D.
Clinical Investigations and Patient Care Branch, National Institute of Dental Research, National Institutes of Health, Building 10, Room 1A06, Bethesda, MD 20892, U. S. A.

BJELLE, Anders O., M. D.
Department of Rheumatology, The Sahlgren University Hospital, Gothenburg 413 45, Sweden

CARSON, Dennis A., M. D.
Department of Basic and Clinical Research, Scripps Clinic and Research Foundation, 10666 North Torrey Pines Road, La Jolla, CA 92037, U. S. A.

CHEN, Pojen, Ph. D.
Department of Basic and Clinical Research, Scripps Clinic and Research Foundation, 10666 North Torrey Pines Road, La Jolla, CA 92037, U. S. A.

CLEARY, Michael L., M. D.
Department of Pathology
Stanford University School of Medicine
Stanford, CA 94305, U. S. A.

CONSTANTOPOULOS, Stavros H., M. D.
Department of Medicine, University of Ioannina Medical School, 453 32 Ioannina, Greece

DANIELS, Troy E., D. D. S.
Department of Oral Pathology, University of California School of Dentistry, San Francisco, CA 94143, U. S. A.

DONG, Yi, M. D.
Department of Medicine, Peking Union Medical College Hospital, Beijing, People's Republic of China

FONG, Sherman, Ph. D.
Department of Basic and Clinical Research, Scripps Clinic and Research Foundation, 10666 North Torrey Pines Road, La Jolla, CA 92037, U. S. A.

FOX, Philip C., D. D. S.
Clinical Investigations and Patient Care Branch, National Institute of Dental Research, National Institutes of Health, Bethesda, MD 20892, U. S. A.

FOX, Robert I., M. D., Ph. D.
Department of Basic and Clinical Research, Scripps Clinic and Research Foundation, 10666 North Torrey Pines Road, La Jolla, CA 92037, U. S. A.

GALILI, Naomi, Ph. D.
Department of Pathology
Stanford University School of Medicine
Stanford, CA 94305, U. S. A.

GREENSPAN, John S., Ph. D.
Department of Oral Biology, School of Dentistry, University of California, San Francisco, CA 94143, U. S. A.

HARLEY, John B., M. D., Ph. D.
Rheumatology Section, Oklahoma Medical Research Foundation, 825 N. E. 13th, Oklahoma City, OK 73104, U. S. A.

HARRIS, Elaine K.
Sjögren's Syndrome Foundation Inc., 29 Gateway Drive, Great Neck, NY 11021, U. S. A.

HOFFMANN, Robert W., D. O.
Department of Medicine, Division of Rheumatology, University of California School of Medicine, Los Angeles, CA 90024, U. S. A.

KASSAN, Stuart S., M. D.
Arthritis and Rheumatic Diseases, Colorado Arthritis Associates, 7760 W. 38th Suite 290, Wheatridge, CO 80033, U. S. A.

Kincaid, Marilyn C., M. D.
Department of Opthalmology, The University of Texas, Health Science Center, San Antonio, TX 78284, U. S. A.

Konda, Susumu, M. D.
Section of Hematology and Immunology, Department of Internal Medicine, Kanazawa Medical University, Uchinada-cho, Kahoku-gun, Ishikawa 920-02, Japan

Levy, Norman, M. D.
Department of Pathology, University of California at Davis, Davis, CA 95617, U. S. A.

Maini, R. N., B. A., M. D., F. R. C. P.
Kennedy Institute of Rheumatology, 6 Bute Gardens, Hammersmith, London W6 7DW, Great Britain

Mann, Dean L., M. D.
Biochemical Epidemiology Section, Laboratory of Human Carcinogenesis, National Institutes of Health, NCI, Bethesda, MD 20892, U. S. A./National Cancer Institute

Medsger, Thomas A., Jr., M. D.
Department of Medicine, University of Pittsburgh School of Medicine, 985 Scaife Hall, Pittsburgh, PA 15261, U. S. A.

Moutsopoulos, Haralampos M., M. D., F. A. C. P.
Department of Medicine, University of Ioannina Medical School, 453 32 Ioannina, Greece

Provost, Thomas T., M. D.
Department of Dermatology, Johns Hopkins University School of Medicine, 60 N. Wolfe Street, Baltimore, MD 21205, U. S. A.

Reichlin, Morris, M. D.
Department of Medicine, Immunology Section, Oklahoma Medical Research Foundation, 825 N. E. 13th Street, Oklahoma City, OK 73104, U. S. A.

Schenker, Steven, M. D.
Department of Medicine, Division of Gastroenterology, The University of Texas Health Science Center at San Antonio, 7703 Floyd Curl Drive, San Antonio, TX 78284, U. S. A.

Shimizu, Shiro, M. D.
Section of Hematology and Immunology, Department of Internal Medicine, Kanazawa Medical University, Uchinada-cho, Kahoku-gun, Ishikawa 920-02, Japan

SKLAR, Jeffrey, M. D., Ph. D.
Department of Pathology, Stanford University School of Medicine, Stanford, CA 94305, U. S. A.

SUGAI, Susumu, M. D.
Section of Hematology and Immunology, Department of Internal Medicine, Kanazawa Medical University, Uchinada-cho, Kahoku-gun, Ishikawa 920-02, Japan

TALAL, Norman, M. D.
Department of Medicine, Division of Clinical Immunology, The University of Texas, Health Science Center at San Antonio, 7703 Floyd Curl Drive, San Antonio, TX 78284, U. S. A.

TREVINO, Hector, M. D.
Department of Medicine, Division of Gastroenterology, The University of Texas Health Science Center at San Antonio, 7703 Floyd Curl Drive, San Antonio, TX, 78284, U. S. A.

TSIANOS, E. B., M. D.
Department of Medicine, University of Ioannina Medical School, 453 32 Ioannina, Greece

TZIOUFAS, Athanasios G., M. D.
Department of Medicine, University of Ioannina Medical School, 453 32 Ioannina, Greece

WALKER, Sara Ellen, M. D.
Rheumatology Section, Harry S. Truman Memorial Veterans Hospital, 800 Hospital Drive, Columbia, MO 65201, U. S. A.

ZHANG, Nai-Zheng, M. D.
Division of Clinical Immunology and Rheumatology, Department of Medicine, Peking Union Medical College Hospital, Beijing, People's Republic of China

I. Introduction

1. Historical Perspective: The Early Years (1930–1960)

A. Bjelle
(as told by Henrik Sjögren)

Henrik Sjögren participated in the first symposium on Sjögren's syndrome held in his own country in Umeå University Hospital of Northern Sweden in 1976. He was then seventy-seven years old. The following is based on correspondence and meetings since 1976 with Henrik Sjögren (Fig. 1) and his wife and colleague Maria Sjögren.

Henrik Sjögren was born in 1899 in a town just outside Stockholm. He started his medical studies at the Karolinska Institute and received his M. D. degree in 1927.

He started in ophthalmology after a few months as an assistant in the pathology department. In 1930 he observed extreme dryness of the eyes and mouth in a female patient with deforming arthritis. Secretion of tears could not be provoked even by brushing inside the patient's nostrils, and the flow of saliva remained diminished after stimulation. In a report to the Ophthalmological Society, Sjögren realized that this syndrome was unknown among his senior colleagues (Sjögren 1930).

In a review published in Swedish, Sjögren (1965) refers to Stock (1924) in Tübingen, who found keratoconjunctivitis sicca (KCS) in patients with dryness of the mouth. Sjögren also recognizes the earliest report by Leber (1882) on keratitis filamentosa, probably identical with KCS. He mentions a Dutchman, Mulock Houwer (1927), reporting the combined finding of corneal lesions and chronic polyarthritis.

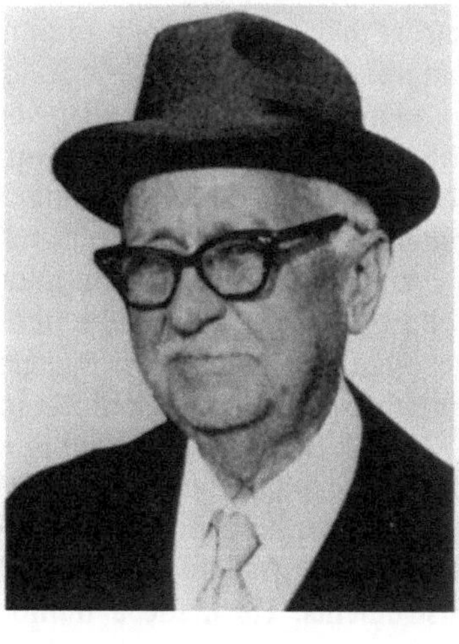

Fig. 1. Henrik Sjögren at the Umeå meeting at age 77

Sjögren reports previous observations on this combined syndrome by Hadden (1888) and by Hutchinson (1888) on single patients with xerostomia, dysphagia, reduced sweat secretion, and complete absence of secretion of tears. Sjögren also includes the reports of Fischer (1889) from Germany on corneal lesions in a woman with arthritis and on the combined symptoms from eyes and mouth.

Sjögren believes his own major contribution to be the recognition of the "sicca syndrome" as a systemic disease. Sjögren's thesis was published in German as was the custom at the time in Sweden. The translation into English by Bruce Hamilton in 1943 was the starting point for a widespread interest into what is now generally recognized as the systemic disease "Sjögren's syndrome."

After his first patient with the sicca syndrome, Sjögren started to look for other patients with similar symptoms. He had great help from his wife Maria, who was working as an ophthalmologist at a nearby Serafimer hospital in Stockholm. This way Sjögren was able to present 19 female patients in his thesis "Zur Kenntnis der Keratoconjunctivitis Sicca" in 1933 (Sjögren 1933). He used Rose Bengal to stain the corneal lesions in a 1% solution causing less harm than other dyes or the stronger solutions of Rose Bengal used previously. He also used the corneal microscope to examine the lesions, and the Schirmer's test after conjunctival and nasal stimulation to measure the flow of tears.

Sjögren found clinical and radiological evidence of arthritic changes in 13 of his 19 cases. Referring to Wissmann (1932) he agrees that "arthritic changes are by no means all of the same kind." He concludes that a close analysis of their type and etiology was outside the scope of his thesis. He also makes the remark that "remaining symptoms that he observed in these patients would take him too far and would exceed the bounds of his present investigations." Later the systemic aspects of keratoconjunctivitis sicca became the focus of Sjögren's interest.

Morphological studies were made in collaboration with the professor of pathology at the Karolinska Hospital, H. Bergstrand. Sjögren emphasizes that they deal with a disease which attacks not only the eyes and lacrimal glands but also the salivary and laryngeal glands. He concludes in his thesis that keratoconjunctivitis sicca is a generalized disease involving not only structures of the eye but also the salivary glands. It presents symptoms from many other organs. The organic change appears earlier than the symptoms of diminished glandular secretion which is of an organic nature.

As in most other European countries, Swedish theses are defended in public. At the time two opponents were appointed by the faculty, in Sjögren's case one ophthalmologist and one pathologist. Sjögren's opponents were not pleased with the pathology microphotographs, referring to them as partly artificial products (Fig. 2). Because of this Sjögren continued his morphology work after his thesis and in the following years published a number of supplementary observations on the microscopy of salivary and lacrimal glands. One important observation was of degenerative changes preceding cellular infiltration.

Henrik Sjögren was asked to establish one of the first ophthalmology units in a county hospital, Jönköping, south of Stockholm in 1935. He continued his interest in keratoconjuntivitis sicca and extended his international contacts. Sjögren also took up corneal transplantation at an early stage and even developed his own instruments. He made a number of other important contributions to his field,

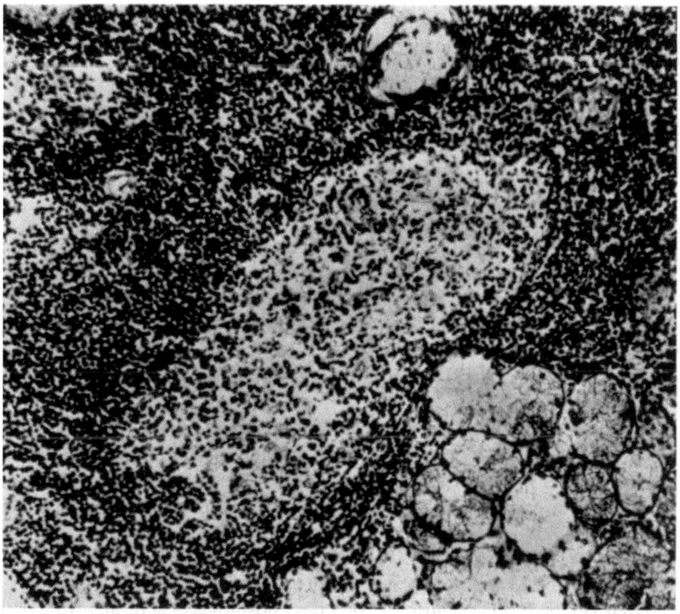

Fig. 2. Photomicrograph from Henrik Sjögren's original studies showing a section from a sublingual gland with "abundant infiltration of round cells"

although his resources for continued scientific studies on the sicca syndrome were limited in the county hospital.

Henrik Sjögren found more interest and understanding for his early observations of keratoconjunctivitis sicca outside Sweden, both among his ophthalmology colleagues and among internists and rheumatologists. As mentioned above, the interest of Bruce Hamilton, an ophthalmologist in Tasmania, Australia, who translated Sjögren's thesis into English and invited him to lecture in Australia, was a great stimulus for Sjögren to continue his work. This led Sjögren to participate in a number of international meetings and to summarize his early findings.

A great reward for Sjögren was to find new important contributions to the further understanding of the systemic nature of Sjögren's syndrome made by an increasing number of scientists. In rheumatology the group at the National Institutes of Health in Bethesda, headed by Bunim (1961), took a particular interest in Sjögren's syndrome. From his early work on systemic aspects of Sjögren's syndrome, the interest has spread with this NIH group (Talal and Bunim 1964). Henrik Sjögren greatly appreciated the monograph by Shearn (1971), which is now a classic in this field.

Henrik Sjögren's pioneering work has increasingly gained recognition, including in Sweden with a docent title from Gothenburg University and later honorary professor (in 1961). At the age of 77 he was pleased to become an honorable member of the Swedish Rheumatology Society and to participate in the first symposium on Sjögren's syndrome within his own country in 1976.

Henrik Sjögren has never expressed any complaints because of the initial indifference to his pioneeing work in his own country and his difficulties in continuing academic work. On the contrary, he took on his work in the county hospital with great enthusiasm. He and his family also participated actively in the social and musical life in his new town. He has viewed his role as helping spread his important observation that permits diagnosis from eye symptoms of a systemic disorder of great clinical and scientific importance.

References

Bunim JJ (1961) A broader spectrum of Sjögren's syndrome and its pathogenetic implications. Heberden Oration Dec 2 1960. Ann Rheum Dis 20: 1

Fischer E (1889) Über Fädchenkeratitis. Graefes Arch 35: 201

Hadden WB (1888) On "Dry Mouth" or Suppression of the Salivary and Buccal Secretions. Transc Clin Soc Lond 21: 176

Hutchinson J (1888) A Case of "Dry Mounth" (Aptyalism) Trans Clin Soc Lond 21: 180

Leber T (1882) Präparate zu dem Vortrag über Entstehung der Netzhautablösung und über verschiedene Hornhautaffektionen. Ophthalm Ges Heidelb. Klin Mbl Augenheilk, p 165

Mulock Houwer AW (1927) Keratitis filamentosa and chronic Arthritis. Trans Ophthal Soc U K 47: 88

Shearn MA (1971) Sjögren's Syndrome WB. Saunders Co Philadelphia

Sjögren H (1930) Keratoconjunctivitis sicca. Hygiea 82: 829

Sjögren H (1965) Siccasyndromet och dess nosologiska stallning. In: Medicinsk årbog VIII, 1965. Munksgaards forlag Copenhagen, p 192

Sjögren H (1933) Zur Kenntnis der Keratoconjunctivitis Sicca. Acta Ophthal Suppl II

Sjögren H (1943) A New Conception of Keratoconjunctivitis Sicca. Australasian Medical Publ Co Ltd Sydney

Stock W (1924) Die Pathologie der Tränenorgane. Graefe-Saemisch Handb d ges Augenheilk, Vol IX, Berlin

Talal N (1966) Sjögren's Syndrome. Bull Rheum Dis 16: 404

Wissmann R (1932) Keratitis filiformis als Teilsymptom innersekretorischer Störungen. Deutsch Med Wschr 58: 1525

2. The Patient's Perspective

E. K. Harris

In August 1970, Hazel F. Kessler, a patient of Dr. Norman Talal's, wrote the following:

Sicca is
having your eyes hurt all the time and your vision slowly deteriorate,
keeping artificial tears wherever you are,
avoiding as much as possible movement of air such as fans, heaters, windows, air-conditioning or sitting or walking in a breeze,
having to leave from anywhere if there is an accumulation of smoke and Heaven help you if you get caught at dinner between two smokers,
having to wear sun glasses when out of doors and finding it nearly impossible to be out on a very bright day,
getting headaches,
not wanting to kiss your husband or anyone else as your mouth feels so dry and adheres to your teeth and gums and so inflexible that you feel that you would be most undesirable,
always wondering if you have bad breath from concentrated food or drink that you were not in a position to wash out,
having to rinse your mouth, gargle and brush your teeth to clear away debri after you have eaten,
having to take a drink of some fluid before you can take that first bite and then having to continue alternating food and fluid or not eat,
having the fillings in your teeth crumble away or fall out and you nearly go steady with your dentist as he uses all his ingenuity to save your teeth as he can't tell for sure if you could support dentures or if they would give you a constant sore mouth,
having a bottle of water in your purse, your pocket, your car and asking your hostess for a glass of water immediately on your arrival so that you can converse – otherwise, your mouth and throat and upper bronchi get drier and drier and soon you cannot talk at all, your words become distorted and you choke,
having by your bed at night a glass of water and a spoon with a little oleo on it – a bit of oleo on the tongue and smoothed around over the teeth and gums will get you about three hours of sleep,
learning techniques in applying lipstick so it does not get all over your teeth when your dry lips drag on your teeth as you talk,

having to put water or saline in your nostrils before you can blow your nose, even when you have a cold,

having to walk to the vestibule of the church with communion in your mouth and get out your water bottle.

Sicca is misery

Although Hazel Kessler wrote her "Sicca Is" poem fifteen years ago, unfortunately all the problems she described still exist for Sjögren's syndrome patients.

In addition to the physical misery she describes, there is still the problem of getting diagnosed, and then, how to deal with it.

The following brief scenario is all too typical of what happens to a Sjögren's syndrome patient.

You are sure that your pains are real, not imagined - the burning eyes, the frequent "hurt all over" feeling, the dry mouth with the mucosa that sticks to the teeth, the stinging tongue, the painful throat, the food that gets stuck as you swallow, the dry vagina, and the swollen glands - but a particular flare-up may no longer be evident by the time you see the doctor. Finally, after having been to a myriad of assorted specialists, you are diagnosed as having Sjögren's syndrome, only to be told, "It is a chronic disease for which there is no cure; but, it is only life-style threatening, not life-threatening." Now you are really upset. How are you going to live with it? The doctor has given you a diagnosis but no guidelines for living with "this thing" that you are afflicted with.

Sjögren's syndrome patients have *several* problems unique to their disease:

1. The difficulty in achieving a diagnosis due to:
   a. The discrete, seemingly unrelated symptoms - how many patients would think of telling their ophthalmologist that they are also suffering from a dry mouth? Or their dentist that they have dry eyes which burn, which are glued together, which "shut down" at night?
   b. The lack of awareness on the part of general practioners about SS and its manifestations.
   c. The great fluctuations in symptoms and their manifestations.
2. The lack of knowledge by many physicians treating SS patients about the practical tips which can help many patients live and function more comfortably.
3. The impracticality of a doctor's being able to take the time to explain the ramifications and background of this disease to a patient because of the vast amount of time involved and the lack of reference material for patients.
4. The inability to communicate with other patients because so few people know about SS; in fact, many who have Sjögren's are not aware that they have it.
5. The need for coordinated medical care so that:
   a. A patient does not have to run from place to place to see the doctors caring for her.
   b. The physicians involved in her care can communicate knowledgeably and quickly, making a group evaluation and recommendations for treatment not only feasible but very practicable.

Every patient must, at some level, come to terms with her illness. The pains and frustrations of having SS, coupled with a fighting spirit and a need to know more about the disease were the forces responsible for my forming *The Moisture Seekers*, now the Sjögren's Syndrome Foundation. This organization, which, with medical and administrative support from three very caring, involved doctors at the Long Island Jewish

Medical Center (James J. Sciubba, Steven Carsons, and Ira J. Udell) and help, particularly in public relations, from the N. Y. Chapter of the Arthritis Foundation, had its first meeting in December 1983. It was formed as a response to several of the needs mentioned previously - to educate SS patients about their disease and to afford them opportunities to communicate with each other, sharing their successes and frustrations in living with this chronic illness. The desperate need of Sjögren's syndrome patients for a mutual aid organization has been more than proven - the SSF (official successor to *The Moisture Seekers*), although just two years old, has already become a multi-chapter national and potentially international organization.

What do patients need from the medical profession? Of course we want a cure; of course for now we'll settle for treatments that will make us more comfortable, treatments in which the side effects will not make us more miserable than we were without the medications.

What we do need now, what the medical profession can do for us now, is:

1. Respect and address the patient's physical problems.
2. Help in finding ways to live more comfortably with the existing condition.
3. Help patients understand more about their disease:
   a. Which symptoms demand medical attention.
   b. Which symptoms, with luck, stamina, forebearance, understanding family and friends, will subside after a period of time; for how long should a patient try to "hold out"? How to hold out?
   c. Alert patients as to SS manifestations which may occur in other parts of the body, and how proper care on the patient's part may prevent damage. Rheumatologists and oral specialists can briefly explain KCS to their patients and the need for regular eye examinations to check for corneal damage, as well as the fact that corneal erosion in many cases can be prevented by the regular use of appropriate lubricants (artificial tears, gels, etc.) rather than using them only when the eyes hurt. Likewise, the ophthalmologists and rheumatologists should explain to the SS patient that her mouth is particularly vulnerable to cavities, periodontal disease, etc., and emphasize that she should see a knowledgeable oral specialist who can advise her on treatments to prevent or at least slow down the damage that can be done by SS and thus, hopefully, save her teeth.
4. Help educate patients and the public about this disease - what is being done in research.
5. Keep informed about new approaches to treating SS so that they are in a position to advise their patients about new treatments that might be helpful, although only to a limited number of people.

The Sjögren's Syndrome Foundation Inc. is helping to meet these needs. The Foundation was incorporated in August 1985 as a not-for-profit organization. The name change from Moisture Seekers to Sjögren's Syndrome Foundation was made so that the public could more easily identify the programs and work of the Foundation with the disease. Because of the strong feeling and bond of the early members with *The Moisture Seekers,* the monthly newsletter published by the Foundation retains the Moisture Seekers title.

Currently (December 1985), in addition to the founding group which meets at the Long Island Jewish Medical Center, New Hyde Park, N. Y. each month, there are chapters in: Boston, meeting at Massachusetts Eye & Ear; Boca Raton, FL meeting at

Boca Raton Community Hospital; Delaware Valley Area (including Philadelphia and Trenton), meeting at St. Mary's Hospital, Langehorne, PA; Seattle, WA, meeting at the Arthritis Foundation; St. Paul-Minneapolis, meeting at Metropolitan Medical Center, MN; and Greater Metropolitan Washington, meeting at the NIH, Bethesda, MD. Chapters are being planned for California, Michigan, Texas, Central Florida, the Pittsburgh, PA area, Canada, and Copenhagen, Denmark. Patient and professional membership is international, with members in places as far away from our headquarters on Long Island, NY, as Australia, Brazil, Denmark, England and Ireland.

The SSF has filled these important needs:

1. Educating patients about their illness in order to help them better manage their illness and continue productively with their work and family life.
2. Providing avenues of communication between patients so that they can help each other by sharing techniques for living more comfortably with their illness.
3. Increasing the awareness of doctors and other health professionals and the public about Sjögren's syndrome, its diagnosis and treatment.

Patients, both diagnosed and undiagnosed, are aided through the following:

1. Monthly meetings with medical specialists from all over the country, knowledgeable about a particular area of SS. Speakers' presentations are taped and available for replay.
2. Sponsorship of an annual symposium on Sjögren's, bringing together practicing medical specialists and researchers so that the patients and their families, doctors and other health professinals can all become better informed about current medical diagnosis and treatment, and research developments that would be of benefit to Sjögren patients. Norman Talal, M. D. was keynote speaker at the first symposium, held in October 1984; Harry Spiera, M. D. was the keynote speaker at the second symposium which took place in November 1985. Participating specialists included: Allan Abramson, M. D., Steven Carsons, M. D., R. Linsy Farris, M. D., Howard Kerpen, M. D., James J. Sciubba, D. M. D., Ph. D., and Ira J. Udell, M. D.
3. Distribution of articles about Sjögren's, KCS and xerostomia to both the public and members. The materials include: 1) Reprints or summaries of articles appearing in the press and scientific articles appearing in the press and scientific journals; 2) Specially prepared articles written by members of our Medical Advisory Board and other qualified professionals.
4. Sending out a monthly newsletter containing summaries of meetings, news of developments in caring for Sjögren's patients, opportunities for patients to participate in programs (e.g., the PhEx-100 clinical investigations by Dr. Farris at Columbia-Presbyterian, New York City, Dr. Lemp at the Center for Sight in Washington, D. C., Dr. deLuise at the Southern New England Regional Eye Center, Waterbury, CT; names of other patients with whom they can communicate - particularly important in less populated communities. The newsletter is currently sent individually to over 1000 patients and doctors plus quantity mailings that are distributed to centers and physicians specializing in the care of Sjögren's syndrome, KCS and xerostomia.

There still is a need for a reference book on Sjögren's which patients can use. To meet this important need for a book that will help patients identify their symptoms, learn how to obtain proper medical treatment, and how to cope with this chronic, debilitating disease, the Sjögren's Syndrome Foundation is currently involved in the development and publication of such a volume, with specially prepared chapters contributed by leading Sjögren specialists, many of whom are represented in this professional book. The book will be entitled, "Sjögren's Syndrome: A Handbook for Patients".

Earlier diagnosis of Sjögren's syndrome and certainly better treatment will take place when coordinated treatment centers for Sjögren patients are available throughout the country. The University of Texas Health Science Center at San Antonio and the University of California Medical Center at San Francisco both have Sjögren's Syndrome Clinics. The New England Medical Center at Tufts University, Boston is currently developing a coordinated treatment center for Sjögren's patients. (This center should be open in early 1986.) Another exists at the medical center attached to the University of Copenhagen in Denmark. Facilities such as these are needed in more locations so that the several specialists involved in a Sjögren's patient's care can communicate, see the patient's chart and be informed about her overall status merely by access to a central chart at the clinic. Perhaps, in the next decade, records of Sjögren's patients throughout the world can be fed into a computer and thus give both practioners and researchers access to more information (both quality and quantity) about the treatment of Sjögren's.

The Foundation would like to be able to sponsor medical teaching about Sjögrens so that specialists, internists and other health professionals will be better informed abut SS, its manifestations, currently approved treatments and treatments under investigation, so that they can better diagnose and advise their patients. Communication between practioners in the United States and practioners and researchers in other parts of the world in regard to work being done on Sjögren's has not been very active. Hopefully, the first International Conference on Sjögren's held in Copenhagen in May 1986, will result in better exchange of information. The SSF was recently responsible for an impromtu meeting between Dr. Prause of Copenhagen and several members of its Medical Advisory Board in the New York Metropolitan area. This meeting generated much interest in theories and treatments not currently under investigation in the New York area. Everything possible must be done to stimulate research specifically on Sjögren's and encourage the exchange of information on causes and treatment.

At the moment the Foundation's sole funds come from membership dues and contributions. As the work of the Foundation becomes better known, it is hoped that funds will be available so that in addition to the services it currently provides (all through volunteers), the Foundation will be able to sponsor research grants and coordinated treatment centers in various places.

SS patients need intelligent, coordinated, improved care; they need doctors who realize that these patients hurt, that they frequently have difficulty in functioning, that their flare-ups may be short-term or long-term, that they need to be able to communicate with someone who understands what they are going through; that although there may be no cure today, they still need ways of "living with Sjögren's", and that they deserve the interest of the medical profession in finding the cause and subsequently a cure for Sjögren's, as well as improved treatment.

As you read this important book on Sjögren's syndrome, please bear in mind that the diagnoses and statistics involved in the investigations in this book represent *real people.*

II. Clinical Spectrum

A. Glandular Findings

1. Oral Manifestations of Sjögren's Syndrome

T. E. Daniels

Oral symptoms

The principal oral symptom of Sjögren's syndrome (SS) is dryness (xerostomia), but not all patients offer this complaint directly. Some may describe difficulty in swallowing food, problems in wearing complete dentures, changes in their sense of taste, a marked increase in dental caries, chronic burning symptoms in their oral mucosa, or inability to eat dry food or to speak continuously for more than a few minutes. These symptoms usually have an insidious onset, but their severity may wax and wane over periods of many weeks or months. A differential diagnosis of xerostomia is presented in Chapter II.E.1.

Extraoral signs

The parotid or submandibular glands in SS may exhibit firm, diffuse, non-tender enlargement, or there may be mild induration of the glands without enlargement. The frequency of visible or palpable changes in parotid glands increases from 25% to 45% of cases in association with increasing severity of flow rate reduction and salivary gland inflammation (Daniels 1984). Many patients with SS report that their salivary gland enlargement occurs in episodes lasting for many weeks or months, whereas other patients will have chronic enlargement, with slow fluctuations in size. The swelling or induration may begin unilaterally but usually becomes bilateral, although often of different magnitude (Fig. 1). Labial angular cheilitis is a common feature of those patients who have oral candidiasis as a result of their xerostomia (Fig. 2), and is discussed later in this chapter.

Intraoral signs

The intraoral signs of SS are non-specific and appear in chronic xerostomia of whatever cause. These signs include 1) dry, sticky oral mucosal surfaces (Fig. 3); 2) dental caries, primarily affecting the necks of the teeth parallel to the gingival margin (root caries) or the incisal edges (Fig. 4); 3) absent or cloudy saliva expressible from the parotid or submandibular ducts; and 4) a predisposition to overgrowth of *Candida* species, producing generalized oral mucosal erythema and, on the dorsal tongue, fissuring and atrophy of the filiform papillae (Fig. 5).

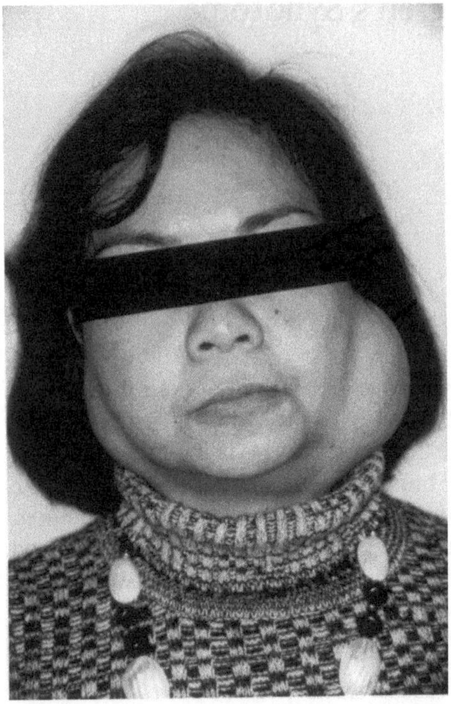

Fig. 1. 45 year old patient with primary Sjögren's syndrome and 14 year history of bilateral parotid gland enlargement which has been slowly progressive. The swellings have never been more than mildly symptomatic, and they are firm and non-tender to palpation

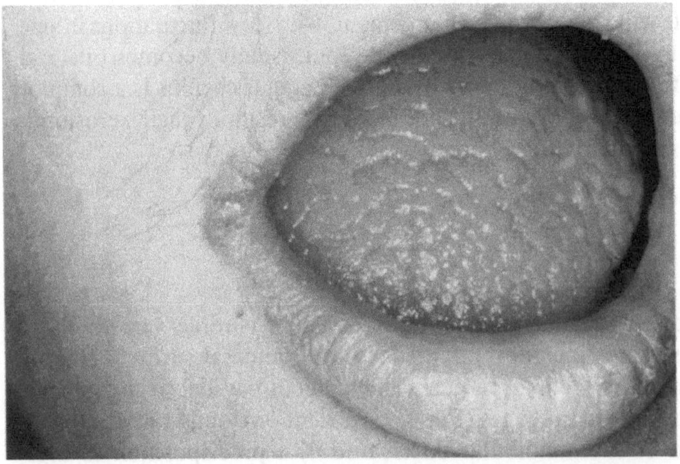

Fig. 2. 28 year old patient with primary Sjögren's syndrome, severe xerostomia, bilateral labial angular cheilitis and chronic atrophic candidiasis of the oral mucosa

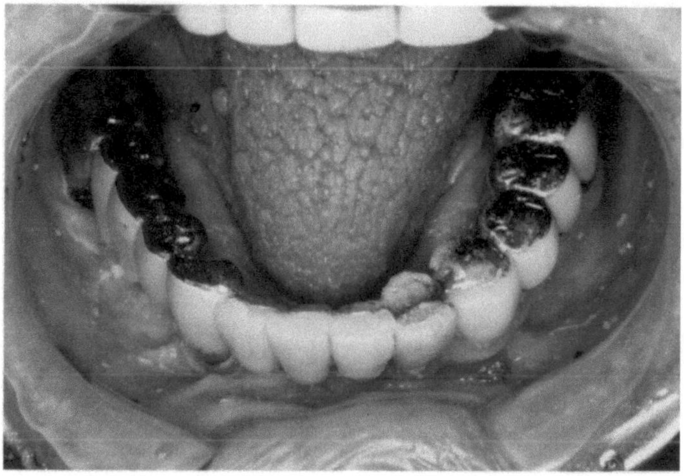

Fig. 3. 69 year old woman with primary Sjögren's syndrome and 15 year history of progressive oral dryness. All teeth have been crowned but most have recurrent marginal caries. Note accumulations of desquamated epithelial cells adhering to the occlusal surfaces of crowns

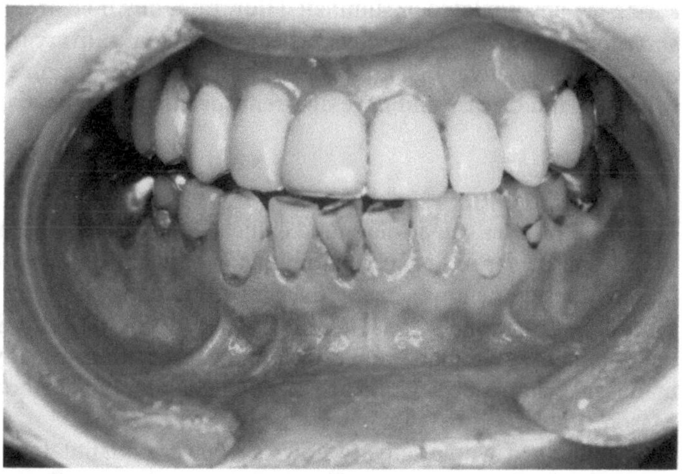

Fig. 4. 74 year old patient with primary Sjögren's syndrome, and caries on the lower teeth at the gingival margins and incisal edges

Diagnosis of the salivary component of Sjögren's syndrome

Although "xerostomia" is part of the traditional definition of SS and is certainly a clinically important component for most patients, it is unsatisfactory as a diagnostic criterion. Its perception by patients is highly subjective, it can be caused by a variety of conditions (reviewed in Chapter II.E.1.), and it is difficult to define objectively.

The various means of assessing the salivary component of SS have included mea-

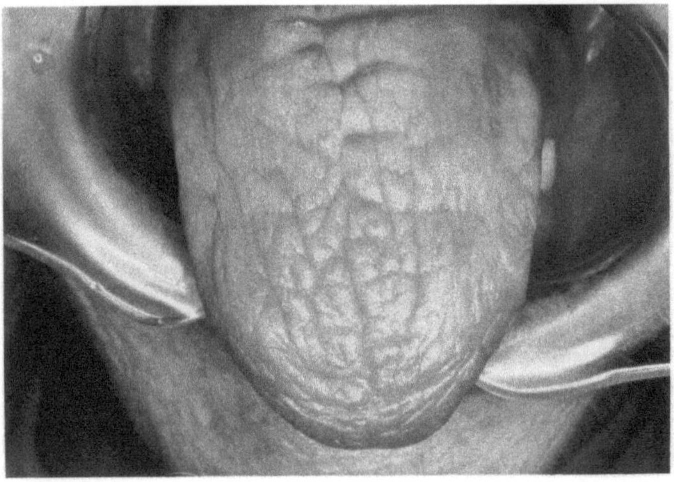

Fig. 5. 68 year old patient with primary Sjögren's syndrome, severe xerostomia (10 minute stimulated parotid flow rate = 0 ml), and chronic atrophic oral candidiasis, showing fissuring and papillary atrophy of the dorsal tongue

suring the unstimulated or stimulated flow rates of whole or separate salivary gland secretions, contrast sialography, nuclear imaging of salivary glands, sialochemistry and accessory salivary gland biopsy. These methods examine different aspects of salivary gland disease and have different specificity for the diagnosis of SS.

Sialometry

Salivary flow rates can be measured clinically for whole saliva or for separate secretions from the parotid or submandibular/sublingual glands, with or without stimulation. Measurement of separate parotid secretion is clinically convenient through the use of a standard Carlson-Crittenden cup (Sproles and Schaeffer 1974), but measurement of submandibular or sublingual secretions usually requires a custom-made collection device for each patient. Sialometric methods are reviewed by Mason and Chisholm (1975).

Unstimulated whole salivary flow rates give a quantitative assessment of a patient's basal salivary secretion. These rates most closely reflect a patient's symptoms of xerostomia and are reduced by diseases directly affecting salivary glands such as SS (Bertram 1967) or sarcoidosis, drug effects (Bahn 1972), depression (Brown 1970), and increasing age, especially in women (Heintze et al. 1983; Ben-Aryeh et al. 1984).

Separate gland flow rates with a gustatory stimulus give an estimate of the gland's secretory capacity, but the maximal secretory rate is directly proportional to the size of the gland and varies greatly between individuals (Ericson 1971). Analysis of the responses of healthy individuals to different kinds of salivary stimuli show weak or even negative correlations between resting secretion, citric acid stimulation and cholinergic stimulation (Ericson 1969). This indicates that individuals have very different responses to various salivary stimuli, and results obtained from sialometric methods using different stimuli may not be comparable. A recent study found no significant differences in parotid flow rate related to age, either unstimulated or with stimulation (Heft and Baum 1984).

Gustatory stimulation overcomes the secretory inhibition caused by parasympatholytic drugs such as atropine (Mandel et al. 1968) but not that caused by neuroleptic drugs (Molander and Birkhed 1981). Combinations of drugs, such as those used for treating hypertension, heart failure or asthma seem to cause symptoms or signs of xerostomia in some patients, but these combined drug effects have not yet been studied. Thus, standardized flow rate assessments provide useful quantitative assessment of an individual's salivary gland function, within the limits described above, and a repeatable, noninvasive method to monitor the course of a chronic disease, but are too variable and non-specific to serve as a diagnostic criterion.

Sialography

Sialography, a radiocontrast method of assessing anatomical changes in the salivary gland duct system, has been widely used to examine patients with SS. In studies using oil-based contrast media and two-phase secretory sialography, several degrees of sialectasis were observed in 85-97% of patients with SS (Bloch et al. 1965; Bertram 1967; Gonzalez et al. 1970). But in studies using water-based media, which are rapidly absorbed, similar degrees of sialectasis were found in only 58-64% of patients with SS (Chisholm et al. 1971; Whaley et al. 1973), and normal sialograms were seen in 20% (Chisholm et al. 1971) and 46% (Whaley et al. 1973) of patients with primary SS - which, by definition, involves the salivary glands. Sialography is a less sensitive indicator of gland abnormality than parotid flow rate measurement (Chisholm et al. 1971) and does not correlate well with parotid gland histopathology (Bloch et al. 1965). Furthermore, sialectasis has been seen in 15-20% of a normal population (Dijkstra 1980), and the sialectasis associated with SS may not be distinguishable from that associated with chronic sialadenitis of other causes (Lowman and Cheng 1976).

Oil-based contrast media provide a more sensitive indication of salivary changes in SS than water-based media, but carry hazards. For example, potentially severe granulomatous reactions may result if an oil-based medium extravasates beyond the duct system (Lowman and Cheng 1976). Or, abnormal glands may retain the medium for weeks or months (Lowman and Cheng 1976; Dijkstra 1980), possibly causing further glandular damage. In SS, therefore, sialography with an oil-based medium is associated with unacceptable side effects, and with a water-based medium is both insensitive and non-specific.

Scintigraphy

Sequential salivary scintigraphy with ^{99m}Tc sodium pertechnetate can be used to assess the function of the major salivary glands by observing the rate and density of label uptake and time of appearance of label in the mouth during the 60-minute period after the radionuclide is intravenously injected. In patients who have SS, uptake of label by the glands is delayed and secretion of labeled saliva into the mouth is delayed or absent (Schall et al. 1971; Daniels et al. 1979). Rectilinear scanning of salivary glands done with the same label is more sensitive than sialography in SS (Alarcon-Segovia et al. 1974), but scintigraphy is more useful than scanning because it repeatedly examines the four major glands simultaneously, over a period of time. Salivary scintigraphic changes correlate with stimulated parotid flow rate measurement (Schall et al. 1971; Daniels et al. 1979), but these changes are not disease-specific for SS.

Sialochemistry

Chemical and immunological investigations of saliva from patients with SS have produced some promising results. So far, most of the observations are unconfirmed or controversial, but ultimately these studies may provide a method for diagnosis of the salivary component of SS. They are discussed in Chapter II.A.3.

Accessory salivary gland biopsy

The use of accessory salivary gland biopsy in SS was introduced in 1966 (Calman and Reifman 1966; Cifarelli et al. 1966) and subsequently has been widely applied in many studies to assess the salivary component of SS. The observation of significant focal sialadenitis in a labial salivary gland biopsy specimen has been shown to be the most disease-specific diagnostic criterion for the salivary component of SS, if the specimen 1) is taken from beneath clinically normal mucosa, 2) includes 5 to 10 glands, separated from their surrounding connective tissue, 3) is interpreted with application of appropriate exclusions, and 4) uses a focus score of greater than 1 focus/4 mm^2 of gland area as a threshold for significance (Daniels 1986). The rationale and details of the labial salivary gland biopsy are presented in Chapter II.A.4.

Sequelae of chronic xerostomia

Dental caries

Although dental caries is one of the most troubling and difficult to manage sequelae of SS, little attention has been given to it in studies of the disease. Bloch et al. (1965) found that 37% of their 62 patients with SS complained of an increased incidence of dental caries, often in the form of recurring breakdown of previous dental restorations. In a study of 34 patients with chronic xerostomia, half of whom had SS, 7 out of 16 patients with remaining teeth had caries in all teeth, mainly in cervical or incisal locations (Bertram 1967). A study of 65 patients with SS found cervical or incisal dental caries at the time of initial diagnosis in 45% of the patients with secondary SS and 63% of the patients with primary SS who had remaining teeth (Daniels et al. 1975). Their mean stimulated parotid flow rates were reduced by 45% and 82%, respectively, as compared with patients who had a connective tissue disease alone.

The dental caries associated with SS, and with other causes of chronic xerostomia, frequently attacks the margins of dental restorations, even those located subgingivally (Figs. 3 and 4). This makes the prevention of caries an important aspect of treatment for all patients with SS who have remaining teeth. Although little is known about the etiology and prevention of root caries, frequent fluoride applications and plaque control have been clearly established as effective in greatly reducing the frequency of post-radiation caries (Dreizen et al. 1977), and these measures seem to be of similiar benefit for patients with SS.

Methods of preventing new and recurrent dental caries in patients with SS need to be individualized according to the severity of a given patient's xerostomia. A reasonable beginning level of prevention for patients with a 50% or greater reduction in salivary flow should include: 1) daily fluoride mouth rinsing (e.g., Phos-flur®) for 1 to 2 minutes before going to bed, 2) discontinuance of all between-meal sucrose, 3) careful daily removal of dental plaque deposits, and 4) regular dental supervision. Patients who comply with these procedures and still develop caries should then be placed on daily use of a tray-applied fluoride gel. The management of dental caries is discussed in detail by Newbrun (1983).

Oral candidiasis

The oral mucosal signs of generalized erythema and dorsal tongue fissuring and papillary atrophy seen in patients with fairly advanced chronic xerostomia are usually caused by overgrowth of *Candida* species, producing chronic atrophic candidiasis (Figs. 2 and 5) (Tapper-Jones et al. 1980; Holmstrup and Bessermann 1983). This condition is usually responsible for the burning mucosal symptoms experienced by some patients. It can be diagnosed by the presence of fungal hyphae in a smear suspended in 10% potassium hydroxide solution. This form of candidiasis usually requires treatment for many weeks, during which progress is monitored by observing improvement in oral symptoms and resolution of the oral mucosal changes to normal appearance. Effective treatment of this form of candidiasis usually provides a significant improvement in patients' oral symptoms. However, since the xerostomia is chronic, recurrence is common, and each case must be followed for reappearance of the mucosal symptoms or signs and retreatment as necessary.

The most generally effective treatment is to have the patient dissolve nystatin vaginal tablets orally for 20 to 30 minutes, beginning at two or three per day. Most patients find these unflavored tablets acceptable for long term use. Patients with very dry mouths usually require periodic sips of water to help the tablets dissolve within 30 minutes. Nystatin oral suspension is usually not an effective form of the drug because it cannot be kept in the mouth long enough. A clotrimazole oral troche has recently been introduced which is flavored with glucose (Mycelex®). Because the dose of drug it provides is low (10 mg), effective treatment requires slowly dissolving five troches per day, but the inclusion of glucose in this antifungal preparation raises the concern that such use may increase dental caries formation in patients with severe xerostomia.

Additional antifungal treatment is necessary for those patients who have dentures. To permit the drug access to all mucosal sites, all dentures must be removed while antifungal tablets are dissolving. The dentures must also be disinfected regularly. The method and frequency of disinfection should be decided in consultation with the patient's dentist, but generally it is sufficient to soak complete dentures overnight in 1% sodium hypochlorite solution, or in benzalkonium chloride (1:750 in water) if they have cast metal frames or clasps. The dentures should be carefully cleaned before soaking and rinsed before reinsertion in the mouth. Daily use of nystatin powder on the fitting surfaces of complete dentures may be a helpful adjunct to treating active oral candidiasis, and its continued use may help prevent recurrence.

Salivary stimulation and replacement

Attempts to relieve symptoms of oral dryness and restore salivary function have taken two approaches: stimulation of additional salivary secretion, and use of saliva substitutes. Gustatory or masticatory stimulation with regular use of sugarless, sour hard candies or sugarless chewing gum can provide a significant increase in saliva, but only during application of the stimulus. The parasympathomimetic drug pilocarpine has been shown to increase saliva production significantly in patients with chronic xerostomia, both over long periods (Greenspan and Daniels 1987) and in the short term, where a single oral dose gives approximately 2 hours of stimulation (Fox et al. 1986). Doses of 5 mg three times per day are usually well tolerated, but side effects of sweating or stomach cramping may be encountered. Pilocarpine is contraindicated in patients with a history of gastrointestinal ulcer, and it should be used with caution in patients with hypertension or other cardiovascular diseases. Effects of its long term use are unknown.

Short term use of the drug trithioparamethoxyphenylpropene, called Sulfarlem® in Europe and Sialor® in Canada, has been shown to be helpful in treating patients with dry mouth. In a double-blind, cross-over trial with placebo, there were significant increases in whole unstimulated salivary flow rate in patients with generally mild chronic xerostomia from SS (Epstein et al. 1983). However, an open study conducted on patients with severe xerostomia from SS, using the same dosage of this drug as the previous study, found no significant improvement in unstimulated whole salivary flow rate or in patient-reported symptoms (Schiødt et al. 1986). This drug's pharmacologic actions are not well understood, it is contraindicated in patients with chronic hepatobiliary disease, and its long term effects on patients with SS are unknown. It is not yet available for use in the United States.

Several methyl-cellulose-based saliva substitutes are available commercially (ADA 1984), some of which also contain fluoride. In controlled studies, these have been found to be more effective than a glycerine mouth rinse for relieving nocturnal oral discomfort (Klestov et al. 1981) or than distilled water (Wiesenfeld et al. 1983) for relieving general symptoms of xerostomia. Use of these preparations may be helpful for patients with severe xerostomia, especially at night and for those wearing complete dentures. Patients with mild or even moderately severe xerostomia may find frequent sips of water as effective, and we have found that most of these patients do not continue using saliva substitutes for very long. Oral lubricants containing lemon flavor and citric acid as a sialogogue have been suggested (Donatsky et al. 1981; Wiesenfeld et al. 1983), but these may have limited usefulness in patients with remaining teeth because of the erosive potential of the acid on dental enamel. Saliva substitutes containing mucin are being tested in Europe (Vissink et al. 1983) and show encouraging results.

Summary

The intraoral symptoms and signs of SS are not specific to SS, being shared with those of chronic xerostomia of any cause. The loss of saliva causes chronic oral discomfort and functional problems, and predisposes patients to dental caries and oral candidiasis. Many methods have been used to objectively assess salivary glands in SS, but so far, a labial salivary gland biopsy specimen showing focal sialadenitis (as described in Chapter II.A.4) provides the best diagnostic criterion for the salivary component of SS, in terms of its disease specificity, convenience, availability and low risk.

The treatment of xerostomia in patients with SS consists of 1) preventing new and recurrent dental caries by frequent and regular application of topical fluoride, careful dental supervision, and discontinuing sucrose (and other metabolizable carbohydrates) between meals; 2) reducing oral symptoms by diagnosing and treating oral candidiasis (repeatedly if necessary); and 3) attempting to replace lost salivary function by stimulating salivary secretion with sialogogues or pilocarpine, or if adequate amounts of saliva cannot be stimulated, using some form of saliva substitute, especially for patients wearing complete dentures.

References

ADA Council on Dental Therapeutics (1984) Accepted Dental Therapeutics, 40th edn. American Dental Association, Chicago

Alarcon-Segovia D, Ibanez G, Hernandez-Ortiz J, Cetina JA, Gonzales-Jimenez Y, Diaz-Jouanen E (1974) Salivary gland involvement in diseases associated with Sjögren's syndrome. I. Radionuclide and roentgenographic studies. J Rheumatol 1: 159-165

Bahn SL (1972) Drug-related dental destruction. Oral Surg 33: 49-54

Ben-Aryeh J, Miron D, Szargel R, Gutman D (1984) Whole-saliva secretion rates in old and young healthy subjects. J Dent Res 63: 1147-1148

Bertram U (1967) Xerostomia: clinical aspects, pathology and pathogenesis. Acta Odontol Scand 25: suppl 49

Bloch KJ, Buchanan WW, Wohl MJ, Bunim JJ (1965) Sjögren's syndrome: a clinical, pathological and serological study of sixty-two cases. Medicine 44: 187-231

Brown CC (1970) The parotid puzzle: a review of the literature on human salivation and its application to psychophysiology. Psychophysiology 7: 66-85

Calman HI, Reifman S (1966) Sjögren's syndrome: report of a case. Oral Surg 21: 158-162

Chisholm DM, Blair GS, Low PS, Whaley K (1971) Hydrostatic sialography as an index of salivary gland disease in Sjögren's syndrome. Acta Radiol [Diagn] (Stockh) 11: 577-585

Cifarelli PS, Bennett MJ, Zaino EC (1966) Sjögren's syndrome: a case report with an additional diagnostic aid. Arch Intern Med 117: 429-431

Daniels TE (1984) Labial salivary gland biopsy in Sjögren's syndrome: assessment as a criterion in 362 suspected cases. Arthritis Rheum 27: 147-156

Daniels TE (1986) Salivary histopathology in diagnosis of Sjögren's syndrome. Scand J Rheum in press

Daniels TE, Silverman S Jr, Michalski JP, Greenspan JS, Sylvester RA, Talal N (1975) The oral components of Sjögren's syndrome. Oral Surg 39: 875-885

Daniels TE, Powell MR, Sylvester RA, Talal N (1979) An evaluation of salivary scintigraphy in Sjögren's syndrome. Arthritis Rheum 22: 809-814

Dijkstra PF (1980) Classification and differential diagnosis of sialographic characteristics in Sjögren's syndrome. Semin Arthritis Rheum 10: 10-17

Donatsky O, Johnsen T, Holmstrup P, Bertram U (1981) Effect of Saliment on parotid salivary gland secretion and on xerostomia caused by Sjögren's syndrome. Scand J Dent Res 90: 157-162

Dreizen S, Brown LR, Daly TE, Drane JB (1977) Prevention of xerostomia-related dental caries in irradiated cancer patients. J Dent Res 56: 99-104
Epstein JB, Decoteau WE, Wilkinson A (1983) Effect of Sialor in treatment of xerostomia in Sjögren's syndrome. Oral Surg 56: 495-499
Ericson S (1969) An investigation of human parotid saliva secretion rate in response to different types of stimulation. Arch Oral Biol 14: 591-596
Ericson S (1971) The importance of sialography for the determination of the parotid flow. Acta Otolaryngol 72: 437-444
Fox PC, van der Ven PF, Baum BJ, Mandel ID (1986) Pilocarpine for the treatment of xerostomia associated with salivary gland dysfunction. Oral Surg 61: 243-245
Gonzalez L, Mackenzie AH, Tarar RA (1970) Parotid sialography in Sjögren's syndrome. Radiology 97: 91-93
Greenspan D, Daniels TE (1987) Effectiveness of pilocarpine in postradiation xerostomia. Cancer (in press)
Heft MW, Baum BJ (1984) Unstimulated and stimulated parotid salivary flow rate in individuals of different ages. J Dent Res 63: 1182-1185
Heintze U, Birkhed D, Bjorn H (1983) Secretion rate and buffer effect of resting and stimulated whole saliva as a function of age and sex. Swed Dent J 7: 227-238
Holmstrup P, Bessermann M (1983) Clinical, therapeutic, and pathogenic aspects of chronic oral multifocal candidiasis. Oral Surg 56: 388-395
Klestov AC, Webb J, Latt D, Schiller G, McNamara K, Young DY, Hobbes J, Fetherston J (1981) Treatment of xerostomia: A double-blind trial in 108 patients with Sjögren's syndrome. Oral Surg 51: 594-599
Lowman RM, Cheng GK (1976) Diagnostic roentgenology. In: Rankow RM, Polayes IM (eds) Diseases of the salivary glands. WB Saunders Co, Philadelphia
Mandel ID, Katz R, Zengo A, Kutscher AH, Greenberg RA, Katz S, Scharf R, Pintoff A (1968) The effect of pharmacologic agents on salivary secretion and composition in man. I. Pilocarpine, atropine and anticholinesterases. J Oral Ther Pharmacol 4: 192-199
Molander L, Birkhed D (1981) Effect of single oral doses of various neuroleptic drugs on salivary secretion rate, pH, and buffer capacity in healthy subjects. Psychopharmacology 75: 114-118
Mason DK, Chisholm DM (1975) Salivary glands in health and disease. WB Saunders, London
Newbrun E (1983) Cariology, 2nd edn. Williams and Wilkins, Baltimore
Schall GL, Anderson LG, Wolf RO, Herdt JR, Tarpley TM, Cummings NA, Zeiger LS, Talal N (1971) Xerostomia in Sjögren's syndrome: evaluation by sequential salivary scintigraphy. JAMA 216: 2109-2116
Schiødt M, Oxholm P, Jacobsen A (1986) Treatment of xerostomia in patients with primary Sjögren's syndrome with Sulfarlem. Scand J Rheum (in press)
Sproles A, Schaeffer LD (1974) An advanced design of the Carlson-Crittenden cup for collection of parotid fluid. Biomat Med Dev Art Org 2: 95-101
Tapper-Jones L, Aldred M, Walker DM (1980) Prevalence and intraoral distribution of *Candida albicans* in Sjögren's syndrome. J Clin Pathol 33: 282-287
Vissink A, 's-Gravenmade EJ, Panders AK, Vermey A, Petersen JK, Visch LL, Schaub RMH (1983) A clinical comparison between commercially available mucin- and CMC-containing saliva substitutes. Int J Oral Surg 12: 232-238
Whaley K, Williamson J, Chisholm DM, Webb J, Mason DK, Buchanan WW (1973) Sjögren's syndrome. I. Sicca components. Q J Med 42: 279-304
Wisenfeld D, Stewart AM, Mason DK (1983) A critical assessment of oral lubricants in patients with xerostomia. Br Dent J 155: 155-157

2. The Eye in Sjögren's Syndrome*

M. C. Kincaid

The classic description of Sjögren's syndrome was written in 1933 by an ophthalmologist who described keratoconjunctivitis sicca and noted that it was a symptom of a systemic disease (Sjögren 1933). Today, we realize that there are two syndromes, primary and secondary. Both include keratoconjunctivitis sicca with or without xerostomia; secondary Sjögren's adds a connective tissue disorder, often rheumatoid arthritis (Moutsopoulos 1980).

It is our purpose in this chapter to review the normal physiology of tears, and to discuss the differential diagnosis of tear disorders. We then discuss the clinical workup and therapy for these unfortunate individuals.

The surface of the cornea and conjunctiva consists of nonkeratinized squamous epithelium, which is normally moistened at all times by the tears. In addition, the cornea, an avascular structure, depends on the tears for nutrition and oxygenation, and for ingress of white cells for repair of wounds. They contain lysozyme to help prevent bacterial infection and also form a smooth clear optical surface for optimal vision (Lemp 1985).

Tears are often thought of as simply salty water, but in fact they are considerably more complex. The tears consist of three layers, the mucous layer, the aqueous layer, and the lipid layer, each secreted by its own set of glands. They are, of course, predominantly water; over 98% of the volume is water. In addition to electrolytes, amino acids, and glucose, other substances present in the tears include immunoglobulins A and G, albumin, lysozyme, lactoferrin, ceruloplasmin, and tear-specific prealbumin (Crandall and Leopold 1979). Other components include complement, properdin, and properdin factor B (Smolin 1985).

The innermost layer is produced by the goblet cells of the conjunctiva. These mucopolysaccharides serve to render the otherwise hydrophobic cell surfaces of the cornea and conjunctiva wettable, and thus to enhance the stability of the tear film. The surface epithelial cells have short microvilli which appear to serve as anchors for the mucin (Lemp 1985). Several components form the mucus, including hyaluronic acid and neuraminic acid (McGhee and Lee 1985).

The second layer is by far the thickest, and accounts for most of the entire 7 micron thickness of the tear film. The aqueous layer is secreted by the main and accessory lacrimal glands. The main lacrimal gland is located superotemporal to the globe in the lacrimal fossa. Also, there are several accessory lacrimal glands located

* Supported in part by a Research to Prevent Blindness Research Development Award and by grants from Fight for Sight and the San Antonio Area Foundation.

in the superior and inferior fornices and at the tarsal margins. It is believed by some (Jones et al. 1985) that these accessory glands are responsible for true basal tear secretion, and that the main gland secretes only in response to irritative or emotional stimuli, but Wright (Wright 1985) finds no evidence to support this view.

The outermost layer is secreted by the tarsal, or Meibomian glands. These unusual sebaceous glands normally have no associated hair follicle, and are located just outside the conjunctival lid margin. The exact composition of the lipid layer is imperfectly understood, but it is known to contain cholesterol and branched fatty acids. It is believed that the thin external coating of oily material helps stabilize the tear film and also prevents evaporation (Tiffany 1985).

In order for tears to perform their function of wetting the external surface of the eye and presenting a smooth clear optical surface, all anatomic and physiologic functions must be intact. It is most helpful to think of tear dysfunctions as falling into one of three groups; that is, abnormalities of the lids which interfere with proper blinking, abnormalities of the ocular surface to be wetted, and abnormalities of the tears themselves. Within this last group would be abnormalities of each of the tear film layers. Therefore, tear disorders can be grouped into five categories (Holly and Lemp 1977).

While it is evident that true keratoconjunctivitis sicca is a disorder of the aqueous layer, it is important to understand this classification, as it determines the rationale of the workup for the complaint of dry eyes. The constituents of the tear film and surfaces interact, so that while one disorder may be primary, other aspects of this functional unit may be affected. Furthermore, an individual patient may have more than one etiology contributing to the dry eyes, and optimal treatment depends on recognition of all of them.

Abnormalities of the lid include those of position and those of function. If normal blinking is interrupted, as in any neuromuscular disease, the tears will not flow across the ocular surface properly. The tear film is normally unstable, so that if proper blinking does not occur, the film will not be replenished (Lemp 1985). The position of the lids is also important. The lids normally become less taut with age, so that the lower lid tends to fall away from its normal position against the globe. This in turn interferes with maintenance of the lacrimal lake and normal blinking function. Other causes of eyelid impairment include malformation or scarring, including symplepharon, or obliteration of the normal fornix by conjunctival scarring. One of the more common diseases responsible for lid dysfunction is ocular cicatricial pemphigoid (Leonard et al. 1985).

Corneal surface irregularities may contribute to abnormalities of tearing. Tears will pool in scars and depressions, sometimes leaving adjacent dry areas. Furthermore, for obscure reasons, an anaesthetic cornea, resulting from an interruption of the ophthalmic branch of the trigeminal nerve, is no longer wet properly. This condition usually occurs secondary to a herpes simplex infection (Holly and Lemp 1977).

The tear abnormalities themselves generally do not occur in a pure state, since each layer affects the others. Nevertheless, it is helpful to think of each type individually, to understand the role of each layer. As might be anticipated, abnormalities of the mucus-secreting glands of the conjunctiva result in poor wetting of the ocular surface. Thus, there may be tears in abundance but the patient is symptomatic.

Causes of decreased mucus secretion include any chronic inflammation, such as Stevens-Johnson syndrome or mucous membrane pemphigoid; toxicity as with chemical burns; and hypovitaminosis A. Interestingly, even though it has been shown that there is a decrease in conjunctival goblet cells, they are still present at about 50% of their normal number (Kinoshita et al. 1983).

Abnormalities of the lipid layer are uncommon, but diseases include familial lack of sebaceous secretion (Muenzler 1986) and chronic blepharitis (Holly and Lemp 1977).

The most common abnormality lies with the aqueous layer. It is normal for there to be some decrease in the tear volume with age; however, this is generally not symptomatic (Seal 1985). Several diseases, including congenital abnormalities of the lacrimal glands, may give rise to keratoconjunctivitis sicca, but the vast majority of cases are in postmenopausal women (Holly and Lemp 1977).

Patients do not generally complain of dry eye per se. In fact, Baum (1985) stated categorically that the only patients who complain of dry eye do so because they are quoting their physician's diagnosis. Instead, the complaint is usually of a sandy feeling under the lids, or a scratchy sensation. Parodoxically, the patient may complain of increasing tearing, since the tears may suddenly gush in a reflex response. Very often, these patients will have increased symptoms on windy days, because of the increased drying effect. We have found that reading and other activities requiring concentration are also likely to elicit symproms because of decreased blinking frequency. Smoke, a suspension of solid material in air, is a major irritant to the dry eye patient (Lamberts 1983). Keratoconjunctivitis sicca patients often become symptomatic at night or upon awakening. This is because tear production is greatly diminished during sleep or with the eyes closed (Baum 1985).

Medications may decrease tear output, including parasympatholytics, sympatholytics, and antihistamines (Crandall and Leopold 1979). Since these patients may be taking a variety of medications for various conditions, the possibility that they may be diminishing the tear secretion should be borne in mind.

There is no single, recognized test to make the diagnosis of keratoconjunctivitis sicca (Lemp et al. 1986). Instead, in addition to the history, there are a number of observations and tests performed by the ophthalmologist to aid in making the diagnosis. First, of course, is simply observation of the position and action of the lids, to assure that the blink reflex is intact, that the lids close completely, and that the lids are in proper alignment. Corneal sensation is checked with a cotton wisp drawn out from a swab.

The Schirmer test to measure tear secretion has come under increasing criticism. It is inexpensive and simple to do, but may be both inaccurate and imprecise. The test is performed with strips of filter paper 30 mm in length, with a notch and rounded margin at one end. This end is bent at the notch, and the paper is slipped beneath the inferior lid, with the remainder of the paper hanging out. The test is usually conducted for five minutes, and the length of paper wet by the tears measured. The wetting curve is an exponential one (Lamberts 1983b). Generally the patient is advised to keep the eyes closed, and the paper is placed so that it does not touch the cornea.

Some authors advocate the use of the Schirmer's test without anaesthetic, stating that it thus reflects the ability of the eye to tear in response to stimuli (Farris et al.

1983, Epstein and Waring 1985). Others use anaesthetic drops to get a better idea of "basal" tear secretion (Muenzler 1986). In fact, there is doubt that such a test really measures basal secretion, since even the instillation of the anaesthetic drops is an irritant (Lamberts 1983 a). Doing the test with the eyes open or closed seems not to matter (Lamberts 1983 b). Other parameters of the test have really not been adequately studied, such as the length the paper strips should be or how long they should remain in the eye.

A modification of the Schirmer test, which promises to be less irritating, is the Hamano thread test (Hamano and Bode 1985). Instead of filter paper strips, the end of a thread impregnated with phenol-red dye is placed under the inferior lid. As the thread is moistened, the dye changes color permanently, so the thread can be saved in the patient's record for future documentation and comparison. Also, the test is complete in 15 seconds rather than five minutes.

Another easily performed test is rose bengal staining. Rose bengal is an aniline dye which, unlike fluorescein, will stain devitalized or damaged epithelium of both the cornea and conjunctiva. Persons with keratoconjunctivitis sicca show a highly characteristic staining pattern across the nasal and temporal conjunctiva which extends in a band across the cornea, sparing those areas normally covered by the lids (Lamberts 1983 b). Others (Farris et al. 1983) found this test much more sensitive than the Schirmer test, with 58% positive results compared to 10%; however clearly it was not sufficiently so. Nevertheless, the characteristic pattern, when present, is diagnostic for keratoconjunctivitis sicca.

Rose bengal also stains filaments, another hallmark of the dry eye in Sjögren's syndrome (Tabbara and Frayha 1983). Filaments are epithelial covered strands of mucus that are attached to the cornea. Their pathogenesis is not understood, but they may be associated with hydrophobic foci on the corneal surface to which lipid-containing mucus becomes attached (Lamberts 1983 b). Traction on the filaments from blinking causes a foreign body sensation.

Tear breakup time is another useful parameter. A drop of fluorescein is instilled, and the time between the last blink and the appearance of dark, nonfluorescent areas in the tear film is measured. Classically, an overly rapid breakup of the tear film, when not seen consistently over the same area and indicating a local surface irregularity, points toward either a mucin or lipid layer abnormality (Holly and Lemp 1977). However, the tear film becomes unstable in aqueous deficiencies as well (Epstein and Waring 1985), because of lipid contamination of the ocular surface (Holly 1985).

Other tests, such as lactoferrin concentration and lysozyme concentration, have been shown to be sensitive (Farris et al. 1983), but they are less easily done in the clinical setting. The enzyme tests have been found to be more reliable than the Schirmer test and are performed using an ELISA (enzyme-linked immunosorbent assay) on tear eluates (Seal 1985). Also, tear osmolarity has been found to be markedly elevated in keratoconjunctivitis sicca patients (Gilbard 1985).

Other newer tests and methods include the study of tear dilution of fluorescein, measured with a fluorophotometer (Lemp et al. 1986). Fluorescein is instilled in the eye, and its disappearance over time measured with the fluorophotometer. It was found that not only is the dye diluted more slowly in patients with keratoconjunctivitis sicca, but also that these eyes were not able to respond to irritative stimuli.

The corneal surface itself can be studied more quantitatively as well. Wide field specular microscopy has been used to study the corneal endothelium, but more recently has been combined with fluorescein and rose bengal application and color photography to study the epithelium (Lemp and Gold 1985). In keratoconjunctivitis sicca, there appears to be greater turnover of surface epithelial cells.

A very important test used in the workup of the patient with Sjögren's syndrome is biopsy of an accessory salivary gland (Tabbara et al. 1974). Clearly, it is imprudent and relatively difficult to biopsy the lacrimal gland itself, but changes in these glands correlate well with the clinical findings and symptoms, and hence presumably with the morphologic changes in the lacrimal gland itself.

The ocular surface is best examined with the slit lamp. Abnormalities in the corneal surface may be readily apparent or may be enhanced with application of fluorescein. The tear lake may also be examined for stability, and also for the presence of debris, an almost universal finding in keratoconjunctivitis sicca (Lemp 1985). Also, there may be sterile infiltrates at the corneal periphery, which are grayish in color. Corneal sensation remains intact, but the overlying epithelium may break down, sometimes leading ultimately to perforation (Pfister and Murphy 1980). These infiltrates consist of immune complexes and neutrophils (Tabbara and Frayha 1983). Ulcerations leading to perforation may also occur more centrally (Pfister and Murphy 1980).

The dry eye is also at higher risk of superficial infection, including blepharitis and conjunctivitis, probably because of the loss of the antibacterial component of normal tears (Lemp 1985). Band keratopathy, or calcium deposition in superficial cornea at the interpalpebral fissure, is also more frequent in patients with keratoconjunctivitis sicca, through an unknown mechanism (Lamberts 1983b).

The patient with Sjögren's syndrome has a chronic, symptomatic disease which can be controlled but not cured. The task of the ophthalmologist is to provide a means of controlling symptoms, and fortunately, recent therapeutic advances may make this job easier.

For the vast majority of patients, tear substitutes are the mainstay of therapy. There are many of these available, with varying degrees of viscosity. Advertisements make much of the particular osmotic and viscotic properties of a given preparation, citing the studies which show that the tears of the keratoconjunctivitis sicca patient have a considerably higher osmolarity (Gilbard 1985; Gilbard and Kenyon 1985). It would seem that the content of the tear substitute prescribed should be tailored to the patient's tear abnormality. However tears, both normal and abnormal, tend to dilute the preparation within minutes (Gilbard 1985, Gilbard and Kenyon 1985). Despite this, these authors found that a half isotonic solution was superior in symptom relief. However, we and others have found that the most effective tear substitute for a patient is the one that the patient prefers (Holly and Lemp 1977). The tear substitute should not, however, contain vasoactive substances which promise to whiten the conjunctiva, since overuse of these preparations leads to a rebound hyperemia. The severely affected patient may find the drops are needed every few minutes.

Ointments can also be effective, and have the advantage of lasting longer. However, because of the marked blurring of vision, they are generally used only at night. Recently, a slow-release tear substitute has been marketed under the trade name Lacrisert (© Merck Sharp & Dohme). It is a polymer of hydroxypropyl cellulose and comes as a cylinder which is inserted below the inferior tarsal margin, where it absorbs tears, slowly dissolves, and releases polymer (Lamberts 1983b). It is particularly useful for moderately severely affected patients, but not all can tolerate it (Muenzler 1986). Some find the presence of the piece of polymer irritating, and some unwittingly lose it.

Some therapeutic failures occur because of sensitivity to preservatives (Wilson 1979). Furthermore, some preservatives, such as benzalkonium chloride and the other quaternary ammonium salts, damage the lipid layer, contributing further to tear instability (Burstein 1985). Some tear substitutes are now available without preservatives, and these or saline solutions can be used (Muenzler 1986). Care is required, however, especially with saline solutions, that they do not become contaminated.

Several new kinds of topical therapy have recently been suggested. One is the use of dilute sodium hyaluronate (Polack and McNiece 1982). This substance was recently developed for anterior segment surgical use, and has gained wide popularity. For topical use, a ten per cent solution is suggested, and several investigators (Polack and McNiece 1982; DeLuise and Peterson 1984; Stuart and Linn 1985) have found good relief of symptoms. The major drawback to this preparation is its expense.

Another group of investigators (Fox et al. 1984) has developed a procedure for taking the patient's own blood, allowing it to clot, and preparing a centrifuged filtered specimen for use as a tear substitute. Preliminary single blind objective and subjective tests have been promising, and the procedure is not difficult. The only problem noted was in one patient, who had increased symptoms when one batch contained a small amount of fibrin. While the objective signs did not disappear completely, the rose bengal staining was considerably lessened.

Gel tears are another recent development (Leibowitz et al. 1984). These are a high molecular weight crosslinked polymer of acrylic acid. Patients in the study were able to decrease their dosage considerably with this preparation. It is not yet commercially available.

Another new tear substitute is all-trans retinoic acid applied topically (Tseng 1985; Tseng et al. 1985). This treatment was originally pioneered for use in vitamin A deficient patients, and has now been extended to those with other tear abnormalities. It was found that even patients with primarily aqueous layer pathology showed a reduced number of goblet cells by impression cytology (Tseng 1985; Tseng et al. 1985). While in theory one would expect topical retinoic acid to work only in patients with primary deficiencies of the mucin layer, clinical results show that patients with aqueous deficiency can also benefit, although the numbers to date have been small (Tseng 1985). By impression cytology, reversal of the epithelial changes was documented, along with subjective improvement in symptoms.

If tear substitutes are insufficient to control symptoms, other steps can be taken in an effort to preserve the tears that the patient does have (Lamberts 1983a, b). Such entities as swimmer's goggles can be very helpful in creating a moist chamber effect by preventing evaporation. The same effect can be achieved with food plastic wrap taped over the eyes (Lamberts 1983b). Commercial "bubble" bandages are also available. While these methods may not be cosmetically very acceptable, they do offer a method of treatment at least for the patient at home.

Soft contact lenses, referred to as bandage lenses, may also be helpful in protecting the cornea, especially when filaments are a problem (Lamberts 1983 b). However, the lenses themselves absorb tears, and the patients must be followed very carefully, since the patients are at increased risk for deposits and infections (Epstein and Waring 1985). Nevertheless, contact lenses are invaluable in the management of the corneal ulcers of Sjögren's syndrome (Pfister and Murphy 1980). A new type of soft lens, made of acrylic rubber, only has a 1% water content, so that it does not compete for tears. Such a lens may prove safer and more effective in these patients (Epstein and Waring 1985).

Surgical means may be tried when nonsurgical methods fail. Punctal occlusion is another method of conserving the tears that remain (Lamberts 1983 a, b). Probably this method should only be considered when the drying is very severe and when it seems evident that there is no likelihood of spontaneous increase in tear flow (Lamberts 1983 a). Stents have been devised as a nonsurgical means of occlusion (Muenzler 1986); this can be a good way to predict the success of surgical occlusion. Tarsorrhaphy, a partial closure of the lid to narrow the palpebral fissure, is another surgical option, used particularly for the corneal sequelae of marginal thinning and melting (Muenzler 1986).

A form of therapy which has been relatively neglected is that of autonomic stimulation of tear flow (Lamberts 1983 b). The sympathomimetics and parasympathomimetics, especially the muscarinics, stimulate tear flow (Crandall and Leopold 1979). Pilocarpine taken orally has been reported to increase tearing, as has bromhexine (Lamberts 1983 a). We have recently seen a dry eye patient who had relief while on neostigmin and who reported increased symptoms when that drug was withdrawn from the market.

In the patient with aqueous deficiency, a relative excess of mucin production, and formation of corneal filaments, a mucolytic agent such as acetylcysteine has been helpful (Lamberts 1983 a, b). However, other investigators (Pfister and Murphy 1980) could not confirm this. It would seem worthwhile to try it in individual patients as needed.

Patients with Sjögren's syndrome have, of course, a chronic inflammatory infiltrate of the lacrimal glands. Therefore, steroid administration has been suggested. Topical steroid use for the corneal ulcers of Sjögren's syndrome was associated with a worsening clinical course (Pfister and Murphy 1980). However, systemic steroids on an alternate day schedule was helpful relatively early in the course of the disease (Tabbara and Frayha 1983).

Sjögren's syndrome represents a chronic disease which may be extremely debilitating. It is important for the physician to stress to the patient that for this and all symptoms of Sjögren's syndrome there is no cure, but that there are many treatment modalities available. It has been our experience that if the patient can be relieved of some of the more distressing dry eye symptoms, he or she will be much better able to cope with the tasks of daily living. These patients may easily become depressed (Lamberts 1983 b), so encouragement and symptom relief are therefore of paramount importance in management.

References

Baum J (1985) Clinical manifestations of dry eye states. Trans Ophthalmol Soc UK 104: 415-423

Burstein NL (1985) The effects of topical drugs and preservatives on the tears and corneal epithelium in dry eye. Trans Ophthalmol Soc UK 104: 402-409

Crandall DC, Leopold IH (1979) The influence of systemic drugs on tear constituents. Ophthalmology 86: 115-125

DeLuise VP, Peterson WS (1984) The use of topical Healon tears in the management of refractory dry-eye syndrome. Ann Ophthalmol 16: 823-824

Epstein RJ, Waring GO (1985) Aging and the cornea. Part 2. Conditions that may lead to visual impairment. Geriatr Ophthalmol 1 (3): 17-23

Farris RL, Gilbard JP, Stuchell RN, Mandel ID (1983) Diagnostic tests in keratoconjunctivitis sicca. The CLAO J 9: 23-28

Fox RI, Chan R, Michelson JB, Belmont JB, Michelson PE (1984) Beneficial effect of artificial tears made with autologous serum in patients with keratoconjunctivitis sicca. Arthritis Rheum 27: 459-461

Gilbard JP (1985) Tear film osmolarity and keratoconjunctivitis sicca. The CLAO J 11: 243-250

Gilbard JP, Kenyon KR (1985) Tear diluents in the treatment of keratoconjunctivitis sicca. Ophthalmology 92: 646-650

Hamano H, Bode D (1985) The phenol-red thread test for measuring lacrimation. Scientific poster, presented at American Academy of Ophthalmology, San Francisco

Holly FJ (1985) Physical chemistry of the normal and disordered tear film. Trans Ophthalmol Soc UK 104: 374-380

Holly FJ, Lemp MA (1977) Tear physiology and dry eyes. Surv Ophthalmol 22: 69-87

Jones IS, Jakobiec FA, Nolan BT (1985) Patient examination and introduction to orbital disease. In: Duane TD, Jaeger EA (eds) Clinical Ophthalmology. Harper and Row, Philadelphia (vol 2, chap 21, p 12)

Kinoshita S, Kiorpes TC, Friend J, Thoft RA (1983) Goblet cell density in ocular surface disease. A better indicator than tear mucin. Arch Ophthalmol 101: 1284-1287

Lamberts DW (1983) Physiology of the tear film. In: Smolin G, Thoft RA (eds) The Cornea. Little Brown, Boston, pp 31-42

Lamberts DW (1983) Keratoconjunctivitis sicca. In: Smolin G, Thoft RA (eds) The Cornea. Little Brown, Boston, pp 293-309

Leibowitz HM, Chang RK, Mandell AI (1984) Gel tears. A new medication for the treatment of dry eyes. Ophthalmology 91: 1199-1204

Lemp MA (1985) Diagnosis and treatment of tear deficiencies. In: Duane TD, Jaeger EA (eds) Clinical Ophthalmology, Harper and Row, Philadelphia (vol 4, chap 14, pp 1-10)

Lemp MA, Gold JB (1985) An in vivo study of the corneal surface in keratoconjunctivitis sicca. Trans Ophthalmol Soc UK 104: 436-438

Lemp MA, Mahmood MA, Guimaraes RQ (1986) Lacrimal function in patients with dry eyes. Geriatr Ophthalmol 2 (2): 9-12

Leonard JN, Wright P, Haffenden GP, Williams DM, Griffiths CEM, Fry L (1985) Skin diseases and the dry eye. Trans Ophthalmol Soc UK 104: 467-476

McGhee CNJ, Lee WR (1985) Quantification and enzymic identification of conjunctival surface mucus. Trans Ophthalmol Soc UK 104: 446-449

Moutsopoulos HM, Chused TM, Mann DL, Klippel JH, Fauci AS, Frank MM, Lawley TJ, Hamburger MI (1980) Sjögren's syndrome (sicca syndrome). Current issues. Ann Int Med 92 (part 1): 212-226

Muenzler WS (1985) The dry eye. A working outline of etiology, symptoms, diagnosis, and treatment. Geriatr Ophthalmol 2 (1): 19-23

Pfister RR, Murphy GE (1980) Corneal ulceration and perforation associated with Sjögren's syndrome. Arch Ophthalmol 98: 89-94

Polack FM, McNiece MT (1982) The treatment of dry eyes with Na hyaluronate (Healon). Cornea 1: 133-136

Seal DV (1985) The effect of ageing and disease on tear constituents. Trans Ophthalmol Soc UK 104: 355-362

Sjögren H (1933) Auf Kenntnis der Keratoconjunctivitis sicca (Keratitis filiformis bei Hypofunction der Tränendrüsen). Acta Ophthalmol 11 (suppl 2): 1-151
Smolin G (1985) The defense mechanism of the outer eye. Trans Ophthalmol Soc UK 104: 363-366
Stuart JC, Linn JG (1985) Dilute sodium hyaluronate (Healon) in the treatment of ocular surface disorders. Ann Ophthalmol 17: 190-192
Tabbara KF, Frayha RA (1983) Alternate-day steroid therapy for patients with primary Sjögren's syndrome. Ann Ophthalmol 15: 358-361
Tabbara KF, Ostler HB, Daniels TE, Sylvester RA, Greenspan JS, Talal N (1974) Sjögren's syndrome. A correlation between ocular findings and labial salivary gland histology. Trans Amer Acad Ophthalmol Otolaryngol 78: 467-478
Tiffany JM (1985) The role of meibomian secretion in the tears. Trans Ophthalmol Soc UK 104: 396-401
Tseng SCG (1985) Topical retinoid treatment for dry eye disorders. Trans Ophthalmol Soc UK 104: 489-495
Tseng SCG, Maumenee AE, Stark WJ, Maumenee IH, Jensen AD, Green WR, Kenyon KR (1985) Topical retinoid treatment for various dry-eye disorders. Ophthalmology 92: 717-727
Wilson FM (1979) Adverse external ocular effects of topical ophthalmic medications. Surv Ophthalmol 24: 57-88
Wright P (1985) Normal tear production and drainage. Trans Ophthalmol Soc UK 104: 351-354

3. Chemistry of Saliva

B.J. BAUM and P.C. FOX

Introduction

A hallmark of Sjögren's Syndrome (SS) is salivary gland dysfunction (Chisholm and Mason 1973; Daniels et al. 1975). A variety of subjective complaints or objective tests have been employed to diagnose the salivary component of SS, but at present there is no universally utilized, unequivocal test(s) which distinguishes disease-specific salivary involvement (Fox et al. 1985). Many studies have even employed such a minimal criterion as the verbal affirmation of oral dryness as evidence of salivary dysfunction. Thus, although an enormous literature exists citing salivary complications in SS, there are, in fact, few studies dealing with gland secretions per se and with the chemistry of saliva. It is the purpose of this chapter to 1.) critically review available salivary chemical data (both published studies as well as some of our own unpublished work) and 2.) discuss the implications of these findings for understanding the functional status of glandular cells in the SS patient.

Review of Previously Published Studies

An exhaustive literature search yielded only nine peer-reviewed articles published in the last twelve years focusing on aspects of salivary chemistry in SS. Of these, only four studies examined single gland secretions, in each case the parotid gland, and no study has examined submandibular/sublingual gland function. The paucity of information, which is surprising in light of increasing interest in other aspects of SS over the last several years, is likely the result of a number of factors. First, it is difficult to characterize a homogenous population to study the salivary component of SS. There is a wide range in salivary performance of SS patients. Where present, salivary involvement is usually a chronic feature of the syndrome leading to progressive diminution of function. Second, as noted above, this situation is complicated by the great variability in diagnostic criteria employed to assess salivary function. There is no clear agreement on what constitutes "definite" salivary involvement, although histologic evaluation of labial minor salivary glands is most frequently employed (Greenspan et al. 1974). Finally, it is also clear that in a good number of SS patients salivary chemistry is simply irrelevant as there is no remaining gland function. This number is, at present, unknown and will, of necessity, vary depending on how early a diagnosis can be assigned. Based on recent studies (Stuchell et al. 1984; our own unpublished work), we estimate that perhaps 50–70% of patients have some level of salivary gland secretory function at the time when a diagnosis can initially be made. Salivary performance ranges from minimal to essentially normal. This great variability complicates assigning patients a diagnosis. Thus, the "typical" salivary involvement of a SS patient is difficult to describe. In the context of this section studies by several investigators, using different evaluation procedures, will be reviewed and discussed together. It is also essential to remember that patients not secreting saliva, who represent a significant number of individuals with SS, are not included.

A summary of the four published reports on parotid salivary chemical findings in SS is given in Table 1. Two points should be made initially about these studies. Each involves only stimulated parotid secretions and the two most extensive studies were performed by the same laboratory, albeit eight years apart. The studies show agreement on certain general findings. First is the fact that most patients studied had significantly decreased fluid output following gustatory stimuli. Second, these parotid secretions had increased concentrations of Na^+ and Cl^- and normal quantities of K^+ and total protein. Finally, there were elevations of specific proteins, most notably IgA.

To appreciate these results, a general understanding of the mechanism of saliva secretion is needed. Briefly, salivary fluid flow (water movement) occurs only across acinar epithelial tissue (Young and van Lennep 1979). At present it is felt that water transport is driven primarily by a loop-diuretic sensitive, $Na^+/K^+/Cl^-$ cotransport system located in acinar cell basolateral membranes (Young 1982; Martinez and Cassity 1983). Undirectional fluid movement occurs because Cl^- exits from the apical membrane via a specific Ca^{2+}-dependent channel (Findlay and Petersen 1985). Na^+ is thought to travel paracellularly to provide electrical neutrality. This initial isotonic acinar secretion is termed "primary saliva". It is extensively modified as it traverses the duct system and enters the mouth as a hypotonic fluid (Young and van Lennep 1979; Baum et al. 1984). Most notably, Na^+ and Cl^- are extensively resorbed during normal secretion. This is suspected to occur in the striated duct

Table 1. Summary of Salivary Chemistry Data Previously Reported For the Stimulated Parotid Gland[a]

Study	SS Group[b]	Flow	Na^+	Cl^-	K^+	Protein	IgA	Albumin	Lz[c]	Lf[d]
1. Mandel, Baurmash, 1976	2°	↓70%	↑3×	↑3×	=	=	↑60%	=	–	–
2. Moutsopoulous et al. 1980	1°	↓to =	–	–	–	=	–	–	↑2.5×	–
3. Benedek-Spat et al. 1980	1° + 2°	↓60%	–	–	–	↑50%	–	–	–	–
4. Stuchell et al. 1984	1°	↓40%	↑3×	↑3×	=	=	↑3×	↑7×	–	↑10×

[a] General symbols used in table are ↑, increase; ↓, decrease; =, no change (all relative to controls presented within study); –, not determined
[b] SS Group = Sjögren's Syndrome classification as either 1° (primary) or 2° (secondary)
[c] Lz = lysozyme
[d] Lf = lactoferrin

region along with active K^+ secretion. Most (> 85%) salivary proteins are produced and secreted by acinar cells. These are released by a specific exocytotic process (amylase is an example). The remaining proteins are released from a number of duct cell types. It is also important to recall that large serum proteins are excluded from gland salivas and are not a normal constituent of the secretion. They are apparently "filtered out" at the acinar level. Though clearly some minimal leak can occur, significant quantities of serum components are only seen during acute inflammatory states and represent a loss of gland integrity.

In light of these observations, some of the data on salivary chemistries in SS are conflicting. First examination supports a view that these glands are chronically inflamed, evidenced by increased levels of Na^+ and Cl^-, high levels of albumin and elevated lactoferrin reported by some. In contrast, there was no change in K^+ and impressively no change in total protein. The latter is particularly important because serum protein concentration is much greater (~10×) than that of saliva. One would expect greatly increased protein levels if leakage of serum due to inflammation were responsible for the elevated concentrations of Na^+ and Cl^-. At this stage, we must conclude from these earlier studies that the compromise in the integrity of the parotid salivary unit with SS must be different than occurs with a frank parotitis. There is clear evidence of dysfunction, although the specific sites or mechanisms of damage are still unknown.

Besides these studies on stimulated parotid gland function, there are also five published studies which have examined aspects of salivary chemistry in SS employing unstimulated whole saliva (Table 2). To a considerable extent, studies of whole saliva composition are difficult to interpret and not necessarily informative about gland function. This is because whole saliva may contain (besides gland secretions) food debris, bacteria and bacterial products, cells and serum components from gingival crevicular exudate, bronchial secretions, desquamated cells, and, in the presence of mucosal ulceration or irritation, serum products and whole blood (Mandel 1980). In the absence of severe oral mucositis, oral fluid output likely represents salivary gland fluid transport capabilities. However, whole saliva chemical analyses should be viewed with caution. Thus, the meaning of the increases in both Na^+ and K^+ levels in unstimulated whole saliva is uncertain. Of the data presented in Table 2, most striking are changes in IgA and IgG levels. As shown by Ben-Aryeh et al. (1983) and Elkon et al. (1983), the IgA alteration reflects changes in secretory

Table 2. Summary of Major Findings Previously Reported for Unstimulated Whole Saliva[a]

Study	SS Group[b]	Flow	Na^+	K^+	IgA[c]	IgG	IgM	Albumin
1. Ben-Aryeh et al. 1981, 1982, 1983	1° + 2°	↓70%	↑2.5×	↑2×	↑7×	–	–	–
2. Elkon et al. 1983	2°	ng	–	–	↑75%[d]	↑2.5×[d]	=[d]	=

[a] General symbols used in table are ↑, increase; ↓, decrease; =, no change (all relative to controls presented within study); –, not determined; ng, not given
[b] SS Group = Sjögren's Syndrome classification as either 1° (primary) or 2° (secondary)
[c] IgA values reflect changes in secretory IgA
[d] In study 2, when the relative concentrations of immunoglobulins were compared to albumin levels, in both serum and saliva, only IgG in saliva was elevated

(glandular), not serum, IgA. Elkon et al. (1983), by comparing albumin and immunoglobulin levels, determined a relative concentration ratio of immunoglobulins in serum and in saliva. This ratio was markedly significant for IgG. The authors interpret this finding as being evidence of increased local immunoglobulin synthesis in gland tissue. This may represent another manifestation of immune hyper-reactivity observed in many SS patients. Also an interesting study by Konttinen et al. (1984, not given in Table 2) reported elevated total protein and lactoferrin levels in unstimulated whole saliva. This is consonant with the findings of Stuchell et al. (1984) described above for parotid saliva. However since there was no correlation between labial biopsy results and lactoferrin levels (Konttinen et al. 1984), the interpretation of the findings is not yet clear.

Current Salivary Chemical Studies of Sjögren's Syndrome Patients

A possible explanation for the existing data conflicts might lie with the diagnostic variations utilized by different investigators. We have initiated a series of studies examining salivary gland function in both primary and secondary SS patients. All patients have had an extensive diagnostic evaluation (Fox et al. 1985) and have been assigned to various subject groups based on the criteria outlined in Table 3.

In Table 4, data are shown on salivary gland fluid output by parotid and submandibular/sublingual glands, under resting (unstimulated) and stimulated conditions. It is clear that no major differences were seen in salivary flow rates between the control groups of healthy subjects and patients admitted with oral complaints unrelated to salivary performance. However, in patients with SS, significant differences were seen for each secretion. In general, 50-60% reductions in flow rates were noted, but changes in unstimulated secretions, especially from secondary SS patients, were most dramatic. In this group, resting parotid secretion was negligible, while resting submandibular/sublingual secretion was decreased > 70%. Another very important point, illustrated in Table 4, is that the fluid secreting capabilities of SS patients are extremely variable. With the exception of unstimulated parotid secretion from sec-

Table 3. Diagnostic Criteria Employed in Assigning Patients To Sjögren's Syndrome Groups[a]

Criterion	Primary	Secondary
Salivary flow rate	normal→absent	
Salivary scintigraphy	minimally: delayed secretion, normal uptake	
Labial minor salivary gland histology	minimally: evidence of focal inflammatory infiltrate[b]	
Connective tissue disease	absent	present
Lacrimal dysfunction	present	±
Extraglandular manifestations	±	

± = present or absent

[a] Further discussion of diagnostic criteria differentiating primary from secondary SS may be found in Fox et al. 1984

[b] Equal to grade 3 of Chisholm et al. (1970) or focus score 1 of Greenspan et al. (1974)

Table 4. Salivary Gland Fluid Secretion in Healthy Subjects and Patients ± Sjögren's Syndrome[a]

	N	Unstimulated		Stimulated	
		Parotid	SM/SL[b]	Parotid	SM/SL
Healthy Subjects	8	0.076 ± 0.014 (0.008 – 0.115)	0.104 ± 0.015 (0.043 – 0.162)	0.511 ± 0.075 (0.211 – 0.811)	0.336 ± 0.068 (0.093 – 0.623)
Non-Salivary Gland Patients	9	0.057 ± 0.018 (0.0 – 0.155)	0.128 ± 0.035 (0.033 – 0.367)	0.549 ± 0.145 (0.35 – 1.21)	0.397 ± 0.137 (0.042 – 1.365)
Primary SS	9	0.030 ± 0.015 (0.0 – 0.128)	0.066 ± 0.024 (0.0 – 0.196)	0.260 ± 0.046 (0.0 – 0.481)	0.237 ± 0.072 (0.0 – 0.654)
Secondary SS	7	0.004 ± 0.004 (0.0 – 0.028)	0.031 ± 0.027 (0.0 – 0.193)	0.254 ± 0.084 (0.052 – 0.621)	0.141 ± 0.075 (0.006 – 0.45)

[a] Data are presented as the mean ± SEM of values determined for the number (N) of persons indicated in each category. The range of values observed for each subject category is given in parentheses. Values for flow rates are expressed as ml/min-gland. Saliva was collected as described (Fox et al. 1985). Stimulation was achieved with 2% citrate. Primary Sjögren's Syndrome (SS) patients presented with evidence of lacrimal and salivary dysfunction alone (sicca syndrome). Secondary SS patients presented with the sicca syndrome plus evidence of a connective tissue disease. Patients in both groups had a variety of extraglandular manifestations of SS. Non-salivary gland patients were individuals admitted with oral complaints (eg. altered taste, oral motor dysfunction) unrelated to salivary performance. No individual, in these study groups, presented with detectable levels of albumin (lower limits of detection = 10 μg/ml) in any gland secretion

[b] SM/SL = submandibular/sublingual

ondary SS patients, each group included individuals with fluid transport capabilities well into the normal range.

In Table 5, the concentrations of several salivary constituents in stimulated parotid saliva are shown. It is impossible, and indeed generally unnecessary, to be concerned with salivary composition of resting secretions, as too many SS patients exhibit no resting fluid output. Two important points can be made about these data. First is that, in general, these SS patients and controls displayed similar salivary chemical values for all components studied (total protein, Na^+, K^+, Cl^-, lysozyme). There were some differences between the SS groups. Second, all groups (patients and healthy subjects) exhibited similar variability in compositional values, reflecting the wide range of "normal" concentrations of salivary constituents.

Table 5. Composition of Stimulated Parotid Saliva in Healthy Subjects and Patients ± Sjögren's Syndrome[a]

	Healthy Subjects	Non-Salivary Gland Patients	Primary SS	Secondary SS
Protein (mg/ml)	2.82 ± 0.63	4.3 ± 0.71	3.9 ± 0.56	3.85 ± 0.95
Na^+ (meq/l)	14.8 ± 4.9	8.5 ± 4.8	9.6 ± 5.2	18.7 ± 5.6
K^+ (meq/l)	20.3 ± 1.6	23.6 ± 2.1	24.7 ± 2.6	33.8 ± 6.3
Cl^- (meq/l)	16.4 ± 3.7	22.3 ± 4.7	18.0 ± 3.5	40.8 ± 9.2
Lysozyme (μg/ml)	5.8 ± 0.5	4.4 ± 0.3	5.4 ± 0.5	5.8 ± 0.7

[a] All subjects had no detectable albumin in their saliva (as in Table 4). Results are expressed as the mean ± SEM

Table 6. Composition of Stimulated Submandibular/Sublingual Saliva in Healthy Subjects and Patients ± Sjögren's Syndrome[a]

	Healthy Subjects	Non-Salivary Gland Patients	Primary SS	Secondary SS
Protein (mg/ml)	1.55 ± 0.15	1.21 ± 0.19	1.53 ± 0.24	1.54 ± 0.20
Na^+ (meq/l)	18.7 ± 5.1	13.2 ± 6.7	12.1 ± 2.3	18.4 ± 5.9
K^+ (meq/l)	15.1 ± 1.4	15.4 ± 1.4	17.3 ± 1.3	22.9 ± 3.6
Cl^- (meq/l)	15.3 ± 3.4	18.7 ± 4.2	16.8 ± 1.6	29.1 ± 8.4
Lysozyme (μg/ml)	6.3 ± 0.8	4.5 ± 0.2	4.8 ± 0.3	4.4 ± 0.4

[a] All subjects had no detectable albumin in their saliva (as in Table 4). Results are expressed as the mean ± SEM

Although individual exceptions occur (eg. modestly elevated [K^+] and [Cl^-] in secondary SS patients), it is difficult to describe general chemical characteristics (for those variables examined) of stimulated parotid saliva from SS patients. A similar conclusion may be drawn from the compositional data of stimulated submandibular/sublingual salivas (Table 6).

Conclusions

It is important to restate that there are relatively few data available studying salivary chemistry in SS. With this caveat, certain cautious conclusions can be drawn. A critical point concerning overall salivary gland function in patients with SS is its heterogeneity. SS patients do show a consistent diminution in quantity of secretions (especially unstimulated) but many individuals are seen with normal stimulated fluid output. In general, saliva composition is only modestly altered and is often within normal limits. The data support a conclusion that if gland acinar parenchymal cells are present and capable of fluid movement, remaining cells will function in a "reasonably normal" fashion. Obviously, further studies with standardized assay methods from well-defined populations are necessary to adequately substantiate this point.

The only salivary chemical alteration seen reproducibly, which is apparently unique to SS, is an elevated level of secretory IgA. This has been observed by several investigators. A second, possibly useful salivary marker of SS, is an elevated lactoferrin level. An extensive salivary chemical study by Stuchell et al. (1984) suggested that SS patients display markedly increased amounts of lactoferrin in stimulated parotid saliva. Konttinen et al. (1984) also reported high lactoferrin levels in salivas from SS patients, but more data on this point are required to clarify any diagnostic role. Other salivary changes have not been found by all groups. This may be related to methods of sample collection or of patient selection. The data thus far fail to support the general notion that salivary compositional changes are consistent with glandular inflammation (Mandel and Baurmash 1976; Ben-Aryeh et al. 1981; Stuchell et al. 1984). Our own data and the work of Elkon et al. (1983) also reject such a general conclusion. We have only rarely seen significant albumin levels (i.e. > 10μg/ml) in gland secretions of SS patients.

The overall impression gained given the data available is that salivary glandular alterations in SS are extremely variable. No sweeping conclusions can be drawn at present about either specific diagnostic advantages of salivary chemistry in SS or what salivary chemistry can tell us about the etiology (focal parenchymal cell site) of this disorder.

References

Baum BJ, Costa PT Jr, Izutsu KI (1984) Sodium handling by aging human parotid glands is inconsistent with a two-stage secretion model. Am J Physiol 246: R35-R39

Ben-Aryeh H, Spielman A, Szargel R, Gutman D, Scharf J, Nahir M, Scharf Y (1981) Sialochemistry for the diagnosis of Sjögren's syndrome in xerostomic patients. Oral Surg 52: 487-490

Ben-Aryeh H, Szargel R, Gutman D (1983) Salivary IgA in Sjögren patients. Int J Oral Surg 12: 120-123

Benedek-Spat E, Puskas M, Rajki J (1980) Electrophoretic protein pattern of human parotid saliva in Sjögren's syndrome and sialosis. Acta Otolaryngol 90: 275-282

Chisholm DM, Mason DK (1973) Salivary gland function in Sjögren's syndrome. Brit Dent J 135: 393-399

Chisholm D, Waterhouse J, Mason D (1970) Lymphocytic sialadenitis in the major and minor glands: A correlation in postmortem subjects. J Clin Pathol 23: 690-696

Daniels TE, Silverman S Jr, Michalski JP, Greenspan JS, Sylvester RA, Talal N (1975) The oral component of Sjögren's syndrome. Oral Surg 39: 875-885

Elkon KB, Gharavi AE, Patel BM, Hughes GRV, Frankel A (1983) IgA and IgM rheumatoid factors in serum, saliva and other secretions: relationship to immunoglobulin ratios in systemic sicca syndrome and rheumatoid arthritis. Clin exp Immunol 52: 75-84

Findlay I, Petersen OH (1985) Acetylcholine stimulates a Ca^{2+}-dependent Cl^- conductance in mouse lacrimal acinar cells. Pflugers Arch 403: 328-330

Fox PC, van der Ven PV, Sonies BC, Weiffenbach JM, Baum BJ (1985) Xerostomia: evaluation of a symptom with increasing significance. JADA 110: 519-525

Fox RI, Howell FV, Bone RC, Michelson P (1984) Primary Sjögren's syndrome: Clinical and immunopathologic features. Sem Arthritis Rheum 14: 77-105

Greenspan JS, Daniels TE, Talal N, Sylvester RA (1974) The histopathology of Sjögren's syndrome in labial salivary gland biopsies. Oral Surg 37: 217-229

Konttinen YT, Kulomaa M, Malmstrom M, Kilpi A, Reitamo S (1984) Lactoferrin in Sjögren's Syndrome. Arthritis Rheum 27: 462-467

Mandel ID (1980) Sialochemistry in diseases and clinical situations affecting salivary glands. CRC Crit Rev Clin Lab Sci 12: 321-366

Mandel ID, Baurmash H (1976) Sialochemistry in Sjögren's syndrome. Oral Surg 41: 182-187

Martinez JR, Cassity N (1983) Effect of transport inhibitors on secretion by perfused rat submandibular gland. Am J Physiol 245: G711-G716

Moutsopoulos HM, Karsh J, Wolf RO, Tarpley TM, Tylenda A, Papadopoulos NM (1980) Lysozyme determination in parotid saliva from patients with Sjögren's syndrome. Am J Med 69: 39-42

Spielman A, Ben-Aryeh H, Lichtig C, Szargel R, Gutman D, Scharf J, Nahir M, Scharf Y (1982) Correlation between sialochemistry and lip biopsy in Sjögren's syndrome patients. Int J Oral Surg 11: 326-330

Stuchell RN, Mandel ID, Baurmash H (1984) Clinical utilization of sialochemistry in Sjögren's syndrome. J Oral Path 13: 303-309

Young JA, van Lennep EW (1979) Salivary and salt glands. In: Giebisch G, Tosteson DC, Ussing HH (eds) Membrane Transport In Biology. Springer, Berlin, pp 563-674

Young JA (1982) Is Na/Cl cotransport the basis of transepithelial transport in absorptive and secretory epithelia? In: Case RM, Garner A, Turnberg LA, Young JA (eds) Electrolyte and Water Transport Across Gastrointestinal Epithelia. Raven, New York, pp 181-198

4. Histopathology of Sjögren's Syndrome

T. E. Daniels, Th. B. Aufdemorte, and J. S. Greenspan

A common feature of all organs affected by Sjögren's syndrome (SS) is a potentially progressive lymphocytic infiltration. These infiltrates presumably cause functional changes in the affected organs and the diverse clinical features of this syndrome. The pathologic findings can include: 1) focal lymphocytic adenitis of salivary, lacrimal, eccrine and mucosal glands; 2) primary biliary cirrhosis, sclerosing cholangitis, pancreatitis and atrophic gastritis; 3) interstitial nephritis; 4) lymphocytic interstitial pneumonitis; 5) peripheral vasculitis; and 6) progression to pseudolymphoma or a B-cell lymphoma.

Benign lymphoepithelial lesion of salivary glands

Thus far, the salivary glands are the best studied organs in SS because they are readily accessible, produce prominent clinical symptoms and signs, and are affected in almost all patients. In many patients, the major salivary glands become enlarged and microscopic examination usually reveals a benign lymphoepithelial lesion (BLEL). This lesion, which was first described by Mikulicz (1892) and named by Godwin (1952), is characterized by lymphocytic replacement of the salivary epithelium and by the presence of so-called epimyoepithelial islands, which are helpful in distinguishing this benign lesion from lymphoma (Morgan and Castleman 1953) (Fig. 1). However, these islands are not always present; they were found in only 43% of the major salivary gland specimens from patients who had generally severe SS (Bloch et al. 1965). The cells actually making up the epimyoepithelial islands have never been clearly identified. Recently it was shown that these islands are mainly composed of keratin-containing epithelial cells, and do not contain cells with the immunohistochemical or ultrastructural characteristics of myoepithelial cells (Saku and Okabe 1984). In contrast, another recent study showed the presence of myoepithelial cells in the islands by electron microscopy, but only in the early stages of island development (Chaudry et al. 1986). Epimyoepithelial islands are seen very uncommonly in accessory salivary glands from patients with SS (Fig. 2). In the past, the term "Mikulicz disease" or "Mikulicz syndrome" has been applied to salivary or lacrimal gland swelling caused by SS and a variety of other conditions. These terms are so ambiguous and ill-defined that they should no longer be used (Batsakis 1982).

The progression of SS to extraglandular B-cell lymphoma is well documented (Anderson and Talal 1972; Kassan et al. 1978; Zulman et al. 1978) and discussed in Chapter II.C.1. Fortunately, it is fairly uncommon, considering the number of pa-

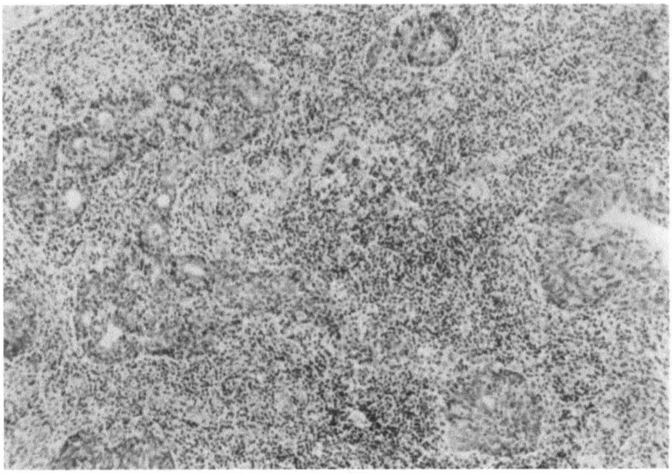

Fig. 1. Benign lymphoepithelial lesion with epimyoepithelial islands. Original magnification ×19

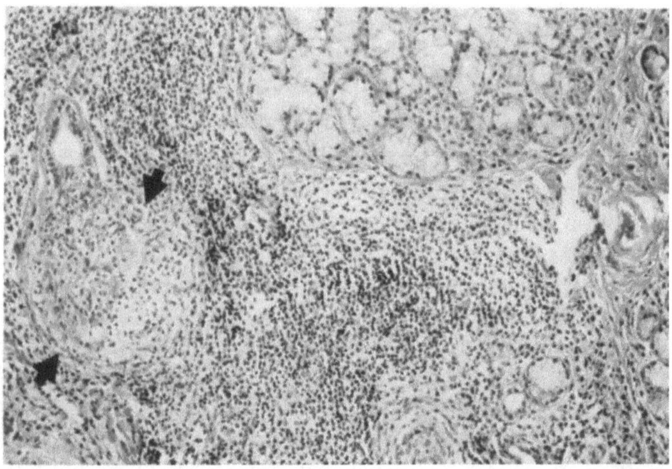

Fig. 2. Labial salivary gland showing focal sialadenitis. Epimyoepithelial island (arrows) is an uncommon finding in accessory salivary glands. Focus score of entire specimen is 6 foci/4 mm^2. Note normal-appearing acini adjacent to inflammatory infiltrate. Original magnification ×40

tients who have SS. Even less frequently, bilateral lymphomas have developed in the salivary glands of SS patients previously diagnosed as having BLEL (Lichtenfeld et al. 1976; Fye et al. 1980; Askari et al. 1985).

Existence of the salivary BLEL as a localized parotid tumor in patients who do not have a connective tissue disease has been discussed by several authors (Redondo et al. 1981; Batsakis 1982; Schmid et al. 1982; Nagao et al. 1983). These uncommon cases may occur in men or women and are sometimes unilateral. Rarely, a unilateral salivary carcinoma has been reported arising in a BLEL; more than half of the 27 reported cases of this apparent transformation have been in Eskimos (reviewed by Redondo et al. 1981). While BLEL may perhaps occur separately from SS as a limited salivary gland disease, the studies describing these patients do not always make clear that the diagnosis of primary SS was excluded. Since far more patients have BLEL in association with SS than separately, the diagnosis of a salivary BLEL should suggest the presence of SS, and additional diagnostic steps should be taken accordingly.

Major salivary gland biopsy in Sjögren's syndrome

Major salivary glands in SS may not show the full features of the BLEL, but instead contain various degrees of focal lymphocytic infiltration, defined as focal aggregates of 50 or more lymphocytes and histiocytes (Waterhouse and Doniach 1966). It is not known whether this focal lymphocytic infiltration represents an early stage that will eventually develop into a BLEL; parotid glands are generally biopsied only if enlarged, and rarely more than once, as the procedure carries potential surgical risks of damage to the facial nerve, cutaneous fistula, and scarring. In addition, diagnosing the salivary component of SS from major salivary gland specimens is problematical in that major salivary glands from persons who do not have SS also commonly contain lymphocytic foci (Batsakis 1979). In 250 sets of postmortem specimens evaluated by semiquantitative focus scoring, lymphocytic foci occurred commonly and equally in submandibular, parotid and lacrimal glands, especially in women over 45 years (Waterhouse 1963). Examination of 500 postmortem specimens of submandibular glands revealed moderate or severe grades of focal lymphocytic inflammation in 23% of females and in 9% of males (Waterhouse and Doniach 1966). Both of these studies found foci in subjects who did not have an antemortem history of rheumatoid arthritis as well as in those who did, but those who did had more extensive inflammation. In postmortem submandibular gland specimens from 96 subjects who had no history of connective tissue disease, focal lymphocytic adenitis was found in most specimens, was not associated with destructive changes in the salivary parenchyma, and had no clear relationship to age or sex (Scott 1976).

When parotid glands are extremely enlarged, partial parotidectomy is occasionally performed to reduce the tumor bulk and improve the patient's appearance. Such a procedure is certainly preferable to low-dose radiation treatment, but the patient must realize that the remaining glandular tissue usually undergoes further enlargement and the clinical problem may return, although it may be less severe. In cases where a malignant tumor is suspected, performing fine-needle aspiration cytology before an open biopsy may be helpful in planning the extent of, or need for, further surgery (Kline et al. 1981).

Minor salivary gland biopsy in Sjögren's syndrome

The need for a practical and objective way to define and assess the salivary component of SS led to the introduction of accessory salivary gland biopsy (Calman and Reifman 1966; Cifarelli et al. 1966), and subsequent studies established the basis for its use as a diagnostic criterion for the salivary component of SS. In contrast to postmortem studies of major salivary glands, most similar studies on labial salivary gland (LSG) specimens confirmed that, after lobes with duct dilation and extravascular polymorphonuclear leukocytes are excluded, significant focal sialadenitis is not found in LSGs unless a connective tissue disease is present (Figures 3 A and 3 B) (Chisholm and Mason 1968; Chisholm et al. 1970; Cifarelli et al. 1966; Davies et al. 1973; Greenspan et al. 1974).

Chisholm and Mason (1968) applied a semiquantitative inflammatory focus scoring method (Waterhouse 1963) to assess inflammation in LSG biopsy specimens from 40 patients with rheumatologic diseases and in 60 postmortem specimens. Using this method to grade the inflammation, they found that more than 1 focus of lymphocytes per 4-mm^2 area of gland was seen only in patients with SS and was not present in postmortem specimens. In a subsequent study of LSGs and submandibular glands from 116 consecutive postmortem subjects, excluding only those specimens showing evidence of salivary infection or neoplasia, there was a high prevalence of lymphocytic foci in the submandibular glands but these foci were not observed in any of the LSG specimens (Chisholm et al. 1970). Furthermore, these investigators suggest that LSGs reflect the status of salivary gland inflammation as a whole, based on the correlation between the extent of non-focal lymphocytic infiltration in LSGs and focal sialadenitis in submandibular glands. In clinical SS, there was histopathological agreement between LSG and parotid gland biopsy specimens from each of 12 patients examined (Bertram and Hjørting-Hansen 1970).

Later, focal lymphocytic sialadenitis was demonstrated in 82% of minor gland specimens from the palate of 80 patients with various connective tissue diseases, and in 6% of those from 80 healthy subjects (Eisenbud et al. 1973). However, this study only considered the presence or absence of lymphocytic foci, not their size, frequency or distribution. Greenspan et al. (1974) examined the histopathologic features of 75 labial salivary glands, 43 of them coming from patients with SS. They modified the Chisholm and Mason (1968) grading criteria to enumerate focus scores of from 1 to 12 foci/4 mm^2 and found that there was a significant positive correlation between higher focus score and larger foci, and that within the foci the proportion of pyroninophilic cells (plasma cells or activated lymphocytes) decreased sharply as focus size increased. An interpretation and comparison of Chisholm and Mason's grading system with this more quantitative focus scoring method has recently been published (Daniels 1986).

Another study grading 86 LSG specimens by qualitative criteria found more and larger lymphocytic foci in patients with primary SS than in those with both SS and rheumatoid arthritis (secondary SS) (Tarpley et al. 1974). Other investigators, examining a series of 111 LSG biopsies, observed focal sialadenitis in 81% of specimens from patients with SS, in 36% of those from patients with another connective tissue disease, and in none of those from patients with other diseases; however, their diagnostic criteria for SS were not reported (Takeda 1980). Whaley et al. (1973), who used xerostomia (as indicated by the absence of salivary pooling) to diagnose the salivary component of SS, biopsied LSGs in 71 of 171 patients defined as having SS and found focal sialadenitis in 68% of them. As noted in the chapter on diagnosis of SS, diagnostic criteria define the set of patients given a syndrome diagnosis, and clearly, different criteria define different sets of patients.

The histopathological characteristics of LSGs in SS are those of a primary lymphocytic infiltrate in otherwise generally normal-appearing glands, and include: 1) focal aggregates of at least 50 (usually more) lymphocytes, plasma cells and macrophages, adjacent to and replacing normal-appearing acini (Fig. 2, 3 A, 3 B and 3 C); and 2) consistent presence of these foci in all or most of the glands in the specimen, but with variability in the number of foci per gland (Fig. 4 C). Larger foci often exhibit formation of germinal centers (Fig. 3 C), but structures resembling epimyoepithelial islands are uncommon (Fig. 2).

Diagnostic specificity of focal sialadenitis in labial salivary glands

Because focal sialadenitis in accessory salivary glands is strongly associated with the presence of SS (as noted above), and because xerostomia is difficult to assess and is not specific to SS, focal sialadenitis in an LSG biopsy specimen was introduced as the diagnostic criterion for the salivary component of SS (Daniels et al. 1975). This study examined 100 patients suspected of having SS, confirmed the diagnosis in 65 of them and observed higher focus scores and lower parotid flow rates in the patients with primary SS than in those with secondary SS.

Questions about the disease specificity of focal sialadenitis in LSG biopsy specimens have arisen because of the presence of focal sialadenitis in minor glands taken from areas where the overlying mucosa shows chronic inflammation or in glands showing diffuse acinar atrophy, and the presence of foci in some postmortem studies.

Although no prospective studies are available to quantify the relationship, pathologists regularly observe various degrees of focal sialadenitis in minor salivary glands when the overlying mucosa is affected by a condition causing chronic inflammation, such as lichen planus, cheek biting or a mucocele. Hence the need to obtain LSG biopsy specimens from clinically normal-appearing mucosa.

Inflammatory cell infiltration associated with diffuse acinar atrophy, duct dilation and fibrosis (Figures 3 D and 3 E) have commonly been observed in all postmortem studies of LSGs. Scott (1980) observed interstitial or focal infiltration in all of 70 postmortem LSG specimens from adults of all ages who had no antemortem diagnosis of SS or other rheumatic diseases. He found that the density of infiltration was not uniform from one gland to another in the same specimen, but was related to the severity of adjacent acinar atrophy and interstitial fibrosis. He observed focal collections of more than 50 lymphoreticular cells in 18 specimens; however, in all but 2 of the specimens, the foci were associated with adjacent acinar atrophy. Another postmortem study (Takeda and Komori 1986) used Chisholm and Mason's grading criteria (1968) on 190 LSG specimens, after excluding those from subjects affected by connective tissue diseases. These authors observed grade 4 inflammation without atrophic epithelial changes in 2/134 specimens from males and 2/56 specimens from females. The 6 specimens in these two studies that showed focal sialadenitis are in apparent contrast to results from the other postmortem studies. Assuming they were not taken from areas of mucosal inflammation, they may indicate the antemortem presence of early, incomplete or unrecognized SS, or may be exceptions to the association of focal sialadenitis with SS. In the worst case, these

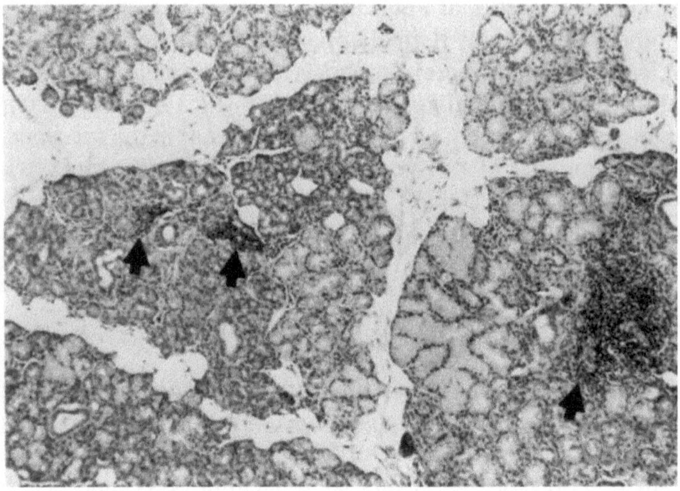

Fig. 3 A

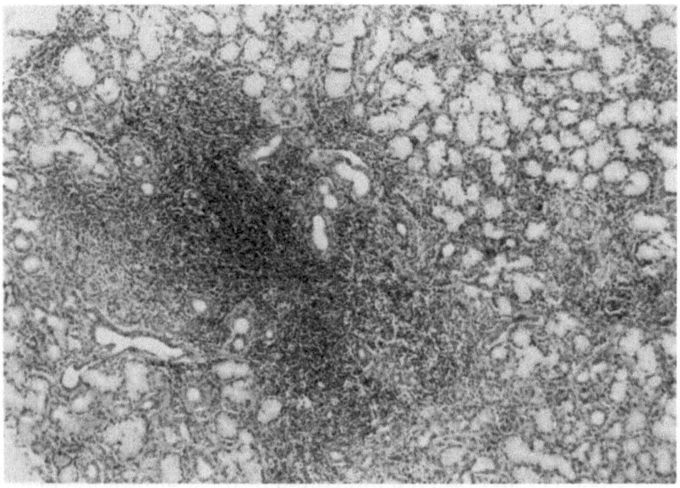

Fig. 3 B

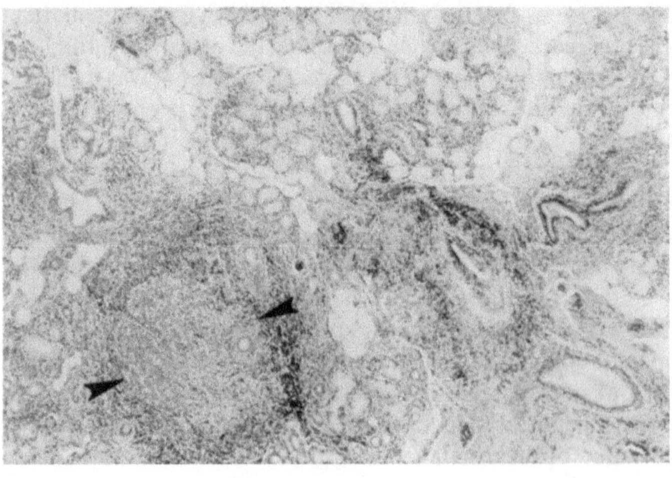

Fig. 3 C

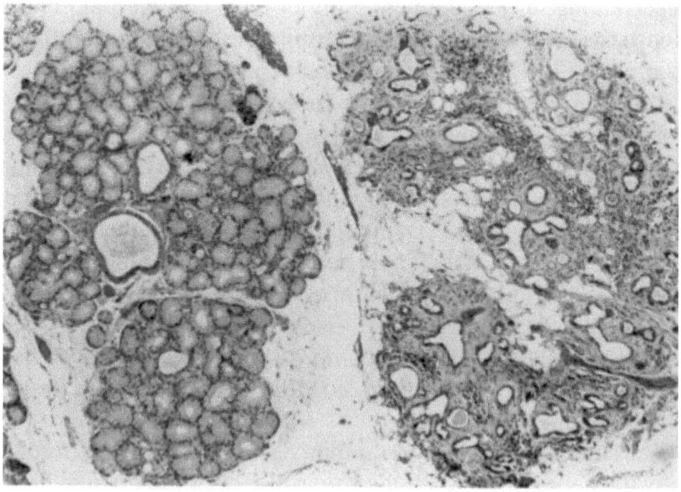

Fig. 3 D

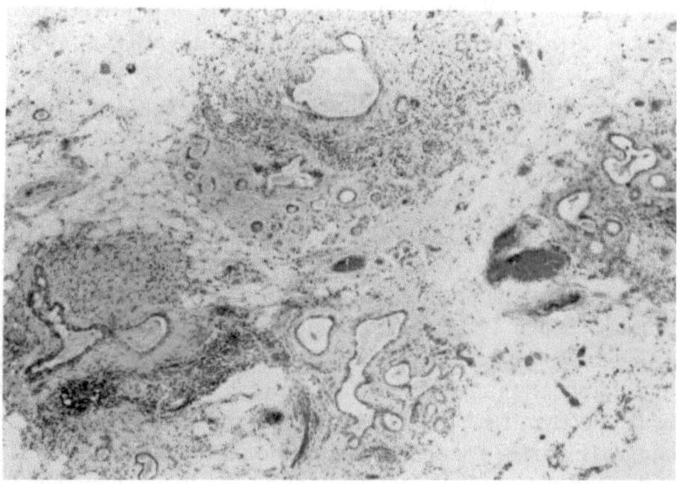

Fig. 3 E

Fig. 3 A–E. Patterns of inflammation in labial salivary gland biopsy specimens (original magnification ×16). **A** Focal sialadenitis in a specimen from a patient with keratoconjunctivitis sicca, rheumatoid arthritis, and a focus score of 2 foci/4 mm^2 (entire specimen) with small and moderate-sized foci (arrows). **B** Focal sialadenitis in a specimen from a patient with keratoconjunctivitis sicca and a focus score of 6 foci/4 mm^2 (entire specimen) with large foci. **C** Focal sialadenitis in a patient with keratoconjunctivitis sicca and a focus score of 7 foci/4 mm^2 (entire specimen). Note germinal center (arrows) and mild fatty replacement at periphery. **D** Portion of a specimen including a gland lobe with diffuse parenchymal atrophy and scattered inflammatory cell infiltration, excluded from scoring. The normal appearing lobe is representative of the remainder of the specimen. Focus score of entire specimen equals 0. **E** Labial salivary gland specimen from a patient who had xerostomia but no connective tissue disease or keratoconjunctivitis sicca. Representative lobes show severe parenchymal atrophy with fibrous and fatty replacement, and both interstitial and focal inflammatory cell infiltration. Focus score of entire specimen equals 0. This appearance is not suggestive of the salivary component of Sjögren's syndrome. Figures A, B, D, and E are reprinted from Arthritis and Rheumatism Journal, copyright 1984, used by permission observations suggest the possibility of false-positive LSG biopsies in 3% of cases. Hence the need to have the diagnostic threshold at greater than 1 focus/4 mm^2 and to apply the LSG biopsy criterion only to the salivary component of SS, not as a single criterion for the entire syndrome.

There are few studies comparing the specificity of various methods of salivary assessment to the diagnosis of SS. One study assessed LSG biopsy specimens after lobes or entire glands showing duct dilation, interstitial fibrosis and diffuse acinar atrophy were excluded (Daniels 1984). This study then examined the correlations between LSG focal sialadenitis and the other components of SS (keratoconjunctivitis sicca [KCS] and another connective tissue disease) and compared them with the correlations for other means of assessing the salivary component of SS. Focal sialadenitis correlated significantly more strongly with KCS, or with KCS and another connective tissue disease, than did either reduced parotid flow rate or the presence of xerostomia symptoms.

The suggestion that long-standing SS results in diffuse fibrous or fatty atrophy of salivary glands, leaving little or no evidence of the original highly cellular lymphocytic infiltration (Whaley and Alspaugh 1985), is not supported by longitudinal data. As noted above, atrophic changes in LSGs are common observations in postmortem specimens from subjects who had no history of connective tissue disease, and these changes increase with age, are associated with inflammation, and affect females earlier than males (Scott 1980). Furthermore, many patients with long-standing primary SS continue to exhibit intense lymphocytic infiltrates in LSG specimens. Therefore, diffuse acinar atrophy of a lobe or entire gland with any pattern of inflammatory cell infiltration must be considered a nonspecific event and should not serve as a diagnostic criterion for the salivary component of SS.

In summary, the pathologic lesion of SS is indeed a distinctive but not pathognomonic chronic lymphocytic sialadenitis (Batsakis and Howard 1982). However, an LSG biopsy specimen can be very disease-specific for SS if it is obtained through normal-appearing mucosa; includes 5 to 10 glands separated from their surrounding connective tissue; is interpreted after lobes or glands showing non-specific changes (Figures 3 D and 3 E) are excluded; demonstrates focal sialadenitis in all or most of the glands in the specimen; and has a focus score that provides a diagnostic threshold (i.e., greater than 1 focus/4 mm^2). LSG biopsy can also provide tissue diagnosis for conditions that can resemble SS clinically, particularly sarcoidosis and amyloidosis.

While there is no perfect diagnostic criterion for the salivary component of SS as yet, observation of focal sialadenitis in an LSG specimen as described above examines the characteristic pathologic lesion of SS and provides the best single criterion in terms of its disease specificity, convenience, availability and low risk.

Fig. 4 A-C. Labial salivary gland biopsy. **A** Initial incision through mucosa, revealing individual ▶ salivary glands. **B** Separate labial salivary glands before fixation and processing. **C** Midplane section through the same specimen. Focus score = 10 foci/4 mm^2 (original magnification ×4). Reprinted from Arthritis and Rheumatism Journal, copyright 1984, used by permission

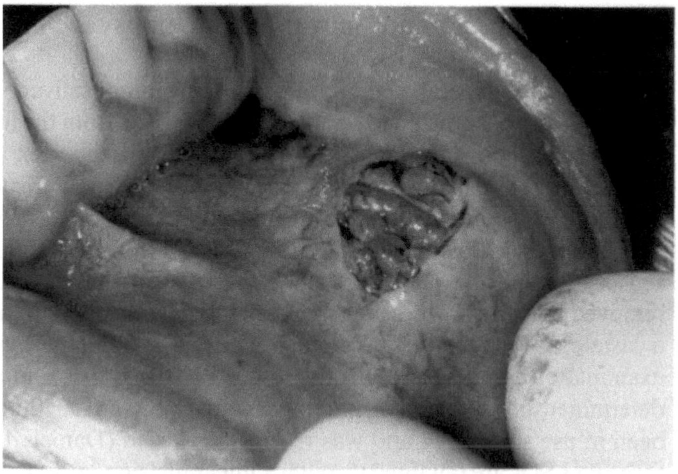

Fig. 4 A

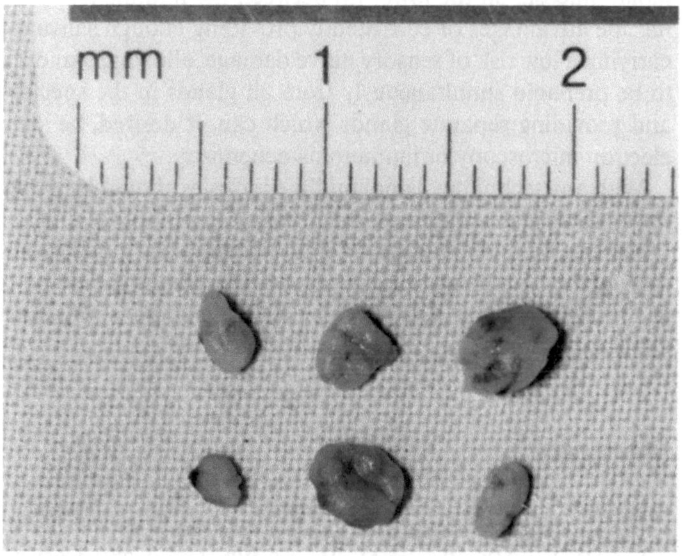

Fig. 4 B

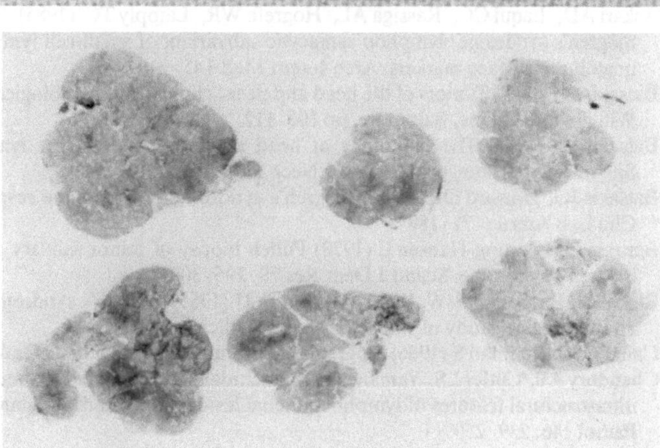

Fig. 4 C

A comparison of minor salivary gland biopsy techniques

There are three general methods of performing minor salivary gland biopsies. Using a skin trephine ("punch") to remove a core of tissue from the lip (Meskin et al. 1964; Bertram and Hjorting-Hansen 1970) or palate (Eisenbud et al. 1973) is rapid and easily done, but usually provides little glandular tissue for examination. Removing an ellipse of labial mucosa that includes all tissue above the obicularis oris muscle (Chisholm and Mason 1968; Davies et al. 1973; Tarpley et al. 1974) may damage sensory nerves that are at or below the level of the glands. Because the glands removed by either of these techniques remain embedded in their connective tissue, a histologic section will reveal each gland at a different level, if at all, requiring examination of many sections to see most of the glands and making a focus score determined on one section unrepresentative. A third method of LSG biopsy has been in use since 1972 and was recently reviewed (Daniels 1984). By this method separate LSGs are obtained through a linear incision in clinically normal-appearing labial mucosa, on the lower lip between the midline and commissure (Fig. 4 A). It has the advantages of consistently providing enough salivary glands for diagnosis, carrying a low risk of sensory nerve damage, allowing a midplane histologic section to be prepared simultaneously from all glands in the specimen (Fig. 4 B and 4 C), and providing separate glands which can, if desired, be separately processed for electron microscopy or immunohistochemistry.

With any technique, labial midline biopsies should be avoided because there are fewer LSGs in the midline of the lip. Histological processing of the small, individual LSGs can be facilitated by folding a foam biopsy pad around the glands before placing them in the processing casette. The glands should be embedded in paraffin at a level such that a section can be cut through the approximate mid-plane of each gland for examination.

References

Anderson LG, Talal N (1972) The spectrum of benign to malignant lymphoproliferation in Sjögren's syndrome. Clin Exp Immunol 10: 199-221

Askari AD, Laqui CC, Rassiga AL, Hogrefe WR, Laipply TC (1985) Small-cell lymphoma and Sjögren's syndrome: lymphoplasmacytic subvariant of small-cell lymphoma with IgA/k immunoglobulin surface markers. Arch Intern Med 145: 935-937

Batsakis JG (1979) Tumors of the head and neck: clinical and pathological considerations, 2nd edn. Williams & Wilkins, Baltimore, pp 105-112

Batsakis JG (1982) The pathology of head and neck tumors: the lymphoepithelial lesion and Sjögren's syndrome, part 16. Head Neck Surg 5: 150-163

Batsakis JG, Howard DR (1982) Sjögren's syndrome: An immune response associated disorder. Clin Lab Ann 1: 171-188

Bertram U, Hjørting-Hansen E (1970) Punch biopsy of minor salivary glands in the diagnosis of Sjögren's syndrome. Scand J Dent Res 78: 295-300

Bloch KJ, Buchanan WW, Wohl MJ, Bunim JJ (1965) Sjögren's syndrome: a clinical, pathological and serological study of sixty-two cases. Medicine 44: 187-231

Calman HI, Reifman S (1966) Sjögren's syndrome: report of a case. Oral Surg 21: 158-162

Chaudhry AP, Cutler LS, Yamane GM, Satchidanand S, Labay G, Sunderraj M (1986) Light and ultrastructural features of lymphoepithelial lesions of the salivary glands in Mikulicz's disease. J Pathol 146: 239-250

Chisholm DM, Mason DK (1968) Labial salivary gland biopsy in Sjögren's syndrome. J Clin Pathol 21: 656-660
Chisholm DM, Waterhouse JP, Mason DK (1970) Lymphocytic sialadenitis in the major and minor glands: a correlation in postmortem subjects. J Clin Pathol 23: 690-694
Cifarelli PS, Bennett MJ, Zaino EC (1966) Sjögren's syndrome: a case report with an additional diagnostic aid. Arch Intern Med 117: 429-431
Daniels TE (1984) Labial salivary gland biopsy in Sjögren's syndrome: assessment as a diagnostic criterion in 362 suspected cases. Arthritis Rheum 27: 147-156
Daniels TE (1986) Salivary histopathology in diagnosis of Sjögren's syndrome. Scand J Rheum in press
Daniels TE, Silverman S, Michalski JP, Greenspan JS, Sylvester RA, Talal N (1975) The oral component of Sjögren's syndrome. Oral Surg 39: 875-885
Davies JD, Berry H, Bacon PA, Issa MA, Schofield JJ (1973) Labial sialadenitis in Sjögren's syndrome and in rheumatoid arthritis. J Pathol 109: 307-314
Eisenbud L, Platt N, Stern M, D'Angelo W, Sumner P (1973) Palatal biopsy as a diagnostic aid in the study of connective tissue diseases. Oral Surg 35: 642-648
Fye KH, Daniels TE, Zulman J, Michalski JP, Jaffe R, Talal N (1980) Aplastic anemia and lymphoma in Sjögren's syndrome. Arthritis Rheum 23: 1321-1325
Godwin JT (1952) Benign lymphoepithelial lesion of the parotid gland (adenolymphoma, chronic inflammation, lymphoepithelioma, lymphocytic tumor, Mikulicz disease): report of eleven cases. Cancer 5: 1089-1103
Greenspan JS, Daniels TE, Talal N, Sylvester RA (1974) The histopathology of Sjögren's syndrome in labial salivary gland biopsies. Oral Surg 37: 217-229
Kassan SS, Thomas TL, Moutsopoulos HM, Hoover R, Kimberly RP, Budman DR, Costa J, Decker JL, Chused TM (1978) Increased risk of lymphoma in sicca syndrome. Ann Intern Med 89: 888-892
Kline TS, Merriam JM, Shapshay SM (1981) Aspiration biopsy cytology of the salivary gland. Am J Clin Pathol 76: 263-269
Lichtenfeld JL, Kirschner RH, Wiernik PH (1976) Familial Sjögren's syndrome with associated primary salivary gland lymphoma. Am J Med 60: 286-292
Meskin LH, Bernard B, Warwick WJ (1964) Biopsy of the labial mucous salivary glands in cystic fibrosis. JAMA 188: 82-83
Mikulicz J (1892) Über eine eigenartige symmetrische Erkrankung der Tränen- und Mundspeicheldrüsen. Beitr z Chir Fetscr f Theodor Billroth, Stuttgart pp 610-630
Morgan WS, Castleman B (1953) A clinicopathologic study of "Mikulicz disease". Am J Pathol 29: 471-503
Nagao K, Matsuzaki O, Saiga H, Akikusa B, Sugano I, Shigematsu H, Kaneko T, Katoh T, Kitamura T, Asano Y, Okamoto M (1983) A histopathologic study of benign and malignant lymphoepithelial lesions of the parotid gland. Cancer 52: 1044-1052
Redondo C, Garcia A, Vasquez F (1981) Malignant lymphoepithelial lesion of the parotid gland. Cancer 48: 289-292
Saku T, Okabe H (1984) Immunohistochemical and ultrastructural demonstration of keratin in epimyoepithelial islands of autoimmune sialadenitis in man. Arch Oral Biol 29: 687-689
Schmid U, Helbron D, Lennert K (1982) Development of malignant lymphoma in myoepithelial sialadenitis (Sjögren's syndrome). Virchows Arch [Pathol Anat] 395: 11-43
Scott J (1976) The incidence of focal chronic inflammatory changes in human submandibular salivary glands. J Oral Pathol 5: 334-346
Scott J (1980) Qualitative and quantitative observations on the histology of human labial salivary glands obtained postmortem. J Biol Buccale 8: 187-200
Takeda Y (1980) Histopathological studies of the labial salivary glands in patients with Sjögren's syndrome. Part I: light microscopic study. Bull Tokyo Med Dent Univ 27: 9-25
Takeda Y, Komori A (1986) Focal lymphocytic infiltration in the human labial salivary glands: a postmortem study. J Oral Pathol 15: 8386
Tarpley TM, Anderson LG, White CL (1974) Minor salivary gland involvement in Sjögren's syndrome. Oral Surg 37: 64-74
Waterhouse JP (1963) Focal adenitis in salivary and lacrimal glands. Proc R Soc Med 56: 911-918

Waterhouse JP, Doniach I (1966) Post-mortem prevalence of focal lymphocytic adenitis of the submandibular salivary glands. J Pathol Bacteriol 91: 53–64
Whaley K, Alspaugh MA (1985) Sjögren's syndrome. In: Kelley WN, Harris ED, Ruddy S, Sledge CB (eds) Textbook of Rheumatology. WB Saunders, Philadelphia, pp 956–978
Whaley K, Williamson J, Chisholm DM, Webb J, Mason DK, Buchanan WW (1973) Sjögren's syndrome. I. Sicca components. Q J Med 42: 279–304
Zulman J, Jaffe R, Talal N (1978) Evidence that the malignant lymphoma of Sjögren's syndrome is a monoclonal B-cell neoplasm. N Engl J Med 299: 1215–1220

B. Extraglandular Findings

1. Primary Sjögren's Syndrome in the People's Republic of China

N. Z. Zhang and Y. Dong

For many years, Sjögren's Syndrome (SS) was erroneously considered to be a rare disease in China. During the last 3 years, however, 68 cases of primary Sjögren's Syndrome were randomly collected in our Rheumatology Unit. In our patients with rheumatoid arthritis (RA), xerostomia and keratoconjunctivitis sicca were present in 38% and 64% of cases respectively. Twenty-three percent of patients had both. In systemic lupus erythematosus (SLE), xerostomia and keratoconjunctivitis sicca were present in 83.3% and 51.4% of cases respectively.

Diagnosis

We have adopted the diagnostic criteria as advocated by Manthorpe (1981). We find none of the methods for examination of keratoconjunctivitis sicca to be sufficiently specific. Specificity is greatly increased if two or more tests are positive before keratoconjunctivitis sicca is diagnosed (Table 1).

A simple sugar tablet test is performed to detect xerostomia. A tablet of 0.8 g cane sugar is placed at the junction of the anterior and middle thirds of the tongue. Incomplete dissolution of the tablet after 30 minutes is considered abnormal. The sensitivity and specificity of this test are both over 90%. Sialography and biopsy of lower lip mucosa are abnormal in almost all cases of primary SS. The typical changes of the former are dilatation (sialectasis) of ducts of various sizes, especially a punctate dilatation of the peripheral ducts, and dye retention.

We tried radionuclide scanning of the salivary glands using radioactive technetium (99mT_c), but the positive rate in primary SS is only 70%. On the other hand, the false positive rate in normal controls may reach as high as 15%. Thus, this procedure is not entirely satisfactory.

Table 1. Specificity and sensitivity of the 3 methods used for detection of keratoconjunctivitis sicca

	Schirmer test (10 mm/5 min)	B^{U}T (10 sec)	Corneal stain (10 spots/eye)	Two or more examinations positive
False positive (%)	29.7	7.9	1.0	4.0
False negative (%)	25.5	13.6	45.5	9.1
Specificity (%)	70.3	92.1	99	96.0
Sensitivity (%)	74.5	86.4	54.5	91.0

Forty percent of primary SS patients have rampant dental caries with extension to the base of the tooth and spontaneous breaking. This is an important accessory sign of xerostomia. One third of our primary SS patients show parotid gland enlargement, usually bilateral and occuring alternately and repeatedly.

In China, some authors advocate nasal mucosa biopsy instead of lower lip mucosa biopsy because it is most easily carried out and can be performed repeatedly for research purposes (Table 2). In 20 cases of allergic rhinitis, despite chronic periglandular inflammatory cell infiltration, only two patients were scored as grade 2. In these two cases, the moderate amount of polymorphonuclear cell infiltration around the duct and in the glandular lobules was sufficient to differentiate from primary SS. Irrespective of what methods of examination are adopted, it is inappropriate to diagnose xerostomia until at least 2 examinations prove to be abnormal.

The diagnostic rate of primary SS would be improved if more physicians were alert to the disease and if more patients considered dryness of the mouth and eyes as important symptoms. Most patients do not know that these symptoms may have bearing on their chief complaints such as arthralgia, Raynauds phenomenon, skin rash, etc. Very rarely do they mention these complaints to their doctors. Physicians

Table 2. Comparison of nasal mucosa biopsy and lower lip mucosa biopsy in primary SS

	glandular changes				duct changes			mononuclear cell infiltration (grading)				
	atrophy	decrease of lobules	fibrosis	sclerotic changes	dilation	occlusion	metaphasia	0	1	2	3	4
Lower lip biopsy (n=42)	35	21	8	2	5	3	1	0	2	13	18	13
nasal biopsy (n=48)	42	19	18	3	1	2	1	0	0	19	15	20

Table 3. Positive rate of anti-SS-A and anti-SS-B antibodies in Chinese primary SS

	anti-SS-A antibody (%)	anti-SS-B antibody (%)
Primary SS (62)	75.0	59.4
Primary SS with renal tubular acidosis (18)	88.8	72.2
Secondary SS		
- SS and SLE (35)	50.4	16.8
- SS and RA (15)	38.4	15.3
RA (24)	8.3	0
SLE (11)	39.3	10.1
Other connective tissue diseases (22)	0	0
Non-connective tissue diseases (134)	1.5	0
Normal controls (108)	0	0

should actively question patients for these symptoms. The presence of complaints of xerostomia and keratoconjunctivitis sicca in proved cases of primary SS is only 69% of 55% respectively.

Serological examination would, to a certain extent, also help increase the diagnostic threshold. In some of our renal tubular acidosis patients who do not have dryness of the mouth and eyes, the diagnosis of primary SS was made on further investigation after the serological examination showed positive results. The anti-SS-B antibody determination is more specific than anti-SS-A antibody (Table 3). Wil-2 cell antigen is difficult to obtain in large amount, thus hindering its wide application. Human spleen extract antigen is used instead. The correlation rate between these two antigens is 95%. Furthermore, human spleen antigen can also be used for determinations of anti-Sm and anti-RNP antibodies.

Clinical Features Other Than Xerostomia and Keratoconjunctivitis Sicca

Skin. Twenty-two percent of primary SS patients have different kinds of skin rashes. Xeroderma is not common in Chinese patients. Erythema nodosum is a common complaint in many patients. A few cases of hyperglobulinemic purpura were finally proven to be primary SS.

Joint and muscle. Seventy-eight percent of our primary SS patients complain of joint pain but X-ray examinations fail to reveal any pathological changes. Two cases of myositis were seen. We cannot be sure whether the myositis is caused by the primary SS or represents a coexisting condition of polymyositis.

Lung. Although only a few cases show interstitial pulmonary changes or increased lung markings by X-ray examination, seventy percent of patients have abnormalities of pulmonary function rests. Disturbance of small airway functions (72%), of diffusion capacity and restrictive functional changes may occur. Many patients do not have a history of smoking, and only a minority have respiratory symptoms or abnormal chest films. Thus, pulmonary function changes, especially small airway function disturbances, may be considered an early sign of lung involvement in primary SS.

Gastrointestinal involvement. Forty-four cases of primary SS had endoscopic examination, basal and maximal acid output determinations after pentagastrin stimulation, and D-xylose tests for absorptive function of the small intestine. Peroral biopsy of the jejunal mucosa was performed in 18 cases. Thirty-one cases show atrophic gastritis histologically. The other 13 showed slight to moderate degrees of superficial gastritis. The incidence of atrophic gastritis in primary SS is 70%, distinctly higher than the overall incidence of 10% observed among all other endoscopic examinations done in our outpatient GI clinic. Fourteen and thirty-six percent of our patients had either achlorhydria or hypochlorhydria respectively. Among the 18 jejunal biopsies, only 2 showed a moderate degree of villus atrophy. These 2 and another 3 cases had abnormal D-xylose absorptive tests. There was, however, no obvious correlation between the symptoms of dyspepsia and the gastric and intestional changes.

Pancreas. Two cases of chronic pancreatitis were observed. The first case started with diarrhea and developed jaundice a month later. Percutaneous cholangiography revealed narrowing of the common bile duct. Exploratory operation revealed that the entire pancreas was firm in consistency. The head of the pancreas was nodular in appearance with adhesions to the lesser omentum. The wall of the common bile duct was thickened and the ampulla of vater was obstructed due to adhesions. The liver was firm and nodular. Several months after operation, the patient developed enlargement of the sublingual and submandibular glands with symptoms of xerostomia. Further investigation firmly established the diagnosis of primary SS. The second case was operated upon for carcinoma of the pancreas because of a palpable abdominal mass. Chronic pancreatitis was diagnosed after the operation but primary SS was not thought of then. Several years later, the patient developed generalized lymphadenopathy and proved to be a case of primary SS.

Liver. Hepatosplenomegaly occurs in primary SS. Five of our patients had a liver biopsy. The first case with presenting features of renal tubular acidosis showed liver changes compatible with viral hepatitis. The second case had enlargement of liver and spleen with positive blood HBsAg. Liver biopsy showed chronic active hepatitis. The third case was the first case of pancreatitis already mentioned. Liver biopsy revealed degeneration and piecemeal necrosis of parenchymal cells, lymphocytic infiltration and duct hyperplasia in portal areas. The fourth case with presenting features of angio-lymphoblastoid lymphadenopathy showed massive plasma cell infiltration in the liver. Seven histologically proved cases of HBsAg negative chronic active hepatitis were examined for SS; in three, primary SS was finally established with one having renal tubular acidosis. It is our impression that chronic active hepatitis is not uncommon in primary SS. In all cases there was lymphocytic infiltration of various degree in the portal area. Clinically overt hepatic disease or abnormal liver function tests were seen only in 20% of cases of primary SS.

Neurological system. Five cases with different psycho-neurological manifestations were seen. Trigeminal neuropathy, psychosis and delusion of persecution were each present in one case. The other two cases had wide involvement of cerebrum, cerebellum, spinal cord and peripheral nerves with a slowly progressive course. One of the two did not respond to corticosteroid treatment but improved favorably after the addition of azathioprin. It is difficult to be certain whether the improvement was due to treatment or the result of spontaneous remission since the other case also improved simply on general supportive measures.

Lympho-proliferation. Among 68 cases of primary SS, only one developed angio-lymphoblastoid lymphadenopathy. The duration of illness in all these cases was 6 years in average, the longest being 20 years. One case has been followed up for 19 years. It is our preliminary impression that the incidence of true malignant lymphoma in primary SS may be lower in China than in Western countries. This awaits further study.

Renal Tubular Acidosis

Primary SS may affect the kidney. In our 68 cases of primary SS, 20 overt cases of renal tubular acidosis were observed. The incidence of 29.4% seems to be higher than that of Western countries. The age distribution ranged between 18 and 41 years. All except one were females. The duration of illness of renal tubular acidosis varied from 1 to 12 years. Aside from symptoms of dryness of the mouth and eyes, polyuria, polydipsia and generalized weakness, the striking presenting clinical feature was recurrent attacks of periodic paralysis, even to the severe extreme of respiratory failure. Laboratory examinations revealed hypokalemia (1.0-3.2 Meq/L), fixation of specific gravity with persistent urinary pH >6 and blood pH changes compatible with the diagnosis of metabolic acidosis. The blood creatinine and urea nitrogen were normal. All cases showed hypergammaglobulinemia of 34-58% with polyclonal increase of immunoglobulins. The predisposing factors for hypokalemic flaccid paralysis were pregnancy, overfatigue and infections.

To further study the effect of SS on renal tubular function, ten randomly selected cases of SS without overt renal tubular acidosis or renal diabetes insipidus were subjected to ammonium chloride loading tests. Eight cases showed positive results with urine pH persistently above 6; in 3 there was also acidemia. Subsequently, without ammonium chloride loading, the urine pH of these 8 cases was examined repeatedly on 10 occasions. Again all showed persistent urine pH above 6. This phenomenon was not observed in the other two cases who showed negative results in the ammonium chloride loading test. This simple test is of help in detecting subclinical cases of renal tubular acidosis.

Renal biopsies were performed in 4 cases of overt and 2 of incipient renal tubular acidosis. All revealed interstitial changes including degenerative changes of the tubules, focal lymphocytic infiltration, hyperplasia of connective tissue and mesangial cells (mesangial nephritis). It is estimated that 35% of primary SS have renal tubular acidosis of various degrees.

For historical reasons, most of the renal tubular acidosis patients in our hospital were centralized in the department of Endocrinology. Over the past many years, the cause of renal disease in most of them was considered unknown. Since our study on SS, retrospective studies on 32 cases revealed that at least half of them were due to primary SS (Table 4). Apparently, the renal abnormalities may precede other manifestations of SS by a number of years, making it important that this diagnosis be considered in renal tubular or interstitial disease where the underlying etiology is obscure.

Aside from renal tubular acidosis, one case of renal diabetes mellitus and two of glomerular nephritis were seen. One of the latter gave the clinical picture of nephrosis and died of uremia in 2 years time because of a progressive downhill course.

Table 4. Causes of 32 renal tubular acidosis in PUMC Hospital, Beijing

	primary SS	hepato-lenticular degeneration	drug induced	cause unknown
%	56.3	9.3	3.1	31.3

Renal biopsy in this case revealed immune complex nephritis. It is estimated that the overall involvement of the kidney from all conditions would be about 40% in primary SS. The seemingly higher incidence and severity of renal involvement in Chinese primary SS patients than in Western countries awaits further confirmation.

References

1. Manthorpe R et al. (1981) Sjögren's syndrome: A review with emphasis on immunological feature. Allergy 36: 139-153
2. Dong Y, Wu DH, Chen PZ, Zhang NC (1984) Clinical analysis of 36 cases of primary Sjögren's syndrome. Chin J Int Med 23: 597-700
3. Wu DH, Dong Y, Chen PZ, Zhang NC (1984) Determination of anti-SS-A and anti-SS-B antibodies and its clinical significance. Chin Med J 64: 194-196
4. Dong Y, Wu DH, Li ZH, Zhang NC (1983) Sjögren's syndrome with periodic paralysis, a report of 5 cases. Chin J Int Med 22: 685-687
5. Chen SP, Liu TH, Jiang M, Ju ZM (1985) Gastrointestinal involvement in Sjögren's syndrome. Presentation during the Annual Scientific Conference, 1985, Hong Kong Society of Gastroenterology, March 23-24
6. Ke MZ, Hsu TR, Chen ZH et al. (1984) Nasal mucosa biopsy in the diagnosis of Sjögren's syndrome. Chin Med J 64: 226-229
7. Zhao ZL (1985) Ophthalmologic manifestations and diagnosis of SS. Chin J Ophth 21: 222-224
8. Wen ZH, Du TH et al. (1985) Oral examinations of SS. Chin J Stomat 20: 226-228

2. Neuromuscular Complications of Primary Sjögren's Syndrome

E. L. ALEXANDER

Introduction

Primary Sjögren's syndrome is complicated by a vast array of neuromuscular complications which recent evidence suggests have an immunologically mediated basis. Neuromuscular complications include involvement of the central and peripheral nervous systems, as well as the skeletal muscle system. Musculoskeletal complaints in Sjögren's syndrome are common symptoms. Inflammatory myopathy (i.e. myositis) is less common, but well documented, and may be accompanied by vascular inflammation (Table 1), (see Chapter II. B. 6.).

Peripheral neurologic complications of primary Sjögren's syndrome have been reported in approximately 10%-20% of patients (Shearn 1971, Kaltreider and Talal 1969, Pittsley 1980, Alexander 1982c, 1983b). In Henrik Sjögren's monograph published in 1935, he described a patient with bilateral facial nerve palsy and transient sensory changes (Sjögren 1935). Subsequently, other investigators have reported a range of peripheral nervous system involvement (Table 2).

Until our recent reports (Alexander 1981a, b, 1982a-c, 1983a, b, 1986a-h; Molina 1985a, b, 1986; Malinow 1985, 1986), the spectrum of central nervous system involvement as a distinct clinical entity in primary Sjögren's syndrome has been largely unexplored. The first report of central nervous system disease in Sjögren's syndrome was published in 1939 by Sheldon (Sheldon 1939). His description of a patient with primary Sjögren's syndrome, putative cutaneous vasculitis character-

Table 1. Muscle disease in primary Sjögren's syndrome

Author	Year	Muscle Involvement
*Bunim	1961	Focal myositis
*Silberberg	1962	Proximal myopathy
Denko	1969	Myositis
*Kaltreider and Talal	1969	Myositis
*Whitaker	1972	Myositis
Whaley	1973b	Focal lymphocytic myositis without fiber necrosis
Bohan	1977	Polymyositis
*Ringel	1982	Polymyositis
Pittsley and Talal	1980	Progressive myopathy with minimal enzyme elevation
*Alexander	1981	Myositis
*Alexander	1982	Polymyositis
*Molina	1986	Myositis in male patients

* Inflammatory vascular disease within muscle (see Chapter II. B. 6.)

Table 2. Peripheral nervous system in primary Sjögren's syndrome

Author	Year	PNS Manifestation
1. Sjögren	1935	Bilateral facial palsy and transient sensory changes
2. Attwood and Poser	1961	Peripheral neuropathy and multiple cranial nerve palsies (III, V, VII, X, XII)
3. Talal	1967	Peripheral neuropathy
4. Gumpel	1969	Peripheral neuropathy
5. Kaltreider and Talal	1969	Peripheral and trigeminal neuropathy
6. Pittsley and Talal	1980	Peripheral and cranial neuropathy
7. Alexander	1981, 1982	Peripheral sensory and motor polyneuropathy, cranial neuropathy, mononeuritis multiplex, carpal tunnel syndrome
8. Peyronnard	1982	Sensorimotor neuropathy
9. Malinow	1986	Pure sensory neuropathy

ized by lower extremity palpable purpura, and central nervous system involvement is presented below.

"In addition to these features, which form the characteristic Sjögren's syndrome, there have developed during the same period:

1. Mental changes, for which she has been a voluntary inmate in the Staffordshire County Asylum. The symptoms are mostly of a delusional type and are cheerful in character.
2. Epileptic fits.
3. An affection of the skin: ... Over the thighs small reddish raised spots frequently develop which disappear in a few days' time. Both legs show a dark pigmentation which is almost symmetrical, but is rather more marked on the right than the left. It reaches from just below the knees and extends to the dorsum of the feet. The colour has varied somewhat in intensity, but is usually a very dark brown, and at times and in places almost black. It consists of darker points on a less dark background, and is associated with numerous small telangiectases. These appear from time to time, and tend to become covered with thick black crusts ... (Sheldon 1939)."

In retrospect, based on our current knowledge, this patient is a classical prototype for the subgroup of patients we recently have defined with cutaneous vasculitis, affective psychiatric disturbances, and neurologic disease (Malinow 1985). Following Sheldon's report, scattered reports of central nervous system involvement in similar patients with Sjögren's syndrome have appeared in the literature (Table 3). Our experience at the Johns Hopkins Medical Institutions would indicate that central nervous system disease occurs in approximately 25% of primary Sjögren's syndrome patients (CNS-SS) and is more common than appreciated previously. In this chapter, our studies on the neuromuscular complications of primary Sjögren's syndrome are summarized and our observations integrated into the existing literature.

Table 3. Historical documentation of central nervous system involvement in Sjögren's syndrome

Author	Year	CNS Manifestation
1. Sheldon	1939	Seizures
2. Weber	1945	Internuclear ophthalmoplegia, ptosis, mental changes, and seizures
3. Coverdale	1948	Hemiplegia
4. Heaton	1959	Seizures, hemianopsia
5. Kaltreider	1969	Seizures
6. Viala and Masson	1970	Hemiparesis, ataxia
7. Shearn	1971	Perivascular lymphocytic infiltrates
8. Steinberg, Green and Talal	1971	Thrombotic thrombocytopenic purpura
9. Monda	1979	Ataxia, nystagmus
10. Alexander	1981 a, b 1982 a–c 1983 a, b 1985 a, b 1986 a–h	Diffuse multifocal CNS involvement of brain and spinal cord
11. Rutan	1986	Transverse myelitis

Sjögren's Syndrome – The Patient

The Sjögren's patients we have reported in our studies have been well characterized both from the standpoint of their sicca syndrome as well as their neurologic dysfunction. All patients classified as having Sjögren's syndrome meet the following criteria. All patients are symptomatic for the sicca complex with two of the following clinical features: xerophthalmia ("dry eyes"), xerostomia ("dry mouth"), or recurrent or chronic salivary gland enlargement. In addition, at least two of the three following features are required for the diagnosis of Sjögren's syndrome: abnormal Schirmer's test (with anesthesia, less than 5 mm of filter paper moistening within five minutes), keratoconjunctivitis sicca defined by a positive rose bengal dye test (type A or B of Holm) (Holm 1949), or a positive minor salivary gland biopsy (grade 3 or 4 by the criteria of Greenspan and associates (Greenspan 1974; Daniels 1984).

Patients defined as having primary Sjögren's syndrome in these studies did not meet criteria for an additional connective tissue disorder (Tan 1982; Ropes 1958; Masi 1980). In particular, no patient had four or more ARA criteria for systemic lupus erythematosus. It is recognized, however, that some Sjögren's patients may actually have four ARA criteria for lupus erythematosus (such as arthritis, positive anti-nuclear antibody test, cytopenia and neurologic dysfunction (i.e. seizure or psychosis) and clinically not have lupus erythematosus. Nevertheless, such patients were not classified as having primary Sjögren's syndrome, but as Sjögren's/lupus overlap syndromes. Furthermore, there is an interesting subgroup of Sjögren's syndrome patients who at varying times along their disease course develop cutaneous manifestations of lupus erythematosus. These patients form the basis of another chapter in this book (see Provost et al.).

In addition, those patients reported as having primary Sjögren's syndrome in no way resemble patients with systemic lupus erythematosus. No patient reported in our series as primary Sjögren's syndrome manifested the following features of systemic lupus erythematosus at the time of study: malar rash, solar induced, discoid, or subacute cutaneous lesions, polyserositis, glomerulonephritis, or antibodies to native DNA, nRNP, or Sm. In addition, over 95% of patients had autoantibodies to Ro(SS-A) and approximately 90% to La(SS-B) detected by either gel double immunodiffusion (Wilson 1984) or a quantitative ELISA (Harley 1986). Furthermore, greater than 90% of patients had HLA-DRw52, an immunogenetic marker for Sjögren's syndrome (Wilson 1984; Harley 1986).

In evaluating these patients classified as having neurological complications of primary Sjögren's syndrome, other etiologies for their neurologic dysfunction have been excluded rigorously. All patients have been examined by at least one neurologist and the majority by a psychiatrist at our institution. Neuroradiologic and electrophysiologic studies, cerebral spinal fluid analyses, psychiatric evaluations, Minnesota Multiphasic Personality Testing, and cognitive function testing have been performed by standard techniques (Alexander 1981 a, b, 1982 a–c, 1983 a, b, 1986 a–h; Molina 1985 a, b, 1986; Malinow 1985, 1986).

Muscle Disease

Clinical Manifestations

In addition to a transient, episodic, nondeforming, nonerosive, usually asymmetrical polyarthritis, musculoskeletal complaints are very common and prominent symptoms in Sjögren's syndrome. There often is a transient, self-limited, recurrent symptom complex resembling a "flu-like" syndrome which can be very disturbing and disabling to patients. This symptom complex is characterized by low grade fever, fatigue, arthralgias, myalgias, lymphadenopathy and, in some cases, salivary gland enlargement. The pathogenesis of this disorder is unknown. The observation of mononuclear cells infiltrating muscle fibers and vessels in muscle tissue obtained from Sjögren's patients without clinical evidence of myositis (Bunim 1961; Bloch 1965; Whaley 1973) suggests that there may be an inflammatory etiology (see below).

Frank inflammatory myopathies are a feature of Sjögren's syndrome and there is a wide spectrum of clinical presentations. Proximal myopathies are most common. Distal involvement, however, may be prominent (Bunim 1961) and we have observed several cases with an almost exclusive distal distribution (Alexander, unpublished observations). Most commonly, the myopathy is mild and insidious. The muscle enzymes may be normal or only mildly elevated. The electromyogram may be only mildly abnormal. At the other end of the spectrum is a clinical presentation indistinguishable from polymyositis with characteristic serum enzyme elevations and/or electromyographic features (Bunim 1961; Bohan 1977). Muscle biopsy confirms the presence of diffuse or focal mononuclear inflammatory infiltrates.

Muscle fiber necrosis and degeneration, if present, is observed most commonly in areas of inflammation. There is variation in fiber size with internal nuclei.

Inclusion body myositis, has been reported in Sjögren's syndrome (Chad 1982). In addition, a myopathy associated with renal tubular acidosis which causes hypokalemic periodic paralysis has been observed (Raskin 1981).

Limited information is available on the prevalence of inflammatory muscle disease (i. e. myositis) in primary Sjögren's syndrome. A summary of the reported cases of myositis is presented in Table 1. In several series, the prevalence of clinical myositis ranges from 2.5 to 10% (Bloch 1965; Bunim 1961; Shearn 1971; Alexander 1981 a, 1982 c, 1983 b; Molina 1986). The frequency of subclinical histopathologic evidence of muscle inflammation on muscle biopsy, however, is much higher. Bunim (Bunim 1961) reported focal lymphocytic myositis (and inflammatory vascular disease, see below) in 14/19 (74%) Sjögren's patients lacking clinical evidence of myopathy (four, moderate to severe and 11, mild myositis). In the subsequent studies of Bloch and Bunim (Bloch 1965), nine of 23 (39%) patients with primary Sjögren's syndrome without symptoms of muscle disease showed focal "chronic" (mononuclear) myositis. We have reported biopsy documented myositis in five of 30 (17%) patients with primary Sjögren's syndrome, only 2 of whom had clinical features characteristic of myositis (Alexander 1983 b). As mentioned above, this high frequency of lymphocytic inflammatory infiltrates within muscle of Sjögren's patients without clinical or laboratory evidence of a frank myopathy may be related to their prominent musculoskeletal symptoms.

The presence of inflammatory vascular disease within blood vessels in muscle, either alone or in association with myositis, is well established in Sjögren's syndrome (Table 1) and is discussed in detail in Chapter II. B. 6.

Peripheral Nervous System

Clinical Manifestations

The range of clinical manifestations of peripheral nervous system disease is secondary to varying involvement of the sensory and motor components of peripheral nerves at various neuroanatomic points (Table 4). Among the most common peripheral nervous system manifestations of primary Sjögren's syndrome is a distal symmetrical pansensory polyneuropathy which tends to affect the lower more than the upper extremities. The symptoms, predominantly anaesthesia and paresthesia in a stocking-glove distribution, usually are relatively mild and nondisabling.

In the mixed polyneuropathy, there is usually a sensory predominance characterized by painful paresthesias and dysesthesias. There frequently also is a mild "stocking-glove" diminution of all sensory modalities particularly in the lower extremities. If motor involvement predominates, the patients may demonstrate motor dysfunction (e. g. mononeuropathy or mononeuritis multiplex).

Another common peripheral nervous system complication is secondary to what are termed "entrapment syndromes" often in the carpal, ulnar, and tarsal distribution. These abnormalities may occur in the setting of active synovitis, but also in the absence of demonstrable arthritis or obvious inflammation. While these neuropa-

Table 4. Peripheral nervous system disease in primary Sjögren's syndrome

Peripheral Neuropathy
Peripheral Nerve
Sensory/Motor
Motor (Mononeuropathy or mononeuritis multiplex)
Entrapment syndromes
Cranial
Brachial plexopathy
Ganglia
Dorsal root - Pure sensory neuronopathy
Gasserian - Trigeminal neuropathy

thies are presumed to be secondary to nerve entrapment, definitive proof for this etiology is often lacking. While the presumptive entrapment neuropathies usually can be managed by conservative measures (i. e. splints, physical therapy, and salicylates or non-steroidal anti-inflammatory drugs), on occasion, corticosteroids or surgical intervention may by necessary. Brachial plexopathies also have been observed (Alexander 1982c).

Cranial nerve involvement is observed in patients with Sjögren's syndrome and may be peripheral or central (see below). The most well recognized cranial nerve syndrome is a trigeminal sensory neuropathy, which may be the sole neurologic abnormality (Kaltreider and Talal 1969). The symptoms consist of unilateral or bilateral numbness or paraesthesia in the distribution of the maxillary and/or mandibular division of the trigeminal nerve. The ophthalmic division is involved less commonly. Pain may be present, but usually is not severe. Most often the corneal reflex is spared. Motor function is normal. Altered taste perception of the tongue may be detected ipsilaterally. This divisional impairment suggests a peripheral process.

There are practical implications of the presence of trigeminal neuropathy which can exacerbate sicca symptoms by worsening lacrimal and taste deficits. The risk of corneal or lingual ulceration is increased. Taste perception is altered due to loss of pain, touch, and temperature sensation in the mucous membranes (Van Bekesey 1964).

Other cranial nerve deficits, with or without trigeminal sensory neuropathy, may occur. It is often difficult to determine whether such lesions are peripheral and/or secondary to brain stem involvement. Facial nerve involvement may compromise autonomic secretory function and further impair the existing decrement in tear and saliva production. Neurosensory hearing loss and peripheral vestibular dysfunction have been observed in Sjögren's syndrome (Alexander, unpublished observations). Other less common cranial neuropathies include III, X and XII.

Diagnosis

Electrophysiologic Studies. If a patient is suspected clinically of having a neuropathy, electrophysiologic studies including nerve conduction and electromyography should be performed. In the presence of weakness these studies may distinguish, or in addition establish, the presence of myopathic involvement. It should be recognized, however, that these studies become abnormal relatively late in the evolution of neuropathic changes. Therefore, a normal study does not preclude the presence of a neuropathic process.

Since peripheral nervous system disease often antedates or accompanies central nervous system disease in Sjögren's syndrome (Alexander 1981 a; Alexander 1982 c; Molina 1985 a), we recommend that a patient with a neuropathy be carefully evaluated for the presence of concomitant central nervous system disease (see below).

Biopsies. In addition to establishing an etiology for peripheral nervous system dysfunction in Sjögren's syndrome, one of the main reasons to perform a nerve biopsy is to establish a tissue diagnosis of inflammatory vascular disease. In the case of mild peripheral neuropathies, nerve biopsies are not necessary or recommended. Biopsies may be helpful, however, in several clinical settings. In a patient with a neuropathy who has systemic complications suspected to be secondary to vascular inflammation or in patients with central nervous system involvement, a peripheral nerve biopsy may document the presence of peripheral inflammatory vascular disease. A positive biopsy provides indirect, although presumptive, evidence that the systemic complications are occurring in the setting of established vascular inflammation and suggest that it is highly likely that there is systemic vasculitis. This is helpful when it is not possible or safe to obtain tissue from an involved organ. It should be emphasized that because of the potential focal nature of vascular inflammation, a negative nerve biopsy does not exclude the presence of a vasculitic neuropathy or systemic vascular complications.

Pathogenesis

The limited available evidence suggests that peripheral neuropathies in Sjögren's syndrome are secondary to vascular inflammation of small vessels in the epineurum or vasa vasorum. These data are presented in Chapter II. B. 6.

We recently have obtained histopathologic documentation of another type of peripheral nervous system inflammation in Sjögren's syndrome (Malinow 1986). We have now observed four patients with primary Sjögren's syndrome with a pure sensory neuronopathy. In three of these patients in whom dorsal root ganglion biopsies have been obtained, dorsal root ganglion mononuclear (predominantly lymphocytic) infiltrates with neuronal degeneration and fibrosis have been observed. Preliminary data indicate that the majority of these lymphocytes are T lymphocytes, some of which are cytotoxic T cells (Griffin D and Griffin J, unpublished observations). Several of these patients also have had clinical evidence of trigeminal neuropathy and abnormal or absent blink reflexes. It is highly likely that some cases of trigeminal neuropathy may be secondary to similar lymphocytic infiltrates and neuronal destruction within the gasserian ganglia.

Central Nervous System

Spectrum of Neurologic Manifestations

The clinical manifestations of central nervous system disease in Sjögren's syndrome are diverse (Alexander 1981 a, b, 1982 a–c, 1983 a, b, 1986 a–h; Molina 1985 a, b, 1986; Malinow 1985, 1986), and span the entire neuroaxis including the brain and spinal cord (Table 5). The abnormalities may be subtle or protean. Since our initial report of the central nervous system manifestations of Sjögren's syndrome (Alexander 1981 a), it has become increasingly apparent that nervous system disease in Sjögren's syndrome is characteristically multifocal, recurrent, additive, and progressive. While any given episode may be transient and reversible, over time, deficits become fixed and are cumulative.

Involvement of the brain causes focal deficits such as hemiparesis, hemisensory deficits, seizure disorders, and movement disorders. Diffuse manifestations of brain involvement include encephalopathy and aseptic meningoencephalitis, often recurrent. More recently we have appreciated that significant impairment in cognitive function and psychiatric abnormalities in Sjögren's syndrome may have an organic basis (see below) (Malinow 1985).

The spinal cord is commonly involved in Sjögren's syndrome central nervous system disease. Acute transverse myelopathy, often recurrent, and chronic progressive myelopathy can occur. Neurogenic bladder may accompany these clinical presentations or occur alone. Less commonly Brown-Sequard Syndrome has been observed.

It is apparent from the description of the neurologic manifestations of central nervous system disease in primary Sjögren's syndrome that these patients share many clinical characteristics with multiple sclerosis patients. In particular, we have

Table 5. Spectrum of central nervous system involvement in primary Sjögren's syndrome

Neurologic Abnormality
Brain
Focal
Deficits (motor and/or sensory)
Seizure disorder
Movement disorder
Brain stem syndrome
Cerebellar syndrome
Diffuse
Encephalopathy
Aseptic meningitis
Cognitive dysfunction
Dementia
Psychiatric abnormalities
Spinal Cord
Transverse myelitis
Chronic progressive myelopathy
Brown-Sequard syndrome
Neurogenic bladder

observed a subset of patients with primary Sjögren's syndrome whose clinical features, electrophysiologic studies, cerebrospinal fluid parameters, and neuroradiologic assessment are indistinguishable from those observed in multiple sclerosis. The clinical manifestations of this subgroup of patients are presented in Table 6. The results of the neurologic evaluation of these patients will be considered below.

These patients met criteria for the diagnosis of multiple sclerosis and multiple sclerosis was considered the most probable neurologic diagnosis prior to the diagnosis of Sjögren's syndrome. Therefore, it is important to recognize that a subset of patients with Sjögren's syndrome may have neurologic dysfunction which is indistinguishable from multiple sclerosis. This may have practical clinical implications in terms of therapy. Sjögren's syndrome central nervous system disease may be more amenable to immunosuppressive therapy than multiple sclerosis.

Although patients with central nervous system disease secondary to Sjögren's syndrome may be indistinguishable both clinically and neurodiagnostically (see below) from patients with multiple sclerosis, there appear to be immunogenetic differences which may distinguish the two disorders. Patients with primary Sjögren's syndrome have a statistically increased prevalence of HLA-B8, DR3, and DRw52 while patients with multiple sclerosis are HLA-A3, B7, DR2, and DQ1 (Alexander 1986g).

In our initial descriptions of central nervous disease in Sjögren's syndrome, we described patients with well defined neurologic deficits. It soon became apparent to us that a significant proportion of patients also had significant psychiatric or cognitive disturbances. Initially, we were reluctant to regard these more subtle manifestations as part of the spectrum of neurologic involvement in Sjögren's syndrome. Our recent data would suggest, however, that psychiatric and cognitive abnormalities

Table 6. Neurologic manifestations in 20 patients with primary Sjögren's syndrome with central nervous system disease mimicking multiple sclerosis (Alexander 1986e)

Clinical Manifestation	Patients	Events
	n (%)	n
Brain	29 (100)	
Hypesthesia		14
Spasticity, hyperreflexia, or both		12
Monocular visual loss		12*
Ataxia		11
Hemiparesis or hemiplegia		10
Cranial neuropathy		9
Dysarthria		8
Nystagmus		5
Internuclear ophthalmoplegia		3
Spinal Cord	17 (85)	
Paraparesis		13
Acute or subacute transverse myelopathy		11
Chronic progressive myelopathy		3
Neurogenic bladder		10
Brown-Sequard syndrome		2

* Five patients had monocular visual loss involving each eye at different times.

may be early manifestations of organic involvement in Sjögren's central nervous system disease (see below). Furthermore, such patients subsequently often develop specific focal or diffuse neurologic dysfunction.

Affective disturbances, defined clinically and by the use of the Minnesota Multiphasic Personality Inventory, are the most common psychiatric abnormality. The affective disturbance is characterized by hysteria, hypochondriasis, somatization, and depression. In many patients there is a striking dysphoric quality to the affective disorder. Anxiety and panic attacks are common. Psychosis, however, is rare.

On Minnesota Multiphasic Inventory Testing (MMPI), the three highest scales in rank order are, 1 (hypochondriasis) 3 (hysteria), and 2 (depression), characteristic of a "conversion V" (Lachar 1978). The MMPI profiles of the patients with primary Sjögren's syndrome are more abnormal than those reported in studies examining patients with systemic lupus erythematosus (Liang 1984, Kremer 1981) and rheumatoid arthritis (Kremer 1981).

Our recent data would indicate that cognitive dysfunction is also a manifestation of central nervous system involvement in Sjögren's syndrome (Malinow 1985; Selnes 1985). Patients commonly spontaneously complain of recent memory deficits, difficulty in concentration, and impaired intellectual performance in their job, school, or home. In one-half to two-thirds of those patients tested with formal cognitive function tests, mild to moderate deficits, particularly of attention and concentration, are documented. The verbal IQ is decremented significantly more than the performance IQ. These features are characteristic of subcortical dementias (Cummings 1984). In addition, patients with progressive dementia of the Alzheimer's type have been observed.

These abnormalities in cognitive function may occur alone and represent very early manifestations of central nervous system involvement. Alternatively, they may accompany psychiatric and/or specific focal or diffuse neurologic disease. The results of neurodiagnostic studies (see below) indicate that there is an organic basis for psychiatric and cognitive dysfunction in Sjögren's syndrome.

Diagnosis

Clinical Neurologic Evaluation. The current challenge of neurodiagnosis in primary Sjögren's syndrome comes not in documenting obvious or established neurologic deficits, but rather in diagnosing early and subtle evidence of neurologic disease. This requires a high index of suspicion, attention to subtle complaints and abnormalities, careful chronologic observations, and the use of several neurodiagnostic tests (see below).

In our experience, the development of new onset, atypical persistent headaches, a change in psychiatric status including the development of affective disturbances such as dysphoria or depression, an alteration in cognitive performance, or transient ill-defined neurologic syndromes may be early manifestations of central nervous system involvement in Sjögren's syndrome. Thus, the onset of such symptoms should not be ignored. If serial observation indicates that these manifestations are persistent or progressive, an appropriate neurodiagnostic work-up is indicated.

We have found that several neurodiagnostic parameters used together can provide important complementary information about the presence of active central

Table 7. Neurodiagnostic studies in central nervous system disease in primary Sjögren's syndrome

	Approximate Percent Abnormal*
Neuroradiology	
Computed axial tomography	<20
Cerebral angiography	<20
Magnetic resonance imaging	>20
Electrophysiology	
Electroencephalogram	>50
**Evoked response testing	>60
PSVER's	
BAER's	
SSER's	
**Cerebrospinal fluid analysis	>60
Elevated IgG index	
Oligoclonal bands	
Cytology - reactive lymphoid cells	

* In patients with established neurologic disease
** One or more abnormality, focal or diffuse

nervous system involvement in primary SS. These studies also can be used to follow patients serially and monitor response to immunosuppressive therapy. The studies we recommend obtaining are the following: electroencephalography, multimodality evoked response testing, cerebrospinal fluid analysis including IgG index, oligoclonal bands, and cytology, and magnetic resonance imaging (Table 7). It must be emphasized that these tests must be of high technical quality and interpreted by experienced individuals. Laboratory abnormalities should be correlated with the clinical evaluation.

Neuroradiology. The Sjögren's syndrome patients with clinical evidence of neurologic disease we described initially were evaluated with three main neurodiagnostic techniques, depending on the clinical indications. Enhanced computerized axial tomography of the brain was abnormal in less than 20% of patients with well-defined neurologic deficits. When abnormal, cortical atrophy, ventricular dilatation or infarcts were observed. In our hands, double-dose enhanced contrast scanning with delayed imaging, unlike the situation in multiple sclerosis (Barrett 1985), was no more sensitive. In patients with spinal cord involvement, myelography was uniformly negative. Four vessel cerebral angiography has been performed in over 20 individuals and has shown evidence of cerebral vasculitis in only four individuals. Thus, standard neuroradiologic techniques have been relatively insensitive in defining neuroanatomic deficits which correlate with the clinical abnormalities.

Our recent evaluation of SS patients with suspected nervous system disease has employed nuclear magnetic resonance imaging studies of the brain. This noninvasive technique is an extremely sensitive technique in detecting abnormalities and has provided valuable information about the pathogenesis of neurologic disease (Alexander 1986c).

Magnetic resonance imaging is more sensitive than computerized axial tomography or cerebral angiography in detecting abnormalities of the brain in SS patients with nervous system involvement. One or more, usually multiple, small areas of increased spin echo image intensity are observed. These lesions are predominantly in white matter in a subcortical and periventricular location. The neuroanatomic location of lesions correlates with neurologic abnormalities, but in addition, subclinical lesions are observed (i. e., defects seen on magnetic resonance imaging which are not associated with a defined neurologic deficit). Lesions are seen in one-half to two-thirds of patients with focal or diffuse active central nervous system disease, but also in a similar proportion of patients with only cognitive dysfunction or psychiatric impairment. The latter patients tend to have fewer lesions than patients with specific neurologic deficits. We have seen, however, more than 10 lesions in patients with only psychiatric or cognitive dysfunction.

The appearance of the regions of increased spin echo intensity is not specific and may be secondary to infarcts, plaques, or edema. It is important to realize that a region of microinfarction cannot be distinguished from a demyelinating lesion (i. e., plaque). Because of the appearance and distribution of lesions in patients with Sjögren's syndrome and central nervous system involvement, these lesions, in general, cannot be distinguished from those occurring in multiple sclerosis.

Electrophysiologic Studies. Electrophysiologic studies, including electroencephalography and multimodality evoked response testing, are useful adjuncts in the evaluation of central nervous system disease in Sjögren's syndrome. Electroencephalograms are abnormal in approximately one-half of patients with specific neurologic deficits. Patients with focal neurologic deficits may show focal slow wave activity, decreased amplitude, or spikes (sharp waves). In patients suspected of having temporal lobe epilepsy, electroencephalography, including sleep studies, may show seizure discharges. In patients with encephalopathy or progressive dementia, there may be diffuse slow wave activity.

We have determined that multimodality evoked response testing is extremely valuable in detecting evidence of diffuse multifocal central nervous system involvement in Sjögren's syndrome. Evoked response studies have demonstrated one or more abnormalities along the visual (PSVER's, pattern shift visual evoked responses), auditory (BAER's, brain stem auditory evoked responses), somatosensory (median and tibial nerve somatosensory evoked responses) pathways, in approximately two-thirds of patients with active central nervous system disease. Blink reflex studies may demonstrate involvement of the fifth nerve pathway (peripherally or centrally). This study also requires an intact facial nerve. Abnormalities in evoked response studies often correlate with clinical deficits or magnetic resonance imaging studies, but more importantly often define one or more subclinical abnormalities including involvement of the optic nerve(s). The spectrum of observed evoked response abnormalities is indistinguishable from that seen in multiple sclerosis.

It is our impression that evoked response testing may be more sensitive in detecting small abnormalities than magnetic resonance imaging. Thus, it should be used in conjunction with magnetic resonance imaging to document the presence of early organic disease and subclinical lesions suggesting multifocal involvement of the central nervous system.

Cerebrospinal Fluid Analysis. Several cerebrospinal fluid parameters suggest that there is an immunopathogenic basis for central nervous system disease in primary Sjögren's syndrome (Alexander 1986d). The total cerebrospinal fluid protein may be mildly elevated and there may be a mild mononuclear pleocytosis. We have found, however, that three other cerebrospinal fluid modalities are more useful in defining active central nervous system disease in Sjögren's syndrome: the IgG index, oligoclonal banding patterns, and cytology. The IgG index, indicative of the intrathecal synthesis of IgG, is abnormal (i.e. ≥ 0.7) in 70% of Sjögren's patients with active central nervous system disease, but in only 20% of patients without active disease ($p \leq 0.005$). Our preliminary data would indicate that these cerebrospinal fluid parameters are less likely to be abnormal in patients with early neurologic disease or psychiatric or cognitive dysfunction.

Cerebrospinal fluid agarose gel electrophoresis provides additional evidence for the presence of abnormal quantities of IgG within the central nervous system in active disease. Eighty-six percent of patients with active central nervous system disease, in contrast to 17% of patients without active central nervous system disease, have one or more clonal bands which migrate in the region of IgG ($p \leq 0.0005$). The majority of patients with abnormal cerebrospinal fluid electrophoretic patterns have a single discrete band, while approximately a third have two bands. A small number of patients have multiple bands (up to six) whose appearance is identical to the oligoclonal banding pattern seen in multiple sclerosis. All Sjögren's syndrome patients without active central nervous system disease, but with an elevated IgG index or clonal bands, had a remote history of neurologic disease.

Preliminary data suggest that the serial determination of the IgG index and clonal banding patterns may be useful in monitoring disease activity or progression and in assessing response to immunosuppressive therapy. The IgG index and number and intensity of clonal bands decrease with therapy. The latter situation is in contradistinction to multiple sclerosis where the number and pattern of oligoclonal bands remains unchanged despite therapy (Olsson 1976).

Special cytologic examination of the cerebrospinal fluid shows an abnormal number of reactive lymphoid cells in patients with active central nervous system disease. These cells include small round lymphocytes, plasma cells, lymphoblastoid cells which appear activated, and atypical mononuclear cells with large convoluted nuclei, irregular aggregates of chromatin, and scant homogeneous cytoplasm.

The blood-brain barrier, measured by the cerebrospinal fluid serum albumin ratio, remains grossly intact in patients with active disease. Myelin basic protein is almost always within normal limits.

The elevated IgG index and clonal bands, in the presence of grossly intact blood-brain barrier, are indicative of the intrathecal synthesis of IgG by lymphoid cells. Further support for the existence of inflammatory cells within the central nervous system is provided by the presence of reactive lymphoid cells within the cerebrospinal fluid. The potential specificity of antibodies synthesized within the central nervous system and their role, if any, in disease pathogenesis in this disorder are unknown.

Recently, we have demonstrated that SC5b-9, the terminal complement component activation neoantigen, is present in increased amount within the serum (and often cerebrospinal fluid) of Sjögren's patients with active central nervous system disease (Alexander 1986). These findings are similar to those reported in autoimmune mediated neurologic diseases such as multiple sclerosis and Guillain-Barre' Syndrome (Sanders 1986). Whether the activation of the complement pathway plays a primary role in the pathogenesis of central nervous system disease in Sjögren's syndrome is not known. It is known that central myelin can activate the classical pathway of complement in the absence of specific antibody (Vanguri 1982; Cyong 1982). Thus, ischemic injury to the nervous system may release myelin and activate the complement pathway as a secondary phenomenon.

Serologic Studies. There are several important observations regarding the serologic features of patients with Sjögren's syndrome, in general, and patients with central nervous system involvement, in particular. While one half to two-thirds of patients with Sjögren's syndrome are seropositive with respect to one or more autoantibodies, a significant proportion are seronegative by standard techniques (Alexander 1982b, 1983b). The patients tend to divide into two serologically distinct groups. Those who are seropositive are often hyperglobulinemia with a panel of autoantibodies including anti-nuclear antibodies, rheumatoid factor, antibodies to Ro(SS-A) or La(SS-B), cryoglobulins, and circulating immune complexes. Those patients with one autoantibody are more likely to have additional autoantibodies suggesting there is a polyclonal activation of B lymphocytes with an attendant polyclonal gammopathy.

Those patients who are seronegative with respect to these autoantibodies, do not have detectable antibodies to Ro(SS-A) or La(SS-B) detected by gel double immunodiffusion. They do, however, have low titers of these autoantibodies detected by a sensitive ELISA (Harley 1986a).

Both "seronegative" and seropositive individuals have the same HLA-DRw52 phenotype, which has been demonstrated to be associated with Sjögren's syndrome (Wilson 1984; Harley 1986). Autoantibody production in Sjögren's syndrome, however, is associated with other HLA antigens. Patients with HLA-DR3 (Harley 1986a) and those who are heterozygous for DQ1 and DQ2 (Harley 1986b) have a polyclonal gammopathy with the production of high titers of autoantibodies to Ro(SS-A) and La(SS-B) and rheumatoid factor. Thus, disease expression and autoantibody production appear to be associated with different histocompatibility antigens.

The clinical importance of recognizing that a subset of patients with primary Sjögren's syndrome may be "seronegative" by standard techniques is several fold. First, the diagnosis of Sjögren's syndrome is a clinical diagnosis and is not established by the presence of autoantibodies. If patients are seropositive, particularly for anti-Ro(SS-A) or La(SS-B) antibodies, this provides evidence supporting the diagnosis of an autoimmune or connective tissue disorder. If they are seronegative, however, the diagnosis is not excluded.

More importantly, both "seronegative" and seropositive subgroups of Sjögren's patients develop systemic complications, including inflammatory vascular disease and nervous system disease (Molina 1985a). The spectrum of clinical manifestations of vasculitis and nervous system disease in both subgroups of patients is indistinguishable.

Table 8. Central and peripheral nervous system complications: association with inflammatory vascular disease (IVD) in Sjögren's syndrome (Molina 1985b)

IVD type (n)*	No. (%) of patients with nervous system complications		
	Central alone	Peripheral alone	Peripheral and central
NIVD (17)	3 (18)	6 (35)	8 (47)
MIVD (16)	2 (12)	3 (18)	11 (70)
Total (33)	5 (15)	9 (28)	19 (58)

* Total number of patients was 30 in the NIVD group, 20 in the MIVD group; n values refer to numbers of patients with nervous system complications.
NIVD = neutrophilic IVD; *MIVD* = mononuclear IVD.

The main difference between these two patient subgroups appears to be in the serologic associations with inflammatory vascular disease. These differences are discussed in detail in Chapter II. B. 6. Briefly, we have described two distinct histopathologic types of inflammatory vascular disease in Sjögren's syndrome: neutrophilic (i.e. leukocytoclastic vasculitis) or mononuclear vasculitis (Alexander 1983d; Molina 1985b). Patients with neutrophilic inflammatory vascular disease are seropositive, while patients with mononuclear inflammatory vascular disease are seronegative. Patients with neutrophilic inflammatory vascular disease also have higher levels of circulating immune complexes and decreased serum complement levels compared to patients with mononuclear inflammatory vascular disease (see Chapter II. B. 6.).

Patients with peripheral inflammatory vascular disease (i.e. skin, nerve, or muscle) have a high frequency of central and peripheral nervous system complications (Table 8). Both histopathologic types of peripheral inflammatory vascular disease are equally associated with the development of central nervous system disease (Molina 1985a).

Neuropathology

In addition to cerebrospinal fluid abnormalities, histopathologic data obtained from post-mortem and biopsy material support the hypothesis that central nervous system disease in Sjögren's syndrome is mediated immunologically. Previous post-mortem studies on patients with Sjögren's syndrome indicated that cerebral inflammation was common, even in patients without antemortem evidence of neurologic dysfunction (de la Monte 1983).

Subsequently, we have obtained autopsy and biopsy tissue from Sjögren's syndrome patients with active neurologic disease. Several histopathologic abnormalities have been observed (Table 9). Within the brain, the meninges are a common site of inflammatory involvement even in patients without clinical evidence of meningitis. The mononuclear cells infiltrating the meninges are predominantly lymphocytes, but plasma cells, and atypical mononuclear cells are also observed (de la Monte 1983). These latter cells are morphologically identical to those we have

Table 9. Spectrum of observed histopathologic findings in central nervous system involvement in primary Sjögren's syndrome

Pathologic Feature	Central Nervous System		
	Brain		*Spinal Cord*
	Meninges	*Parenchyma*	
Mononuclear (lymphocytic) infiltrates	+	+	NO
Microinfarcts	–	+	NO
Microhemorrhages	+	+	NO
Inflammatory vascular disease			
Mononuclear	+	Mild	NO
Neutrophilic	NO	NO	+
Vasculopathy	+	+++	NO
	Peripheral Nervous System		
	Dorsal Root Ganglia	*Nerve*	*Muscle*
Mononuclear (lymphocytic) infiltrates	+	+	+
Inflammatory vascular disease			
Mononuclear	+	+	+
Neutrophilic	No	Less common	Less common

NO = Not Observed to Date

described in the cerebrospinal fluid of Sjögren's patients with active central nervous system involvement (Alexander 1986d). Similar inflammatory infiltrates have been observed in the choroid plexus (de la Monte 1983). Microhemorrhages (recent and remote) and fibrosis are also seen in the meninges.

Examination of the brain parenchyma may show minute microhemorrhages or microinfarcts. Microscopically there is a spectrum of damage to the small parenchymal blood vessels (predominantly post capillary venules). In general, there is extensive endothelial cell damage with relatively few perivascular mononuclear inflammatory infiltrates. Frank cerebral vasculitis of the type seen peripherally or systemically is conspicuously absent. Thus, we have elected to call this vascular process a cerebral vasculopathy. Because this type of histopathology has been observed in several patients who have died with active central nervous system disease, but were receiving no therapy, and in one patient in whom a brain biopsy was obtained, we are beginning to conclude that these histopathologic changes may represent active ongoing disease, rather than a "burnt out" or healing phase. Interestingly, the small blood vessels of the brain appear to be injured by a very different type of process than the peripheral blood vessels. This is particularly striking when patients dying secondary to active central nervous system disease demonstrate a cerebral vasculopathy, but have concomitant classical mononuclear and/or neutrophilic peripheral inflammatory vascular disease.

We suggest that this cerebral vasculopathy results in multiple minute microinfarcts and/or microhemorrhages. The coalescence of these microscopic lesions into larger lesions may cause abnormal electrophysiologic studies and subsequently result in the abnormal areas of increased signal intensity seen at magnetic resonance imaging. The emergence of clinical deficits is dependent upon the development of sufficiently large lesions in clinically critical regions.

Inflammatory vasculitis of larger vessels can also lead to neurologic dysfunction in Sjögren's syndrome. We have observed a patient who developed a fatal spinal subarachnoid hemorrhage secondary to a necrotizing arteritis of the anterior spinal artery (Alexander 1983 a). A patient with dorsal root ganglionitis (see below) had mononuclear vasculitis of a medium sized muscular artery supplying the posterior root of a thoracic nerve.

Recently, we have observed several patients with pure polysensory neuronopathies in whom mononuclear, predominantly lymphocytic, inflammatory infiltrates have been observed in biopsied thoracic dorsal root ganglia (dorsal root ganglionitis). The lymphocytes surround dorsal root ganglia cells which are damaged and destroyed. Preliminary data indicate that a substantial number of these infiltrating lymphocytes are T cells, some of which bear the cytotoxic phenotype.

Thus, it appears that inflammatory cells, predominantly mononuclear, can gain access to the nervous system and its blood vessels at multiple levels. This observation explains the diffuse multifocal manifestations characteristic of central nervous system involvement in Sjögren's syndrome. We have observed similar multifocal lymphocytic infiltrates within the meninges, choroid plexus, and parenchymal blood vessels of autoimmune MRL/Mp mice which have features of several connective tissue disorders (Alexander 1983 c).

Therapy

Our understanding of the appropriate treatment for Sjögren's syndrome patients with nervous system disease is in evolution. Initially, we were very conservative in our approach to therapeutic intervention (Alexander 1981 a, 1982 c). We observed patients who had self-limited transient neurologic deficits which partially or completely reversed spontaneously. Subsequently, with serial observation it became clear that in some patients multiple neurologic events occurred over time with progressive cumulative neurologic dysfunction.

Our initial therapeutic approach to the management of these patients utilized moderate to high dose corticosteroid therapy. In general, corticosteroid therapy alone was unsuccessful in stabilizing neurologic deterioration. Subsequently we have used additional immunosuppressive therapy.

Azathioprine (up to 4 mg/kg) alone or in combination with corticosteroids, likewise, has been ineffective. Daily dose oral cyclophosphamide (up to 3.5 mg/kg) has been used in some patients, with stabilization or improvement of neurologic disease. We have observed the development of transitional cell carcinoma of the bladder, however, in several patients.

We are now employing intravenous pulse cyclophosphamide therapy. The use of intermittent intravenous, in contrast to daily oral, cyclophosphamide therapy decreases the development of complications such as bone marrow suppression, hemorrhagic cystitis, alopecia, pulmonary fibrosis, infection, and theoretically, the potential for the development of malignancy (Austin 1986). Currently, we are using single bolus intravenous pulse cyclophosphamide therapy (0.75 gm/m^2–1.0 gm/m^2). The drug is administered monthly for six months and then every three months for at least two years. The nadir of the white blood cell count is maintained at approximately 3000 cells/mm^3. Moderate doses of corticosteroids initially are administered concomitantly and then tapered to an alternate day regimen. Whether this regimen will be successful in reversing or arresting disease progression is not known at the present time.

CNS-Sjögren's: Perspective

We have been asked why the neurologic complications that we have observed in primary Sjögren's syndrome have not been recognized previously as a prominent feature of this disorder. There are several reasons why this striking association has not been observed.

On the one hand, the diagnosis of Sjögren's syndrome is often overlooked. Our clinical experience suggests that primary Sjögren's syndrome is a common under-recognized, and therefore under-diagnosed, connective tissue disorder. The glandular manifestations of patients with Sjögren's syndrome may be subtle, insidious in onset and progression, and therefore, unrecognized by the patient and the unsuspecting clinician.

It is our impression that Sjögren's syndrome is probably the most common autoimmune connective tissue or rheumatic disease, outranking rheumatoid arthritis which affects between two to five percent of the adult population over 55 years of age (Hochberg 1981). Recent studies of a retirement home population support this clinical impression (Strickland 1984). In an elderly population of 103 Caucasian women evaluated by ophthalmologic testing and minor salivary gland biopsies, two (2%) had definite (keratoconjunctivitis sicca *and* a positive minor salivary gland biopsy) and twelve (12%) had probable (keratoconjunctivitis sicca *or* a positive minor salivary gland biopsy) Sjögren's syndrome. Nine (9%) patients had antibodies to Ro(SS-A) detected by gel double diffusion. Such autoantibodies are detected in the sera of less than 0.1% percent of patients with no evidence of connective tissue disease (Maddison 1979). In this same population, only one patient had rheumatoid arthritis, and none had systemic lupus erythematosus or scleroderma.

A second reason that the diagnosis of Sjögren's syndrome may be overlooked relates to some misconceptions about the significance of serologic abnormalities in this disorder. We have recognized that a subset of patients with primary Sjögren's syndrome are seronegative by standard techniques. It has been our experience that clinicians often incorrectly dismiss the possibility of the presence of a connective tissue disorder, such as Sjögren's syndrome, in the face of seronegativity. It is not generally recognized that such "seronegative" Sjögren's patients are not immune from developing serious systemic complications including nervous system disease.

There also are several reasons why neurologic dysfunction has not been observed in Sjögren's syndrome. The neurologic abnormalities in Sjögren's syndrome, particularly in the early stages of the disease, may be mild, transient, ill-defined, and may mimic other neurologic disorders such as multiple sclerosis, (Alexander 1986e), carcinomatous polysensory neuronopathy (Malinow 1986), or Alzheimer's dementia (Malinow 1985). It is our experience that patients with Sjögren's syndrome, particularly those with neurologic complaints, often have been dismissed as having functional or psychosomatic complaints without an organic basis. Furthermore, the neurologic manifestations of Sjögren's syndrome may not be recognized as being related to the underlying connective tissue disorder.

Finally, a major factor in our recognition of central nervous system complications of primary Sjögren's syndrome has been the serendipitous interaction or collaboration between several disciplines at our institution. The initial clinical correlation of Sjögren's syndrome with central nervous system involvement was made by a rheumatologist/immunologist (Elaine Alexander) and a neurologist (Garrett Alexander) who were asked to evaluate patients with neurologic dysfunction of unknown etiology. The patients were discovered to have classical features of Sjögren's syndrome and it was proposed, by exclusion, that their neurologic disease was related to their connective tissue disorder (Alexander 1981 a). Dr. Thomas Provost, a dermatoimmunologist, simultaneously began to recognize that Sjögren's patients with cutaneous vasculitis developed serious nervous system disease. Previously, the cutaneous inflammatory vascular disease of these patients had been dismissed by dermatologists as benign and self-limited. The central nervous system problems of these patients usually were either unrecognized or attributed to other etiologies. Historically, many Sjögren's syndrome patients with nervous system disease have an antecedent history of cutaneous vasculitis (Molina 1985 a). Subsequently, we have developed a multidisciplinary interest group consisting of specialists in neurology, psychiatry, neuroradiology, neuropathology, dermatoimmunology, rheumatology, and clinical immunology who are interested in understanding the immunopathogenesis of nervous system disease in Sjögren's syndrome.

Acknowledgements

I would like to express my sincere appreciation to Dr. Thomas T. Provost and my collaborators whose continued support, critical discussions, and enthusiasm have made the continuation of these studies possible, and particularly intellectually rewarding. I would also like to thank Vicky Rogers for her professional clerical assistance.

References

Alexander GE, Provost TT, Stevens MB, Alexander EL (1981 a) Sjögren's syndrome: Central nervous system manifestations. Neurology 31: 1391-1396

Alexander EL, Provost TT (1981 b) Ro(SS-A) and La(SS-B) antibodies. Springer Semin Immunopathol 4: 253-273

Alexander EL, Craft C, Dorsch C, Moser RL, Provost TT, Alexander GE (1982 a) Necrotizing arteritis and spinal subarachnoid hemorrhage in Sjögren's syndrome. Ann Neurol 11: 632-635

Alexander EL, Hirsch TJ, Arnett FC, Provost TT, Stevens MB (1982 b) Ro(SS-A) and La(SS-B) antibodies in the clinical spectrum of Sjögren's syndrome. J Rheumatol 9: 239-246

Alexander EL, Provost TT, Stevens MB, Alexander GE (1982 c) Neurologic complications of primary Sjögren's syndrome. Medicine 61: 247-257

Alexander EL, Josifek L, Provost TT, Alexander GE (1982 d) Myositis/vasculitis in primary Sjögren's syndrome (SS). Arthritis Rheum 25: S15

Alexander EL, Alexander GE (1983 a) Aseptic meningitis in primary Sjögren's syndrome. Neurology 33: 593-598

Alexander EL, Arnett FC, Provost TT, Stevens MB (1983b) Sjögren's syndrome: Association of anti-Ro(SS-A) antibodies with vasculitis, hematologic abnormalities, and serologic hyperreactivity. Ann Intern Med 98: 155-159

Alexander EL, Murphy ED, Roths JB, Alexander GE (1983c) Congenic autoimmune murine models of central nervous disease in connective tissue disorders. Ann Neurol 14: 242-248

Alexander EL, Provost TT (1983d) Cutaneous manifestations of primary Sjögren's syndrome: A reflection of vasculitis and association with anti-Ro(SS-A) antibodies. J Invest Dermatol 80: 386-391

Alexander EL (1986a) Central nervous system (CNS) manifestations of primary Sjögren's syndrome: An overview. Scandinavian J Rheum, In press

Alexander EL (1986b) Immunopathologic mechanisms of inflammatory vascular disease in primary Sjögren's syndrome. Scandinavian J Rheum, In press

Alexander EL, Beall S, Provost TT, Patronas M, McFarland HF (1986c) Magnetic resonance imaging (MRI) in primary Sjögren's syndrome with central nervous system disease (CNS-SS): New clues to pathogenesis. Arthritis Rheum 29: S63

Alexander EL, Lijewski JE, Jerdan MS, Alexander GE (1986d) Evidence for an immunopathogenic basis for central nervous disease in primary Sjögren's syndrome. Arthritis Rheum 29: 1223-1231, 1986.

Alexander EL, Malinow K, Lijewski JE, Jerdan MS, Provost TT, Alexander GE (1986e) Primary Sjögren's syndrome with central nervous system dysfunction mimicking multiple sclerosis. Ann Intern Med 104: 323-330

Alexander EL, Provost TT (1986f) Sjögren's syndrome: Association of cutaneous vasculitis with nervous system disease. Arch Derm, In press

Alexander EL, Provost TT, Bias WB, McFarland HF (1986g) Unique immunogenetic associations distinguish Sjögren's syndrome central nervous system disease (CNS-SS) from multiple sclerosis (MS). Arthritis Rheum 29: S63

Alexander EL, Sanders ME, Frank MM, Joiner KA (1986h) Activated terminal complement (SC5b-9) in the sera of Sjögren's syndrome patients with central nervous system disease (CNS-SS). Arthritis Rheum 29: S37

Austin HA III, Klippel JH, Balow JE, Le Riche NGH, Steinberg AD, Plotz PH, Decker JL (1986) Therapy of lupus nephritis - Controlled trial of prednisone and cytotoxic drugs. N Engl J Med 314: 614-619

Barrett L, Drayer B, Shin C (1985) High-resolution computed tomography in multiple sclerosis. Ann Neurol 17: 33-38

Bloch KJ, Buchanan WW, Wohl JJ, Bunim JJ (1965) Sjögren's syndrome: A clinical, pathological and serological study of 62 cases. Medicine (Baltimore) 44: 187-231

Bohan A, Peter JB, Bowman RL, Pearson CM (1977) A computer-assisted analysis of 153 patients with polymyositis and dermatomyositis. Medicine 56: 255-285

Bunim JJ (1961) A broader spectrum of Sjögren's syndrome and its pathogenetic implications. Ann Rheum Dis 20: 1-10

Chad D, Good P, Adelman L, Bradley WG, Mills J (1982) Inclusion body myositis associated with Sjögren's syndrome. Arch Neurol 39: 186-188

Cummings JL, Benson DF (1984) Subcortical dementia: review of an emerging concept. Arch Neurol 41: 874-849

Cyong JC, Witkin SS, Rieger B, Barbarese E, Good RA, Day NK (1982) Antibody independent complement activation by myelin via the classical complement pathway. J Exp Med 155: 587

Daniels TE (1984) Labial salivary gland biopsy in Sjögren's syndrome. Arthritis Rheum 27: 147-156

De la Monte SM, Hutchins GM, Gupta PK (1983) Polymorphous meningitis with atypical mononuclear cells in Sjögren's syndrome. Ann Neurol 14: 455-461

Greenspan JS, Daniels TE, Talal N, Sylvester RA (1974) The histopathology of Sjögren's syndrome in labial salivary gland biopsies. Oral Surg 37: 217-229

Harley JB, Alexander EL, Bias WB, Fox OF, Provost TT, Reichlin M, Yamagata H, Arnett FC (1986a) Anti-Ro(SS-A) and anti-La(SS-B) in patients with Sjögren's syndrome. Arthritis Rheum 29: 196-206

Harley JB, Reichlin M, Arnett FC, Alexander EL, Bias WB, Provost TT (1986b) Gene interaction at

HLA-DR enhances autoantibody production in primary Sjögren's syndrome. Science 232: 1145-1147
Holm S (1949) Keratoconjunctivitis sicca and the sicca syndrome. Acta Ophthalmol Suppl 33: 13-16
Kaltreider HB, Talal N (1969) The neuropathy of Sjögren's syndrome. Trigeminal nerve involvement. Ann Intern Med 70: 751-762
Kremer J, Rynes R, Bartholomew L et al (1981) Non-organic non-psychotic psychopathology (NONPP) in patients with systemic lupus erythematosus. Semin Arthritis Rheum 11: 182-189
Lachar D (1978) The MMPI: Clinical assessment and automated interpretation. Los Angeles: Western Psychological Services, p 46
Liang MH, Rogers M, Larson M et al (1984) The psychosocial impact of systemic lupus erythematosus and rheumatoid arthritis. Arthritis Rheum 27: 13-19
Maddison PJ, Mogavero H, Provost TT, Reichlin M (1979) The clinical significance of autoantibodies to certain soluble cytoplasmic antigens in systemic lupus erythematosus and other connective tissue diseases. J Rheum 6: 189-195
Malinow KL, Molina R, Gordon B, Selnes OA, Provost TT, Alexander EL (1985) Neuropsychiatric dysfunction in primary Sjögren's syndrome. Ann Intern Med 103: 344-349
Malinow KL, Yannakakis GD, Glusman SM, Edlow DR, Griffin J, Pestronk A, Powell DL, Ramsey-Goldman R, Eidelman BH, Medsger TA, Alexander EL (1986) Subacute sensory neuropathy secondary to dorsal root ganglionitis in primary Sjögren's syndrome. Ann Neurol, 20: 535-537
Masi AT, Rodnan GP, Medsger TA et al (1980) Preliminary criteria for the classification of systemic sclerosis (scleroderma). Arthritis Rheum 23: 581-590
Molina R, Provost TT, Alexander EL (1985a) Peripheral inflammatory vascular disease in Sjögren's syndrome: association with nervous system complications. Arthritis Rheum 28: 1341-1347
Molina R, Provost TT, Alexander EL (1985b) Two histopathologic prototypes of inflammatory vascular disease in Sjögren's syndrome: differential association with seroactivity to rheumatoid factor and antibodies to Ro(SS-A) and with hypocomplementemia. Arthritis Rheum 28: 1251-1258
Molina R, Provost TT, Arnett FC, Bias WB, Hochberg MC, Wilson RW, Alexander EL (1986) Primary Sjögren's syndrome (SS) in men - clinical, serologic and immunogenetic features. Am J Med 80: 23-31
Olsson JE, Link H, Muller R (1976) Immunoglobulin abnormalities in multiple sclerosis: relation to clinical parameters: disability, duration and age of onset. J Neurol Sci 27: 233-245
Peyronnard JM, Charron L, Beaudet F, Couture F (1982) Vasculitic neuropathy in rheumatoid disease and Sjögren's syndrome. Neurology 32: 839-845
Pittsley RA, Talal N (1980) Neuromuscular complications of Sjögren's syndrome. Chapter 19, pp 419-433
Raskin RJ, Tesar JT, Lawless OJ (1981) Hypokalemic periodic paralysis in Sjögren's syndrome. Arch Intern Med 141: 1671
Ringel SP, Forstot JZ, Tan EM, Wehling C, Griggs RC, Butcher D (1982) Sjögren's syndrome and polymyositis or dermatomyositis. Arch Neurol 39: 157-163
Ropes MW, Bennett GA, Cobb S (1958) Diagnostic criteria for rheumatoid arthritis. Bull Rheum Dis 9: 175-176
Rutan G, Martinez AJ, Fieshko JT, Van Thiel DH (1986) Primary biliary cirrhosis, Sjögren's syndrome, and transverse myelitis. Gastroenterology 90: 206-210
Sanders ME, Koski CL, Robbins D, Shin ML, Frank MM, Joiner KA (1986) Activated terminal complement in cerebrospinal fluid in Guillain-Barre Syndrome and multiple sclerosis. J Immunol 135: 1-4
Selnes OA, Gordon B, Malinow K, Alexander EL (1985) Cognitive dysfunction in primary Sjögren's syndrome. Neurology 35 (Suppl 1): 179
Shearn M (1971) Sjögren's syndrome. WB Saunders, Philadelphia
Sheldon JH (1938) Sjögren's syndrome associated with pigmentation and scleroderma of the legs. ProcRoy Soc Med 32: 255-256
Silberberg DH, Drachman DA (1962) Late-life myopathy occurring with Sjögren's syndrome. Arch Neurol 6: 428-438

Sjögren H (1935) Zur Kenntnis der keratoconjunctivitis sicca. II. Allgemeine Symptomatologie und Ätiologie. Acta Ophthal (Kbh) 13: 1-39

Strickland RW, Tesar JT, Berne BH et al (1984) The prevalence of Sjögren's syndrome and associated rheumatic diseases in an elderly population. Arthritis Rheum 27: S45

Tan EM, Cohen AS, Fries JF et al (1982) The 1982 revised criteria for the classification of systemic lupus erythematosus. Arthritis Rheum 25: 1271-1277

Vanguri P, Koski CL, Silverman B, Shin ML (1982) Complement activation by isolated myelin: activation of the classical pathway in the absence of myelin specific antibodies. Proc Natl Acad Sci USA 79: 3290

Von Bekesy G (1964) Duplicity theory of taste. Science 145: 834-835

Whaley K, Webb J, McAvoy BA, Hughes GRV, Lee P, MacSween RNM, Buchanan WW (1973) Sjögren's syndrome. II. Clinical associations and immunological phenomena. Quart J Med 42: 513-548

Whitaker JN, Engel WK (1972) Vascular deposits of immunoglobulin and complement in idiopathic inflammatory myopathy. N Engl J Med 286: 333-338

Wilson R, Provost TT, Bias WB, Alexander EL, Edlow DW, Hochberg MC, Stevens MB, Arnett FC (1984) Sjögren's syndrome: Influence of multiple HLA-D region alloantigens on clinical and serologic expression. Arthritis Rheum 27: 1245-1253

3. The Respiratory System in Sjögren's Syndrome

S. H. Constantopoulos and H. M. Moutsopoulos

Introduction

The respiratory system is the target organ of many autoimmune rheumatic diseases. In some of these, serositis is a common manifestation (rheumatoid arthritis, systemic lupus erythematosus), while in other interstitial lung disease predominates (scleroderma) (Hunninghake and Fauci 1979). Manifestations from the trachea to the pleura have been described in patients with Sjögren's syndrome (SS) (Strimlan 1976; Constantopoulos 1985). They are frequent but rarely clinically important. They can present in different ways; from dry cough secondary to desiccation of tracheobronchial mucosa (xerotrachea) to dyspnea from interstitial disease or airways obstruction. Pneumonia and pleurisy, very frequently noted in the older literature (Shearn 1979) do not seem to constitute a serious problem. The detection of this involvement requires clinical, roentgenological and functional evaluation since not all clinical manifestations have functional equivalent (e.g. xerotrachea) and vice versa (e.g. small airways disease). In this chapter we will describe the respiratory manifestations of SS emphasizing the differences between primary and secondary SS.

Trachea and large airways

Xerotrachea

Dessiccation of the tracheobronchial tree (xerotrachea), a common respiratory manifestation of SS (Constantopoulos et al. 1984), is the result of diminished or absent secretions of the mucous glands in the trachea and bronchi. Xerotrachea is manifested with cough which can vary in intensity from a mild foreign body sensation to exaustive dry cough ending in vomiting. It frequently misleads the clinician to erroneous diagnoses such as chronic bronchitis or asthma since it can be one of the first manifestations of primary SS. It has no functional equivalent and must be differentiated from the cough caused by interstitial involvement in SS which is usually accompanied by dyspnea and is expressed functionally with diminished diffusing capacity. It has been described by Sjögren (1933) and was later named "bronchitis sicca" by Alarcon-Segovia (1978). Xerotrachea has recently been proven on several occasions bronchoscopically and histologically (Newball and Brahim 1977; Bariffi et al. 1984). In our series (Constantopoulos et al. 1985) it was the only pulmonary manifestation in 17% of the patients with primary SS.

Recurrent respiratory infections secondary to bronchial dryness, retained secretions and atelectasis

Recurrent respiratory infections have been considered as a major cause of death of patients with SS (Shearn 1977). The diminished secretion of the bronchial mucous glands with subsequent impairment of the mucociliary escalator appeared as a logical explanation. However, in an elegant study from Brompton Hospital, Fairfax et al (1981) using Technitium^{99} labelled polystyrene particles showed that the mucociliary clearance in patients with SS is normal. Other respiratory components of defense mechanisms, however, could be incriminated, provided that recurrent infections do occur frequently in patients with SS. Papathanasiou et al (1986) studied 40 patients with primary SS and 26 with secondary. No one among these patients had significant history of previous pneumonias nor presented with pneumonia. In other studies pneumonia was either absent or infrequent, at least in patients with primary SS and definitely not a frequent cause of death (Fairfax et al. 1981; Vitali et al. 1985).

Functional impairment; obstructive ventilatory defect

In most large series of patients with SS, obstructive defect is either absent (Strimlan et al. 1976) or infrequent (Bariffi et al. 1984; Constantopoulos et al. 1985; Papathanasiou et al. 1986). There are studies however, where obstruction of large airways is frequent. Thus Newball and Brahim (1977) and Segal et al (1981) reported obstructive defect in almost 50% of their patients with SS. It is interesting that in both studies obstruction was frequent in patients with primary SS. They concluded that obstructive airways disease is a result of SS itself while the restrictive defect is a result of the concomitant rheumatic disorder. We had a different experience (Papathanasiou et al. 1986). In our study comparing 40 patients with primary SS, 26 patients with secondary SS, 40 patients with rheumatoid arthritis without SS and 100 healthy matched controls, we found that obstructive disorder occured in only 20% of patients with primary SS versus 46% of patients with secondary SS and 32.5% of patients with rheumatoid arthritis. Since all types of functional impairment were similar in secondary SS and rheumatoid arthritis without SS, we considered that they represented the result of rheumatoid arthritis on the respiratory system and that secondary SS did not influence this result.

Small airways

Obstruction of small airways (those with 2 mm diameter or smaller) is considered an early manifestation of chronic obstructive ventilatory defect. It is very frequently observed in smokers and it is believed that cessation of smoking will improve it (Guenther and Welch 1982). Thus it represents the first reversible manifestation of obstructive lung disease. There are additional points which have to be considered. First, we do not know whether small airways obstruction procedes always to obstruction of larger airways. Second, most of the studies measuring small airways function are sensitive but quite non-specific with a great variability among normal individuals. Third, anatomically, small airways can be considered part of the so-called "pulmonary interstitium" (Crystal et al. 1984). Thus studies evaluating small airways, like flow/volume loop, are influenced in diffuse interstitial lung disease.

For all these reasons, it is difficult to point out the exact significance of small airways disease in a disorder like SS in which it is known that both airways and pulmonary interstitium are involved. Newball and Brahim (1977) obtained histologic evidence of small airways involvement in SS when they found mononuclear cell infiltration around small airways in lung biopsy of two patients with SS. They suggested that "human airways should be considered another target organ of SS". There are other studies revealing small airways abnormality in SS both primary and secondary (Bariffi et al. 1984; Constantopoulos et al. 1985; Vitali et al. 1985). In none of these studies though a control population was included for comparison. When we compared patients with primary SS and secondary SS with an age and sex matched group, there were no differences in the frequence of small airways disease (Papathanasiou et al. 1986). All our patients as well as our controls were lifelong non-smokers. Studies over a period of years are needed to evaluate the significance of this ventilatory abnormality in SS.

Pulmonary interstitium

Diffuse interstitial lung disease with impaired diffusing capacity is a major manifestation of pulmonary involvement in all autoimmune rheumatic disorders. SS is no exception to this generalization. Most large series (Strimlan et al. 1976; Oxholm et al. 1982; Constantopoulos et al. 1984 and 1985) consider this the commonest pulmonary abnormality in SS. Hunninghake and Fauci emphasize in their review (1979) that it can take two patterns; interstitial fibrosis reflecting the primary rheumatic disease and lymphoid interstitial disease characteristic of SS itself. This does not imply that fibrosis is present only in secondary SS and lymphoid interstitial disease only in primary. In five transbronchial lung biopsies in patients with primary SS we found a wide spectrum of interstitial pathology from dense lymphocytic infiltrates to severe interstitial fibrosis (Constantopoulos et al. 1985). Some of those patients with histologically proven interstitial disease had normal lung diffusing capacity while none of nine patients with functional or histologic evidence of interstitial lung disease had incapacitating dyspnea. Finally, an interesting correlation of interstitial lung disease with low serum complement and cryoglobulinemia was observed in our study (Papathanasiou et al. 1986). These findings suggest that the involvement of the pulmonary interstitium in SS may be patchy, not necessarily interfering with diffusion, at least in early stages. Also, the lack of heavy dyspnea suggests that it is a slow process, unlike other rheumatic disorders, most notably scleroderma (Hunninghake and Fauci 1979). Finally, the correlation of interstitial lung disease with low complement and cryoglobulinemia may suggest immune complex deposition as a mechanism of the interstitial process.

The lymphoid interstitial involvement makes SS one of the major known causes of lymphocytic interstitial pneumonitis (LIP). Liebow and Carrington (1973) suggested that LIP is part of the spectrum of SS with only lung involvement. The etiology of LIP in SS has not been elucidated. There has been one report of "virus-like" particles in bronchiolar epithelium of a patient with SS (Sutinen et al. 1977) but viral cultures confirming this are lacking. Anderson and Talal have described "the spectrum of benign to malignant lymphoproliferation in SS" since 1971. Until today this continues to be a serious diagnostic problem since pulmonary histopathology in LIP can be indistinguishable from lymphomatous involvement of the lung (Vath et al. 1982). Even more difficult is the distinction between lymphoma and pseudolymphoma. The chest roentgenogram can serve as initial differential approach; LIP is most often associated with bilateral reticulonodular opacities while pseudolymphoma and lymphoma usually present as localized lymphoid nodules of the lung (Marchevsky et al. 1983). If hilar, mediastinal or distant lymph nodes are also involved, the diagnosis of lymphoma is more likely. If the only radiologic finding is lung nodules, lung biopsy is required. Infiltrates with mature lymphocytes and other inflammatory cells with germinal centers characterize pseudolymphomas while immature lymphocytes without germinal centers within the lesion suggest true lymphomas which also often extend into pleura and bronchi. This was the original description of Saltztein in 1963. Since then, it has been shown that it is not so easy to differentiate between the two entities since their clinical, radiologic and histologic features tend to overlap. Even with the use of monoclonal antibodies and immunofluorescent techniques, the distinction is not clear cut. Furthermore, the prognosis is not necessarily different since pseudolymphomas are not always benign and malignant lymphomas do not necessarily advance to progressive disease (Marchevsky et al. 1983). These observations have confused the issue of efficacy and need of chemotherapy in patients with lymphoid lung nodules.

In addition to interstitial fibrosis and LIP, amyloidosis (Bonner et al. 1973), sarcoidosis and vasculitis (Fairfax 1981) have been reported to occur in the lung parenchyma of SS patients.

Pleura

None of 40 patients with primary SS and 2/26 with secondary SS in our study had a history of pleural effusion (Papathanasiou et al. 1986). We suggested therefore that pleural involvement is not related to SS but most likely to the underlying rheumatic disorder. In Strimlan's series (1976) 5/18 patients with SS and respiratory manifestations had pleurisy; all had secondary SS. The histologic characteristics of pleural involvement in SS have not been clarified. Thus we have no evidence to support or deny that pleural disease is related to SS itself.

Lymph nodes

Hilar and mediastinal lymph nodes can be involved in SS with lymphomatous or pseudolymphomatous changes. The difficulties in the differential diagnosis between these two entities have been discussed previously.

Summary

The respiratory system is frequently involved in SS but this involvement is rarely clinically significant. The commonest manifestation is diffuse interstitial lung disease, which may be related to immune complex deposition. There are differences between primary and secondary SS and it is likely that the respiratory involvement in secondary SS may be just a reflection of the primary rheumatic disorder. Pneumonia and pleurisy do not seem to be frequent problems. Finally, pseudolymphoma or frank lymphoma should always be considered when lung nodules are seen in chest roentgenograms or hilar/mediastinal lymphadenopathy is present.

References

Alarcon-Segovia D (1978) Airways in rheumatoid disease (Letter to the Editor). The Lancet ii: 1058

Bariffi F, Pesci A, Bertorelli G, Mangenelli P, Ambanelli U (1984) Pulmonary involvement in Sjögren's syndrome. Respiration 46: 82-87

Bonner HJr, Ennir RS, Geelhoed GW, Tarpley TMJr (1973) Lymphoid infiltration and amyloidosis of lung in Sjögren's syndrome. Archieves of Pathology 55: 42-44

Constantopoulos SH, Drosos AA, Maddison PJ, Moutsopoulos HM (1984) Xerotrachea and interstitial lung disease in primary Sjögren's syndrome. Respiration 46: 310-314

Constantopoulos SH, Papadimitriou CS, Moutsopoulos HM (1985) Respiratory manifestations in primary Sjögren's syndrome. Chest 88: 226-229

Crystal RG, Bitterman PB, Rennard SI, Hance AJ, Keogh BA (1984) Interstitial lung diseases of unknown cause: disorders characterized by chronic inflammation of the lower respiratory tract. N Engl J Med 310: 154-166 and 238-244

Fairfax AJ, Haslam PL, Pavia D, Sheahan NF, Bateman JRM, Angew JE, Cerke SW and Turner-Warnich M (1981) Pulmonary disorders associated with Sjögren's syndrome. Quarterly J Med New Series 199: 279-295

Guenther CA and Welch MH (1982) Pulmonary Medicine, Philadelphia, JB Lippincott Company

Hunninghake GW, Fauci AS (1979) State of the art: pulmonary involvement in the collagen vascular diseases. Am Rev Respir Dis 119: 471-503

Liebow AA and Carrington CB (1973) Diffuse pulmonary lymphoreticular infiltrations associated with dysproteinemia. Symposium on chronic respiratory disease. Medical Clinics of North America 57: 809-842

Marchevsky A, Padilla M, Kaneko M and Keinerman J (1983) Localized lymphoid nodules of lung. A reappraisal of the lymphoma versus pseudolymphoma dilemma. Cancer 51: 2070-2077

Newball HH and Brahim SA (1977) Chronic obstructive airways disease in patients with Sjögren's syndrome. Am Rev Respir Dis 115: 295-304

Oxholm P, Bundgaard A, Birk Madsen E, Manthorpe R, Vejlø Rasmussen F (1982) Pulmonary function in patients with primary Sjögren's syndrome. Rheumatol Int 2: 179-181

Papathanasiou MP, Constantopoulos SH, Tsampoulas C, Drosos AA and Moutsopoulos HM (1986) Reappraisal of respiratory abnormalities in primary and secondary Sjögren's syndrome: a controlled study. Chest 90: 370-374

Saltztein SL (1963) Pulmonary malignant lymphomas and pseudolymphomas. Classification, therapy and prognosis. Cancer 16: 928-955

Segal I, Fink G, Machtely I, Gura V, Spitzer SA (1981) Pulmonary function abnormalities in Sjögren's syndrome and the sicca complex. Thorax 36: 286-289

Shearn MA (1977) Sjögren's syndrome. Medical Clinics of North America 61: 271-282

Sjögren H (1933) Zur kenntnis der keratoconjunctivitis sicca (Keratitis filiformis bei hypofunction der Tranendrusen) Acta Ophthalmol (Kbh) 11: 1-151

Strimlan VC, Rosenow EC III, Divertie MB, Harrison EGJr (1976) Pulmonary manifestations of Sjögren's syndrome. Chest 70: 354-361

Sutinen S, Sutinen S and Huht E (1977) Ultrastructure of lymphoid interstitial pneumonia: virus-like particles in bronchiolar epithelium of a patient with Sjögren's syndrome. Am J Clin Pathol 67: 328-333

Vath RR, Alexander BC and Fulmer JD (1982) The lymphocytic infiltrative lung diseases. Symposium on interstitial lung diseases. Clinics in Chest Medicine 3: 619-634

Vitali C, Tavoni A, Viegi G, Begliomini E, Agnesi A and Bombardieri S (1985) Lung involvement in Sjögren's syndrome: a comparison between patients with primary and with secondary syndrome. Ann Rheum Dis 44: 455-461

4. Gastrointestinal and Hepatobiliary Features in Sjögren's Syndrome*

H. Trevino, E. B. Tsianos, and S. Schenker

Introduction

Sjögren's syndrome (SS) is a chronic, inflammatory, systemic, autoimmune disease, characterized by dryness of the eyes, mouth, and other mucous membranes, and frequently associated with rheumatic disease (Machin et al. 1984; Simila et al. 1978). It is the second most frequent collagen disorder, surpassed in prevalence only by rheumatoid arthritis (Shearn 1977). The diagnosis is, however, frequently overlooked. Whaley, et al. (1973) observed that SS had been unsuspected before referral in all 94 patients in whom it coexisted with rheumatoid arthritis.

This disorder can occur alone (primary) or in association with other autoimmune disease (secondary) (Ludwig et al. 1977; Parke et al. 1984; Chisholm et al. 1978; Rutan et al. 1986), mainly rheumatoid arthritis (Machin et al. 1984; Simila et al. 1978) and systemic lupus erythematosus (Alarcon-Segovia et al. 1974; Simila et al. 1978).

There are a number of excellent reviews in the literature regarding the clinical and immunological aspects of this disease (Shearn 1977; Moutsopoulos et al. 1980). However, relatively little has been written about the gastrointestinal and hepatobiliary manifestations of this disorder, even in recent textbooks of gastroenterology (Kraft, Kirsner 1985; Kaunitz, Sleisenger 1983). It seems appropriate, therefore, to review the literature and summarize the current concepts in this area.

The upper gastrointestinal tract, the pancreas and the liver are the main organs which may be affected in patients with SS. Although the pathogenesis is uncertain, one may theorize that the involvement of the gut and pancreas reflects their glandular composition (similar to that of salivary glands), while the hepatobiliary disorders may relate to the frequent participation of the liver and biliary system in autoimmune diseases.

Esophagus in Sjögren's Syndrome

Patients with primary Sjögren's syndrome frequently complain of dysphagia (Hradsky et al. 1967). The symptom has been related to xerostomia (Shearn 1977; Hradsky et al. 1967) or to impairment of esophageal motility (Ramirez-Mata et al.

* Supported in part by NIH (Grant No. NIAAA 7RO1AA05814-01) and from Veterans Administration (Research Service, Audie Murphy Memorial Veterans' Hospital).

1976; Tsianos et al. 1985). The latter appears to be the more plausible explanation for the dysphagia. Ramirez-Mata, et al. (1976) reported the esophageal monometric findings in 10 unselected patients with SS. Nine of them had an abnormal motility pattern consisting of either absence or decrease of contractility in the upper third of the esophagus. Three of the nine patients had spontaneous biphasic and triphasic tertiary contractions in the lower 2/3 of the esophagus. Recently we have examined a larger series of patients with primary Sjögren's syndrome and have found that esophageal motility is altered in approximately one-third of these individuals (Tsianos, et al. 1985). Contrary to the earlier observations, this esophageal dysfunction did not correlate with the parotid flow rate, the degree of inflammatory infiltrate of the minor salivary glands, the presence of Raynaud's phenomenon or other extraglandular manifestations of SS. The presence of autoantibodies to RO (SSA), rheumatoid factor and La (SSB) cellular antigens also did not correlate with esophageal dysfunction. We propose that this esophageal impairment may be due to either the involvement of the exocrine glands of the esophagus or that the esophageal dysfunction may represent a low grade myositis. Future studies are needed to confirm these hypotheses. The association of achalasia and SS also has been reported (Weissman 1958; Simila et al. 1978) but it might be a fortutious finding.

Stomach in Sjögren's Syndrome

Nausea, epigastric pain and dyspepsia are common complaints of patients with Sjögren's syndrome (Maury et al. 1985; Buchanan et al. 1966). The gastric mucosa viewed through the gastroscope looks atrophic (Maury et al. 1985) or may have a cobblestone appearance (Shearn 1977). Gastric biopsy specimens show chronic atrophic gastritis and lymphocytic infiltrates (Buchanan et al. 1966; Van Jebavy et al. 1961). Immunohistochemical staining shows that the cell infiltrates consist mainly of T-lymphocytes. Most of the T-cells are OKT_4-reactive lymphocytes (helper T-lymphocytes) (Kilpi et al. 1983). These immunohistologic findings are reminiscent of those described in the minor salivary gland biopsies in patients with Sjögren's syndrome (Moutsopoulos et al. 1986).

Gastric studies in Sjögren's syndrome patients have revealed decreased volume and acid content of gastric secretions (Buchanan et al. 1966), and hypopepsinogenemia. This is usually combined with elevated serum gastrin (Maury et al. 1982; Mulders et al. 1984), low levels of serum vitamin B_{12} (Maury et al. 1985) and varying frequencies (Buchanan et al. 1966) of parietal cell antibodies. The salivary glands are an important source of epidermal growth factor (EGF), which is known to decrease gastric acid secretion (Elder et al. 1975), as well as influence cytoprotection (Konturek et al. 1981). One wonders if salivary gland disease, seen frequently with SS, may not result in impaired EGF output and this contribute to gastric changes seen. Clearly an autoimmune basis is another explanation of these findings. Studies of epidermal growth factor in SS, however, would be of interest. On a histologic and biochemical basis, Maury et al. (1985) were not able to distinguish the gastric findings in primary Sjögren's syndrome from these in secondary Sjögren's syndrome, nor to distinguish chronic atrophic gastritis associated with Sjögren's syndrome from that independent of it.

Small Bowel in Sjögren's Syndrome

Nutritional deficiencies have been noted in patients with Sjögren's syndrome and the results of laboratory tests in these patients have suggested a primary malabsorption syndrome (Raffle 1950, Henderson 1950). In 1965 Pittman and Holub (1965) reported a female patient with Sjögren's syndrome associated with severe nutritional deficiencies and diarrhea which were shown to be due to adult celiac disease. Another similar case has been reported in 1971 (Lancaster-Smith, Strickland 1971). In 1972 MacLaurin et al. (1972) also reported a female patient who presented with an exacerbation of celiac disease following initiation of treatment for an autoimmune thyroiditis. She also had symptoms of Sjögren's syndrome. In the serum of this patient a lymphocytotoxic factor was found which had some but not all of the characteristics of an autoantibody. The association of two uncommon diseases, such as celiac disease and Sjögren's syndrome, in the same individual, raises the possibility of etiological relationship, but this possibility has not hitherto been proved. Recently, a single case of Crohn's colitis and SS was reported (Gainey et al. 1985).

Pancreas in Sjögren's Syndrome

Deranged pancreatic secretion was reported as a frequent feature in patients with Sjögren's syndrome (Fenster et al. 1964; Dreiling, Soto 1976; Hradsky 1967). These studies were done using secretin (Fenster et al. 1964; Dreiling, Soto 1976) pancreozymin-secretin (Dreiling, Soto 1976) or the NBT-PABA test and RIA trypsinemia (Gobelet et al. 1983). These patients had no clinical manifestations of pancreatic disease, suggesting the presence of a subclinical pancreatic insufficiency. Acute pancreatitis in patients with Sjögren's syndrome has been reported infrequently by several workers (Fenster et al. 1964; Cardell, Curling 1954). Recently, we have found in 6 out of 25 (24%) unselected patients with primary Sjögren's syndrome, a serum hyperamylasemia, due to both P- and S-type isoamylases (Tsianos et al. 1984). These increases in serum amylase were modest and were about evenly distributed between the two isoenzymes. None of these individuals had classical attacks of pancreatitis, or gallbladder disease for at least two months prior to the blood collection, were known to abuse alcohol, or received prednisone. This hyperamylasemia may reflect a subclinical, inflammatory process of the pancreas.

In 1977, Ludwig et al. (1977) found antibodies to pancreatic duct cells in the sera of patients with SS. This information, in addition to the pathologic findings in the pancreas (monocellular infiltrate) point to an autoimmune mechanism for the pancreatic involvement.

Furthermore, four cases of a complex syndrome with coexisted sclerosing cholangitis, chronic pancreatitis, and SS have been reported (Waldram et al. 1975; Montefusco et al. 1984). Interestingly, two of the four patients were siblings. This has been tentatively attributed to an altered immunologic response of lymphocytes to HLA-defined antigens resulting in eventual fibrosis of the salivary and pancreatic glands, as well as of the bile ducts (Montefusco et al. 1984).

Liver

The association of chronic liver disease (CLD) and SS has been known for many years. Liver abnormalities have included hepatomegaly from 25% to 58% of patients (Christianson 1954; Hradsky et al. 1967), and some changes in the liver "function" test, such as increase of alkaline phosphatase (Webb et al. 1975; Voigel et al. 1980) in 25% to 33%, gamma GT in 33% (Hradsky et al. 1976), and increase of BSP retention in 14% of these individuals (Hradsky et al. 1967). Antimitochondrial antibodies also have been found in more patients with SS (6 to 11%) than other collagen diseases, i.e., rheumatoid arthritis (1 to 3%) (Webb et al. 1975; Whaley et al. 1970). The co-existence of some forms of liver disease and "sicca complex" (xerostomia, keratoconjunctivitis sicca) was first suggested by Christianson in 1954. He reported the association between corneal changes and abnormal liver tests in a patient with acute hepatitis. McLenachan, in 1956, collected 45 cases of SS, most of whom had evidence of liver dysfunction, i.e. hepatomegaly, splenomegaly and a marked rise of gamma globulin. Vanselaw et al. (1963) detected hepatomegaly in 18% of their patients with SS. In 1970, Golding et al. studied a total of 63 patients with liver disease for the presence of the components of SS. The "sicca complex" was detected in 42% of patients with chronic active hepatitis (CAH), 72% of patients with primary biliary cirrhosis (PBC) and 38% of those who had cryptogenic cirrhosis. No evidence of SS was found in 7 patients with alcoholic cirrhosis. The findings suggest that "sicca complex" and autoimmune liver disease may be part of a systemic disorder in which immunological mechanisms are involved. It is now known that PBC is the most common autoimmune disorder related to Sjögren's Syndrome (Bodenheimer, Shaffner 1979). The reported incidence of SS in a large series of patients with PBC varies between 69 and 81%. Recently, Epstein et al. (1980) suggested that PBC is part of a disease complex characterized by dry eyes, dry mouth and pancreatic hyposecretion. "It is a dry gland syndrome" resulting from damage to ductular epithelium (Epstein et al. 1980). Alarcon-Segovia et al. (1973) investigated prospectively with a complete battery of tests the "sicca component" of SS in 14 consecutive patients with biopsy-proved PBC. They found that all the patients with PBC had at least one ocular or salivary feature of SS, but none of them had a positive assay for rheumatoid factor. The presence or degree of sicca components of SS did not correlate with the duration or the degree of liver disease, the presence of autoantibodies or the levels of immunoglobulins.

The association among SS, collagen disease, PBC, atrophic gastritis, etc., have been important factors suggesting that SS is an autoimmune disease. Recently, Penner and Reichlin (1982) described a patient with PBC and SS who also had evidence of circulating and tissue deposited Ro/anti Ro immune complexes. Finally, Manthorpe et al. (1979) have found the presence of liver-cell membrane antibody (LMA) in 20% of patients who have SS. Other forms of liver disease associated with SS (Shearn 1977) have been reported in the literature. Some of these have been induced, by foreign substances (Okano et al. 1984) or drugs (Rex et al. 1983; Fink et al. 1979).

Autoimmune disease has been precipitated by the injection of foreign substances like silicone and parafin which may act as adjuvants (Okano et al. 1984). In 1984 Okano et al. reported a patient who developed scleroderma, PBC and SS after silicone injections. They speculated that these conditions may represent a "human adjuvant disease". Thiabendazole (Mintezol, Merck, Sharp and Dome) is a widely prescribed, relatively safe antinematodal agent, which induces minor side effects but serious toxocity is rare (Robinson et al. 1969). There are, however, six cases of intrahepatic cholestasis reported in the literature in whom thiabendazole has been implicated as the offending agent (Rex et al. 1983; Fink et al. 1979; Jalota, Freston 1974). Three of these also had features of "sicca complex". The critical course of thiabendazole-induced jaundice is, in general, self-limited but in one of the reported cases, illness lasted seven months.

The information, previously reviewed, indicates that chronic liver disease (CLD), particularly PBC, is frequently seen in patients with either "sicca complex" or SS. Therefore, such patients should be evaluated using biochemical and serological markers of hepatic dysfunction, mainly alkaline phosphatase and antimitochondrial antibodies. If alkaline phosphatase is higher than normal and antimitochondrial antibodies are positive, early PBC is likely and might be documented by liver biopsy. If antimitochondrial antibodies are negative in the presence of high alkaline phosphatase, sclerosing cholangitis is a possibility and might be diagnosed by endoscopic retrograde cholangiography.

Summary

Sjögren's syndrome is a chronic, inflammatory, systemic autoimmune disease which may be associated with pathological changes and/or altered function of the esophagus, stomach, small intestine, pancreas and liver. It is presumed that the pathophysiological derangements in these organs are also due to an altered immune status, although the precise mechanism(s) is unknown. In the interim, awareness of this association is needed and treatment is directed to the functional support of these organs.

References

1. Alarcon-Segovia D, Diaz-Jovanen, Fishbein E (1973) Features of Sjögren's syndrome in primary biliary cirrhosis. Ann Int Med 79: 31-36
2. Alarcon-Sevogia D, Gonzalez-Jimenez Y, Garza LR, et al (1971) Radioisotopic evaluation of salivary gland dysfunction in Sjögren's syndrome. Am J Roentgenol Radium Ther Nucl Med 112: 373-379
3. Alarcon-Segovia D, Ibanez G, Valazquez-Forero F, Hernandez-Ortiz J, Gonzalez-Jimenez Y (1974) Sjögren's syndrome in systemic lupus erythematosus. Ann Int Med 81: 577-583
4. Bodenheimer HC, Shaffner F (1979) Primary biliary cirrhosis and the immune system. Am J Gastro 72: 285-296
5. Buchanan WW, Cox AG, Harden RMcG, Glen AIM, Anderson JR, Gray KG (1966) Gastric studies in Sjögren's syndrome. Gut 7: 351-354
6. Cardell BS, Curling KJ (1954) Observation on the pathology of Sjögren's syndrome. J Pathol Bact 68: 137-146
7. Chisholm DM, Mason DK (1968) Labial salivary gland biopsy in Sjögren's disease. J Clin Pathol 21: 656-660
8. Christiansson J (1954) Corneal changes in a case of hepatitis. Acta Ophthalmol 32: 161-164
9. Crowe JP, Christensen E, Butler J, Wheeler P, Doniach D, Keenan J, Williams R (1980) Primary

biliary cirrhosis: the prevalence of hypothyroidism and its relationship to thyroid autoantibodies and sicca syndrome. Gastroenterology 78: 1437-1441
10. Dreiling DA, Soto JM (1976) The pancreatic involvement in disseminated "collagen" disorders. Studies of pancreatic secretion in patients with scleroderma and Sjögren's "disease". Am J Gastroenterol 66: 546-553
11. Elder JB, Ganguli PC, Gillespie IE, et al (1975) Effect of urogastrone on gastric acid secretion and plasma gastrin levels in normal subjects. Gut 16: 887-893
12. Epstein O, Thomas HC, Sherlock S (1980) Primary biliary cirrhosis is a dry gland syndrome with features of chronic graft-versus-host disease. Lancet 1 (2): 1166-1168
13. Fenster LF, Buchanan WW, Laster L, Bunim JJ (1964) Studies of pancreatic function in Sjögren's syndrome. Ann Int Med 61: 498-507
14. Fink AI, MacKay CJ, Cutler SS (1979) Sicca complex and cholangiostatic jaundice in two members of a family probably caused by thiabendazole. Ophthalmology 86: 1892-1896
15. Gainey R, Rooney PJ, Alspaugh M (1985) Sjögren's syndrome and Crohn's disease. Clin Exp Rheum 3: 67-69
16. Gobelet C, Gerster JC, Rappoport G, Hiroz CA, Maeder E (1983) A controlled study of the exocrine pancratic function in Sjögren's syndrome and rheumatoid arthritis. Clin Rheum 2: 139-143
17. Golding PL, Brown R, Mason AMS, Taylor E (1970) "Sicca complex" in liver disease. Br Med J 4: 340-342
18. Henderson JW (1950) Keratoconjunctivitis sicca. A review with a survey of 121 additional cases. Amer J Ophthalmol 33: 197-203
19. Hradsky, Bartos V, Keller O (1967) Pancreatic function in Sjögren's syndrome. Gastroenterologica 108: 252-260
20. Hradsky M, Hybasek I, Cernoch V, Sazmova V, Juran J (1967) Oesophageal abnormalities in Sjögren's syndrome. Scand J Gastroenterol 2: 200-203
21. Jalota R, Freston JW (1974) Severe intrahepatic cholestasis due to thiabendazole. Am J Trop Med Hyg 23: 676-678
22. Kauntiz JD, Sleisenger MH (1983) Effects of systemic and extraintestinal disease on the gut. In: Sleisenger MH, Fordtran JS (eds) Gastrointestinal Disease, 3rd edn. WB Saunders Company, Philadelphia, p 369-404
23. Kilpi A, Bergroth V, Konttinen YT, Maury CPJ, Reitamo S, Wegelius O (1983) Lymphocyte infiltrations of the gastric mucosa in Sjögren's syndrome. Arthritis Rheum 26: 1196-1200
24. Konturek SJ, Radecki T, Brzozowski T et al (1981) Gastric cytoprotection by epidermal growth factor: role of endogenous prostaglandins and DNA synthesis. Gastroenterology 81: 438-443
25. Kraft SC, Kirsner JB (1985) Immunology in Gastroenterology. In: Berk JE, Haubrich WS, Kalser MH, Roth JLA, Schaffner F (eds) Bockus Gastroenterology, 4th edn WB Saunders Company, Philadelphia, p 4487-4524
26. Lancaster-Smith MJ, Strickland ID (1971) Autoantibodies in adult coeliac. Lancet i: 1244-1247
27. Ludwig H, Schernthaner G, Scherak O, Kolarz G (1977) Antibodies to pancreatic duct cells in Sjögren's syndrome and rheumatoid arthritis. Gut 18: 311-315
28. Machin ND, Chard MD, Paice EW (1984) Serum angiotensin converting enzyme in Sjögren's syndrome. A case report and study of 21 further cases. Postgrad Med J 60: 270-271
29. MacLaurin BP, Matthews N, Kilpatrick JA (1972) Coeliac disease associated with auto-immune thyroiditis, Sjögren's syndrome and a lymphocytotoxic serum factor. Aust NZ J Med 4: 405-411
30. Manthrope R, Permin H, Tage-Jensen U (1979) Auto antibodies in Sjögren's syndrome with special reference to liver-cell membrane antibody (LMA). Scand J Rheumatol 8: 168-172
31. Maury CPJ, Rasanen V, Teppo A-M, Helve T, Wegelius O (1982) Serum pepsinogen I in rheumatic diseases: reduced levels of Sjögren's syndrome. Arthritis Rheum 25: 1059-1063
32. Maury CPJ, Tornroth T, Teppo A-M (1985) Atrophic gastritis in Sjögren's syndrome. Morphologic, biochemical and immunologic findings. Arthritis Rheum 28: 388-349
33. McLenachan J (1956) New aspects of the aetiology of Sjögren's syndrome. Trans Ophthalmol Soc UK 76: 413-426
34. Montefusco PP, Geiss AC et al (1984) Sclerosing cholangitis, chronic pancreatitis, and Sjögren's syndrome: A syndrome complex. Am J Surg 147: 822-826
35. Moutsopoulos HM et al (1980) Sjögren's yndrome (sicca syndrome) Current issues. Ann Int Med 92: 212-226

36. Moutsopoulos HM, Hooks JJ, Chan CC, Dalavanga YA, Skopouli FN, Dietrick B (1986) HLA-DR expression by labial salivary gland tissues in Sjögren's syndrome. Ann Rheum Dis (in press)
37. Mulders AV, Van Den Bergh H, Dequeker J, Peeters TL, Vantrappen G (1984) Hypergastrinemia in rheumatoid arthritis related to Sjögren's syndrome. Letter to the Editor. J Rheumatol 11: 246-247
38. Okano Y, Nishikai M, Sato A (1984) Scleroderma, primary biliary cirrhosis and Sjögren's syndrome after cosmetic breast augmentation with silicone injection: a case report of possible human adjuvant disease. Ann Rheum Dis 43: 520-522
39. Parke AL, Fagan EA, Chadwick VS, Hughes GRV (1984) Coelic disease and rheumatoid arthritis. Ann Rheum Dis 43: 378-380
40. Penner E, Reichlin M (1982) Primary biliary cirrhosis associated with Sjögren's syndrome: evidence for circulation and tissue: deposited RO/anti RO immune complexes. Arth Rheumatism 25: 1250-1253
41. Pittman FE, Holub DA (1965) Sjögren's syndrome and adult celiac disease. Gastroenterology 48: 869-876, 1965
42. Raffle RB (1950) Sjögren's disease associated with a nutritional deficiency syndrome. Brit Med J 1: 1470-1472
43. Ramirez-Mata M, Pena-Ancira FF, Alarcon-Segovia D (1976) Abnormal esophageal motility in primary Sjögren's syndrome. J Rheumatol 3: 63-69
44. Rappaport PM (1963) Acinar units and the pathophysiology of the liver. In: Roulier CH (ed) The Liver, Morphology, Biochemistry, Physiology. Academic Press, New York, p 265-328
45. Rex D, Lumeng L, Eble J, Rex L (1983) Intrahepatic cholestasis and sicca complex after thiabendazole. Report a case and review of the literature. Gastroenterology 85: 718-721
46. Robinson HJ, Silber RH, Graessle OE (1969) Thiabendazole: toxicological, pharmacological and antifungal properties. Tex Rep Biol Med 27: 537-560
47. Rutan G, Martinez AJ, Fieshko JT, Van Thiel DH (1986) Primary biliary cirrhosis, Sjögren's syndrome and transverse myelitis. Gastroenterology 90: 206-210
48. Shearn MA (1977) Sjögren's syndrome. Med Clin No Amer 61: 271-282
49. Simila S, Kokkonen J, Kaski M (1978) Achalasia sicca-juvenile Sjögren's syndrome with achalasia and gastric hyposcretion. Eur J Pediatr 129: 175-181
50. Sjögren I, Wengle B, Korsgren M (1979) Primary sclerosing cholangitis associated with fibrosis of the submandibular glands in the pancreas. Acta Med Scand 205: 139-141
51. Tsianos EB, Chiras CD, Drosos AA, Moutsopoulos HM (1985) Oesophageal dysfunction in patients with primary Sjögren's syndrome. Ann Rheum Dis 44: 610-613
52. Tsianos EB, Tzioufas AG, Kita MD, Tsolas O, Moutsopoulos HM (1984) Serum isoamylases in patients with autoimmune rheumatic diseases. Clin Exper Rheumatol 2: 235-238
53. Vanselaw NA, Dodson VN, Angell DC, Duff IF (1963) A clinical study of Sjögren's syndrome. Ann Int Med 58: 124-135
54. Voigel C, Wittenborg A, Reichart P (1980) The involvement of the liver in Sjögren's syndrome. J Oral Surg 50: 26-29
55. Von Jebavy M, Hradsky M, Herout V (1961) Gastric biopsy in patients with Sjögren's syndrome. Zschr Med Lab Diagn 16: 930-940
56. Waldram R, Kopelman H, Tsantoulas D, Williams R (1975) Chronic pancreatitis, sclerosing-cholangitis and sicca complex in two siblings. Lancet 1: 550-552
57. Webb J, Whaley K, MacSween R, et al (1975) Liver disease in rheumatoid arthritis and Sjögren's syndrome: prospective study using biochemical and serological markers of hepatic dysfunction. Ann Rheum Dis 34: 70-81
58. Weissmann G (1958) Sjögren's syndrome. Review of the literature and report of a case with achalasia of the esophagus. Am J Med 24: 475-481
59. Whaley K, Williamson J, Chisholm DM, et al (1973) Sjögren's. I. Sicca components. Q J Med 42: 279-304
60. Whaley K, Williamson J, Dick WC, et al (1970) Liver disease in Sjögren's syndrome and rheumatoid arthritis. Lancet 1: 861-863

5. Renal Disease with Sjögren's Syndrome

S. S. Kassan and N. Talal

Introduction

Sjögren's syndrome (SS) is a systemic lymphoproliferative and autoimmune disease whose extraglandular manifestations may include focal or diffuse lymphocytic and plasma cell infiltration of almost any organ [1]. Extraglandular lymphoid infiltrates may be found in lung [12], liver [8], muscle [24], skin [1], and kidney [29]. The degree of infiltration as well as individual cell characteristics define whether the process becomes clinically significant and is judged relatively benign or malignant [2].

The renal involvement in primary SS, well documented in the literature [3, 10, 21, 22, 29], may be overt or latent [22] and consists primarily of interstitial disease with interstitial infiltration by lymphocytes, tubular atrophy and fibrosis [29]. The clinical presentation may be hyposthenuria [22, 29], overt or latent distal renal tubular acidosis (RTA) (Type I) [22] and less commonly, the Fanconi syndrome [21] with proximal RTA (Type II). Other less common forms of renal involvement include immune complex glomerulonephritis [6] often associated with mixed cryoglobulinemia [9, 18]. In patients with secondary SS, renal disease may develop as a result of the underlying associated connective tissue disease (e.g. systemic lupus erythematosus and scleroderma) and is typical of that disease process [3, 25].

Clinical and Histologic Studies

Interstitial Nephritis

Interstitial nephritis is the most common renal lesion reported in SS. Many of the patients manifest clinical syndromes of hyposthenuria, renal tubular acidosis (Type I) (distal) and uncommonly the Fanconi syndrome. Often, coexistant hypergammaglobulinemia and/or dysproteinemias have been noted in these patients.

Renal tubular acidosis is characterized by hyperchloremic acidosis and an inability to excrete a highly acid urine. The impaired acid excretion is out of proportion to a reduction of glomerular filtration rate [22]. Proximal RTA (Type II) is characterized by an abnormality in resorption of bicarbonate by the proximal nephron; hydrogen ion transport by the distal nephron is normal [7]. Distal RTA (Type I) results from an abnormality of hydrogen ion transport at the distal nephron site. Severe potassium depletion and acidosis is often present in the untreated patient. Other common clinical findings in distal RTA include an inability to reduce the urine pH below 5.5, nephrocalcinosis, renal stones, and low urinary citrate concentrations.

Various hypergammaglobulinemic states have been associated with distal RTA and include SS [16], SLE [28], primary biliary cirrhosis [8], chronic active hepatitis [8], fibrosing alveolitis [15], autoimmune thyroid disease [14], hypergammaglobulinemic purpura [5], idiopathic hypergammaglobulinemia [19] and cryoglobulinemia [13]. SS, however, has been present in over half of the reported cases of overt or latent RTA associated with hyperglobulinemia [26]. Other cases are reported in disease states that often co-exist with SS as noted above.

RTA may be present in 22% [27] to 30% [22] of SS patients. Many of the cases have been latent and detected only by means of an acid loading test performed in SS patients lacking overt evidence of acid-base disturbances. In one study [22], three of ten patients tested by ammonium chloride loading showed definite impairment in acidification of urine with urinary pH values all 5.45 or higher. Talal et al [27] noted impairment of urinary acidification overtly in three SS patients and subclinically in two of nine SS patients without evidence for acid-base abnormalities.

The tubular dysfunction may also become manifest as an abnormality in the urine concentrating mechanism [7]. Nephrogenic diabetes insipidus was reported in ten of 62 SS patients by Block et al [3]. It is unclear, however, whether this is a result of RTA indirectly (i.e., the effect of hypokalemia on tubular function) or a direct result of the interstitial inflammatory process [7]. Proximal RTA (Type II) with or without manifestations of the Fanconi syndrome (i.e., glycosuria, aminoaciduria, phosphaturia and uricosuria) have been reported less frequently in SS. In those reported with Fanconi's syndrome [21], extensive pathologic changes including marked tubular atrophy and fibrosis were noted in the kidneys.

The pathophysiology for the development of RTA has been debated in the literature [17, 23, 26]. A causal effect of hyperglobulinemia has been proposed as one reason for the development of RTA in many patients with SS and/or related diseases. Two hypotheses have been presented in favor of this argument [23]. The first argues that filtered immunoglobulin causes renal tubular dysfunction when it reaches the renal tubule. This hypothesis is countered by the data of Shioji et al. [20, 23] in patients with SS and RTA. They found the renal IgG clearance to be increased and the electrophoretic appearance of urinary proteins to show a "tubular pattern". This pattern is characterized by a small albumin fraction of less than 20% of total urinary proteins, 2 or 3 distinct bands in the region and a post-gamma protein. In addition, proteinuria disappeared completely when the metabolic acidosis and hypokalemia were corrected by the use of alkalinizing agents. The proteinuria returned when treatment was withheld and metabolic acidosis and hypokalemia worsened [20]. Renal tubular dysfunction remained unchanged despite successful treatment of the proteinuria. Thus, it was argued that tubular proteinuria may be related to the reversible defect in renal tubular resorption of proteins mediated by metabolic acidosis and/or hypokalemia.

This study also found no significant difference in degree of hypergammaglobulinemia or degree of increase in serum immunoglobulins between cases of SS with RTA and those without RTA. Thus, by this data, this "tubular pattern" of proteinuria seemed to be the result of RTA rather than its cause.

The second hypothesis for the pathogenesis of RTA in patients with hypergammaglobulinemia is based on disturbances in the peritubular circulation. Histologic studies [23] in patients with SS and RTA have revealed no significant vascular abnormalities in renal biopsy specimens. The possibility that elevated serum viscosity may alter peritubular blood flow is also possible in hypergammaglobulinemic states. However, in one of four cases of SS with RTA reported by Shioji et al. [23], no evidence for hypergammaglobulinemia was present. Also, other studies [22, 28] have failed to show a correlation between the level of serum gamma globulin elevation and degree of alteration of acid excretion. Thus, from the foregoing arguments, it seems unlikely that hypergammaglobulinemia or its concommitant increase in blood viscosity is the major cause for the development of RTA in SS and/or related disorders.

Alternatively, the frequently observed renal tubular impairment in SS may be immunologically mediated [26]. In these patients, renal histologic changes reveal lymphocytic and mononuclear cell interstitial infiltrates resembling the infiltrates seen in the exocrine glands. It was postulated that these changes were part of the characteristic multiple organ/extraglandular involvement of SS-all potentially related to a disturbed immunoregulatory system. Other studies [19, 23, 27, 30] have also suggested the concept that lymphocytic and plasma cell infiltrates surrounding renal tubules are associated with and may cause a renal tubular defect.

Sjioji et al. [23] identified two groups of patients with SS, four with renal tubular acidosis (Group I) and ten without this complication (Group II). No differences were noted between the two groups with respect to patient age, duration of disease, degree of hypergammaglobulinemia or serological reactivity. Renal biopsies demonstrated interstitial lymphocytic infiltrates in three of four Group I patients and no lymphocytic infiltration in renal biopsy specimens from four of the Group II patients despite the presence of hypergammaglobulinemia in both groups.

In the study of Pasternack and Linder [19], similar renal histologic findings were noted in four patients. In addition, C3 and immunoglobulin were identified by immunofluorescence techniques in renal tubular cells. Talal et al. [27] reported renal biopsies in patients with primary SS where all of these patients exhibited renal acidification defects. Interstitial infiltrates were noted in all and a focal glomerulonephritis was found in one patient. Using an anti-human IgG antiserum, two patients showed an unusual granular fluorescence of the cytoplasm in tubular epithelial cells.

Gerhardt et al. [6] showed immunofluorescence with IgG antiserum in the renal interstitial infiltrate in one patient with SS. Winer et al. [30] demonstrated in one patient focal deposits composed of IgG and C3 in the renal tubular basement membrane with interstitial inflammation. Glomeruli contained no such deposits in this patient. They proposed that local or in situ formation of immune complexes may be one of the mechanisms for the development of tubulointestinal disease in SS. Thus, support for an immune pathogenesis for the interstitial nephritis and RTA in SS appears to be the presence of immunocompetent cells in the interstitium and the finding of immunoglobulin and complement in the tubular cell cytoplasm and/or in the interstitial cells of patients with SS.

Kaltreider and Talal [11] re-evaluated three previously reported patients with SS and related diseases. Their findings of the inconsistent contribution of various factors to the development of impaired renal acidification (RTA) support the complexity of the pathogenesis of RTA. In some of their patients, elevated gamma globulin, interstitial cellular infiltration, auto-antibodies, and vasculitis may have played a role, but these findings proved to be present in some and not in others, which underscores the multifactorial nature of this abnormality.

The role of analgesic usage in SS has been addressed as possibly altering tubular function and contributing to the development of the interstitial nephritis seen in these patients. However, the drug histories of SS patients in one study [22] showed only inconsistent or no analgesic use among SS patients found to have renal involvement.

In some patients, SS symptoms may be subclinical or may post-date the onset of RTA. In the study by Tu et al. [29], three patients volunteered sicca symptoms only after careful questioning and in two patients, renal lesions actually preceded the onset of clinical disease. This finding makes it mandatory that evidence for SS be sought in every patient with unexplained RTA, proteinuria and/or interstitial nephritis.

Findings other than RTA resulting from interstitial nephritis in SS may also be seen. These changes include necrosis of renal tubules with resultant hyalinization of glomeruli and renal insufficiency [6]. Others [29, 30] have reported interstitial inflammatory infiltrates with renal insufficiency and no evidence of RTA.

Urinary findings have been unimpressive in reports of patients with SS and interstitial nephritis [11, 2, 29]. Most commonly, findings consist of mild proteinuria, a few leukocytes and occasional granular or hyaline casts. Mild azotemia is also reported and seems to correspond with the severity of the interstitial disease [29].

Immune Complex Glomerulonephritis

Glomerulonephritis in SS has been described in a limited number of case reports [18, 29]. Various modes of pathogenesis have been proposed in these cases where glomerulonephritis has been associated with immune complex deposition, cryoglobulinemia and macroglobulinemia. Both membranous, membranoproliferative and proliferative glomerulonephritis have been recognized in these SS patients.

In the study by Moutsopoulos, et al. [18], three cases of glomerulonephritis were reported where on renal biopsy, two had membranoproliferative glomerulonephritis and one had membranous glomerulonephritis. In two cases, interstitial infiltrative changes were also noted. All three patients had considerable amounts of immune complexes in their serum detected by Clq binding at the time when glomerulonephritis was diagnosed. The levels of immune complexes decreased somewhat in association with treatment and subsequent improvement in renal function. In two of three patients, mixed cryoglobulins were detected. In one patient, this cryoglobulinemia was also associated with a low C3 level. All three patients manifested clinical symptoms of profound extraglandular involvement with vasculitic skin lesions and/or purpura, marked hypertension, and urinary findings of hematuria and proteinuria. In addition, high titers of rheumatoid factors and moderate ANA titers were noted in all patients.

Proliferative glomerulonephritis has been described in cases of mixed cryoglobulinemia in SS [9, 16] where the clinical syndrome is often similar to that described by Meltzer et al. [16]. Here, the clinical picture may be associated with vasculitis, epistaxis, myocarditis, lymphadenopathy, hepatosplenomegaly, Raynaud's phenomenon and both peripheral and central nervous system manifestations. In these cases, circulating high molecular weight (22S) complexes have been found [9]. The cryoglobulins are most often mixed and some cases of mixed cryoglobulins with one monoclonal component have been seen [4]. Most of these patients have hypocomplementemia and local deposition of IgG, IgM and complement at sites of tissue injury [4, 16].

The pathophysiology of immune complex glomerulonephritis in SS is not fully understood. Perhaps an increased level of immune complexes can overwhelm the clearance mechanisms of the glomerular mesangium and/or the reticuloendothelial system [18]. Alternatively, other unknown properties of immune complexes may allow or enhance local deposition in glomeruli or elsewhere resulting in tissue injury [9].

The pathogenic role of cryoglobulins also remains unclear. It is possible that their effect is similar to that of immune complexes whose deposition at various sites results in the fixation of complement and tissue injury.

References

1. Alexander EL, Arnett FC, Provost TT, Stevens MB (1983) Sjögren's syndrome: association of anti-Ro (SSA) antibodies with vasculitis, hematologic abnormalities and serologic hyperreactivity. Ann Intern Med 98: 155-159
2. Anderson LG, Talal N (1972) The spectrum of benign to malignant lymphoproliferation in Sjögren's syndrome. Clin Exp Immunol 10: 199-219
3. Bloch KH, Buchanan WW, Wohl MJ, Bunim JJ (1965) Sjögren's syndrome. A clinical, pathological, and serological study of sixty-two cases. Medicine 44: 198-231
4. Brouet JC, Clauvel JP, Danon F, Klein M, Seligmann M (1974) Biological and clinical significance of cryoglobulins: a report of 86 cases. Am J Med 57: 775-783
5. Cohen A, Way BJ (1962) The association of renal tubular acidosis with hyperglobulinemic purpura. Australas Ann Med 11: 189-194
6. Gerhardt RE, Loebl DH, Rao RN (1978) Interstitial immunofluorescence in nephritis of Sjögren's syndrome. Clin Nephr 10 (5): 201-207
7. Glassock RJ, Feinstein EE, Tannen R, Blau R, Koss M (1984) Metabolic acidosis in a young woman. Am J Nephrol 4: 58-65
8. Golding PL, Smith M, Williams R (1973) Multisystem involvement in chronic liver disease. Studies on the incidence and pathogenesis. Am J Med 55: 772-782
9. Hardin JA (1975) Case records of the Massachusetts General Hospital 2292: 1285-1290
10. Kahn M, Merritt AD, Wohl MJ, Orloff J (1962) Renal concentrating defect in Sjögren's syndrome. Ann Intern Med 56: 883-895
11. Kaltreider HB, Talal N (1969) Impaired renal acidification in Sjögren's syndrome and related disorders. Arthritis Rheum 12 (5): 538-541
12. Karlish AJ (1969) Lung changes in Sjögren's Syndrome. Proc R Soc Med 62: 1042-1043
13. Lo Spalluto J, Dorward B, Miller W Jr, Ziff M (1962) Cryoglobulinemia based on interaction between a gamma macroglobulin and 7s gamma globulin. Ann J Med 32: 142-147
14. Mason AMS, Golding PL (1970) Renal tubular acidosis and autoimmune thyroid disease. Lancet ii: 1104-1107
15. Mason AMS, McIllmuray MD, Golding PL, Hughes DTD (1970) Fibrosing alveolitis associated with renal tubular acidosis. Br Med J iv: 596-599
16. Meltzer M, Franklin EC, Ellias K, McCluskey RT, Cooper N (1966) Cryoglobulinemia. A clinical and laboratory study. II cryoglobulins with rheumatoid factor activity. Am J Med 40: 837-856
17. McCurdy DK, Cornwell GG III, DePratti VJ (1967) Hyperglobulinemic renal tubular acidosis. Report of two cases. Ann Intern Med 67: 110-117
18. Moutsopoulos HM, Balow JE, Cawley TJ, Stahl NI, Autonovych TT, Chused TM (1978) Immune complex glomerulonephritis in sicca syndrome. Am J Med 64: 955-960

19. Pasternack A, Linder E (1970) Renal tubular acidosis. An immunopathological study on four patients. Clin Exp Immunol 7: 115-123
20. Saito H, Furuyama T, Shioji, Onodera S, Sasaki Y, Ito H: Polyacrylamide gel electrophoretic and immunochemical studies on urinary proteins in Sjögren's syndrome with special reference to tubular proteinuria. Tohoku J Exp Med 101: 205-214
21. Shearn M, Tu W (1965) Nephrogenic diabetes insipidus and other defects of renal tubular function in Sjögren's syndrome. Am J Med 39: 312-318
22. Shearn MA, Tu WH (1968) Latent renal tubular acidosis in Sjögren's syndrome. Ann Rheum Dis 27: 27-32
23. Shioji R, Furuyama T, Onodera S, Saito H, Ito H, Sasaki Y (1970) Sjögren's syndrome and renal tubular acidosis. Am J Med 456-463
24. Silberberg DH, Drachman DA (1962) Late-life myopathy occurring with Sjögren's syndrome. Arch Neurol 6: 428-438
25. Sobel JD, Taylor Z, Alroy G, Lichtig C, Valero A (1977) Systemic lupus erythematosus, Sjögren's syndrome and glomerular nephritis. Postgrad Med J 53: 97-101
26. Talal N (1971) Sjögren's syndrome, lymphoproliferation and renal tubular acidosis. Ann Intern Med 74: 633-634
27. Talal N, Zisman E, Schur P (1968) Renal tubular acidosis, glomerulonephritis and immunologic factors in Sjögren's syndrome. Arthritis Rheum 11 (6): 774-786
28. Tu W, Shearn MA (1967) Systemic lupus erythematosus and latent tubular dysfunction. Ann Intern Med 67: 100-108
29. Tu WH, Shearn MA, Lee JC, Hopper (1968) Interstitial nephritis in Sjögren's syndrome. Ann Inter Med 69 (6): 1163-1170
30. Winer RL, Cohen AH, Sawhney AS, Gorman JT (1977) Sjögren's syndrome with immune-complex tubulointerstitial renal disease. Clin Immunol Immunopathol 8: 494-503

6. Inflammatory Vascular Disease in Sjögren's Syndrome

E. L. ALEXANDER

Introduction

Inflammatory vascular disease (i.e. vasculitis) as a complication of primary Sjögren's syndrome is well documented, but generally is incorrectly considered to be a benign condition which predominantly affects only the skin. There is a growing awareness, however, that primary Sjögren's syndrome patients with peripheral (i.e., involving the skin, peripheral nerve, or muscle) inflammatory vascular disease may have systemic complications. Peripheral inflammatory vascular disease occurs in 20 to 30% of patients with primary Sjögren's syndrome (Bloch 1965; Mason 1973; Bunim 1963; Alexander 1983a; Molina 1985a; Molina 1985b).

Historically, cutaneous vasculitis is the most frequently recognized manifestation of inflammatory vascular disease in primary Sjögren's syndrome. Classically, purpuric or petechial lesions, usually involving the lower extremities, have been observed (Strauss 1959; Kyle 1970). Clinically these lesions are indistinguishable from those described by Waldenstrom as benign hyperglobulinemic purpura (Waldenstrom 1943). The association of primary Sjögren's syndrome with hyperglobulinemic purpura is well established (Strauss 1959; Kyle 1970). Recently, it has been appreciated that these purpuric lesions, as well as other cutaneous manifestations of vasculitis, may herald systemic disease in Sjögren's syndrome (Alexander 1983c; Molina 1985).

Our laboratory has been studying the immunopathogenesis of inflammatory vascular disease in primary Sjögren's syndrome. We have elected to study inflammatory vascular disease using primary Sjögren's syndrome as a prototype of autoimmune rheumatic disorders for several reasons. First, Sjögren's syndrome is a very common connective tissue disorder. Second, peripheral inflammatory vascular disease is sufficiently common that serum and biopsy samples can be obtained for analysis. Third, the majority of primary Sjögren's syndrome patients, in general, and those with isolated cutaneous vasculitis, in particular, usually have not been treated with immunosuppressive therapy. Thus, the natural history of peripheral vasculitis and the possible development of systemic complications can be observed. Finally, from available evidence it is highly likely that the immunopathologic mechanisms operative in vascular inflammation in Sjögren's syndrome are applicable to vasculitis in other clinical settings.

Our observations on inflammatory vascular disease primarily have focused on patients with well documented primary Sjögren's syndrome in whom the presence of a second connective tissue disorder has been rigorously excluded (see Chapter II. B.2). Briefly, patients we characterize as having primary Sjögren's syndrome, in addition to meeting rigorous clinical and laboratory criteria for Sjögren's syndrome, do not have the following features characteristic of systemic lupus erythematosus: malar rash, discoid, subacute cutaneous or solar induced skin lesions, polyserositis, glomerulonephritis, or antibodies to double stranded DNA, nRNP, or Sm. We have observed, however, a subgroup of Sjögren's syndrome patients who at varying times in their clinical courses have developed cutaneous manifestations of lupus erythematosus. The clinical, serologic, and immunogenetic features of these unique patients are presented in Chapter III. 4.

This chapter will outline the clinical manifestations of the spectrum of inflammatory vascular disease seen in Sjögren's syndrome. It will emphasize that peripheral, particularly cutaneous, vasculitis may identify those Sjögren's syndrome patients at risk for the development of systemic disease, especially involving the nervous system. Two distinct histopathologic types or inflammatory vascular disease will be described [i.e. neutrophilic inflammatory vascular disease (NIVD) and mononuclear inflammatory vascular disease (MIVD)]. Evidence will be presented that each of the two histopathologic types of inflammatory vascular disease observed in Sjögren's syndrome can cause frank vessel damage and give rise to end-organ dysfunction. The distinct serologic correlates of these two types of vasculitis will be presented. Our observations on vascular inflammation in an autoimmune murine model of connective tissue disease, with features of Sjögren's syndrome, will be discussed. Based on these observations in human patients with Sjögren's syndrome and an autoimmune murine model, an hypothesis of the immunopathogenesis of inflammatory vascular disease in Sjögren's syndrome will be presented.

Clinical Documentation of Inflammatory Vascular Disease

Skin

The skin is the most common target organ for the expression of peripheral inflammatory vascular disease in Sjögren's syndrome (Alexander 1983c; Molina 1985b). The cutaneous manifestations of vasculitis may be subtle and, in our experience, often have been overlooked. The cutaneous features of vasculitis in a group of

Table 1. Cutaneous manifestations in primary Sjögren's syndrome patients with inflammatory vascular disease of two histopathologic types (*NIVD* neutrophilic inflammatory vascular disease, *MIVD* mononuclear inflammatory vascular disease) (Molina 1985a)

Cutaneous manifestations	No. (Percent)		
	NIVD (n=25)	MIVD (n=16)	Total (n=41)
Purpura	12 (48)	4 (25)	16 (39)
Urticaria	7 (28)	4 (25)	11 (27)
Erythematous lesions	4 (16)	7 (44)	11 (27)
Subcutaneous nodules	2 (8)	1 (6)	3 (7)

45 patients with Sjögren's syndrome (35 with primary and 10 with secondary) and biopsy documented peripheral inflammatory vascular disease are presented in Table 1 (Molina 1985b).

The most common cutaneous vasculitic manifestations of Sjögren's syndrome are palpable purpura and petechial lesions, generally involving the lower extremities (Fig. 1). These lesions may be aggrevated by dependency and activity. The lesions frequently are asymptomatic. The development of lesions is episodic and they tend to occur in showers or crops. The lesions may leave residual hyperpigmentation (secondary to hemosiderin deposition) which may not be recognized as the sequelae of previous vascular inflammation.

The second most common type of vasculitic skin lesions in primary Sjögren's syndrome are urticaria-like lesions which may or may not contain petechiae (Fig. 2). Characteristically these erythematous, edematous lesions usually persist for more than 24 hours, in contrast to transient common urticaria whose duration is generally less than 4 to 6 hours. These urticaria-like vasculitic lesions generally are non-pruritic, but may be associated with a burning sensation. The application of light touch or pressure to the lesions may produce hyperpathia.

A third, but less frequent, category of Sjögren's syndrome vasculitic skin lesions includes erythematosus macular and papular lesions, some of which may be rather subtle and nondescript. In this category also are classical erythema multiforme

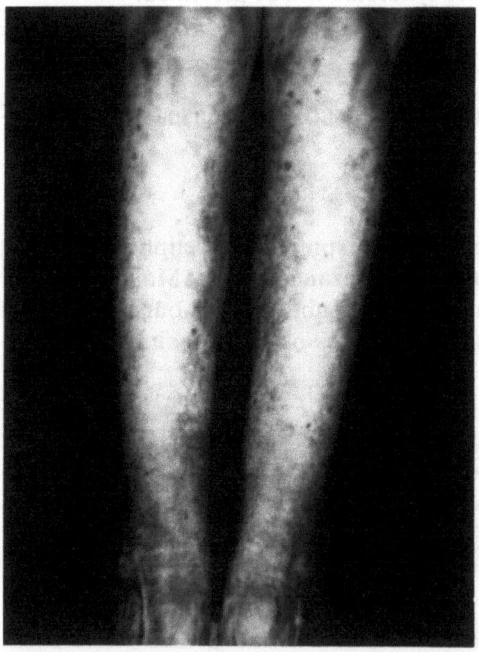

Fig. 1. Lower extremity palpable purpura and petechiae secondary to cutaneous vasculitis in a patient with a long history of primary Sjögren's syndrome. Fresh erythematous purpuric lesions are seen among the brawny discoloration which represents the residual hyperpigmentation of previous vasculitic lesions

lesions (persistent erythematous macules, papules, with target or iris lesions) which have been seen in a small subset of Sjögren's patients. Another less common cutaneous manifestation of vasculitis is subcutaneous nodules, some of which resemble erythema nodosum lesions. Necrotizing panniculitis, secondary to vasculitic lesions involving the subcutaneous adipose tissue, also has been noted occasionally. A rare patient has had digital infarcts, ulcers, or gangrene.

These manifestations of cutaneous vasculitis are not specific or unique to Sjögren's syndrome, but represent the spectrum of lesions that can be produced by vasculitic involvement of the skin. Recognition of their significance as lesions of vasculitis and potential markers for possible systemic disease in patients with Sjögren's syndrome, however, are important (see below).

Peripheral nerve

Peripheral nervous system involvement in Sjögren's syndrome is well recognized (Kaltreider and Talal 1969; Pittsley and Talal 1980; Alexander 1982c). Several forms of neuropathy have been observed and are described in Chapter II.B.2.

Limited evidence suggests that the etiology of at least some forms of neuropathies in Sjögren's syndrome is related to inflammatory vascular disease of the vasa nervorum. The limited available evidence suggests that peripheral neuropathies in Sjögren's syndrome are secondary to vascular inflammation of small vessels in the epineurum or vasa nervorum. Kaltreider and Talal described 10 cases of neuropa-

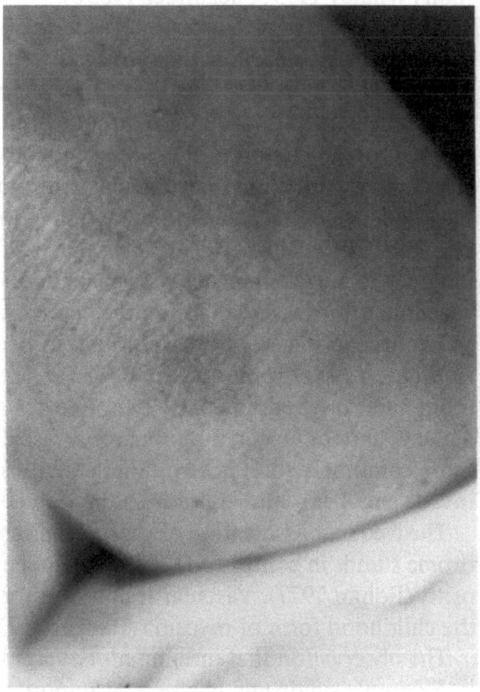

Fig. 2. Urticaria-like lesion on the inner thigh of a patient with primary Sjögren's syndrome. Such lesions may persist for days and demonstrate hyperpathia. The cutaneous lesions seen in Figures 1 and 2 can be caused by either neutrophilic or mononuclear inflammatory vascular disease

thy in Sjögren's syndrome (Kaltreider and Talal 1969). Nerve biopsies were performed in 4 patients two of whom showed vasculitis. We have reported 10 patients with Sjögren's syndrome in whom nerve biopsies showed vascular inflammation (Alexander 1981 a, 1982 c, 1983 a; Molina 1986; Malinow 1986). Peyronnard (Peyronnard 1981) reported a patient with Sjögren's syndrome who had a severe sensorimotor neuropathy secondary to epineural vasculitis. There was a loss of both myelinated and non-myelinated fibers. Thus, the inflammatory vascular changes appear to result in ischemia which causes axonal degeneration.

Interestingly, the most common histopathologic type of inflammatory vascular disease in these patients with peripheral nerve vasculitis demonstrated on biopsy, by our group and others, is mononuclear inflammatory vascular disease (see Chapter II. B. 2.; Molina 1985 a, 1985 b, 1986). These observations document that mononuclear vascular insults, as well as the better recognized neutrophilic inflammatory vascular disease (i.e. leukocytoclastic vasculitis), can result in sufficient vascular compromise to induce ischemia and nerve damage. This concept will be discussed in detail subsequently.

Muscle

Patients with primary Sjögren's syndrome often have muscle involvement (see Chapter II. B. 2). Briefly, classical myositis, with proximal muscle weakness, striking elevation of muscle enzymes, and characteristic electromyographic changes, is relatively uncommon (Shearn 1971). In our experience, however, a smoldering myopathy with focal lymphocytic infiltrates and minimal or no myonecrosis is more common (Whaley 1973; Alexander 1982 b).

The presence of inflammatory vascular disease within muscle blood vessels either alone or in association with myositis is well established in Sjögren's syndrome (see Chapter II. B. 2., Table 1). In 1961, Bunim reported 3 patients with primary Sjögren's syndrome who had vasculitis on random muscle biopsies, two of whom had peripheral neuropathy (Bunim 1961). Subsequently, there have been over 50 muscle biopsies reported in primary Sjögren's syndrome, approximately two-thirds of which had evidence of vascular inflammation (Bloch 1965; Whitehouse 1967; Kaltreider and Talal 1969; Shearn 1971; Whitaker 1972; Ringel 1982; Alexander 1982 b). The majority of muscle biopsies with myositis also had vascular inflammation, although vasculitis alone was seen in some specimens. Both histopathologic types of vascular inflammation that we have described in peripheral inflammatory vascular disease in Sjögren's syndrome (Molina 1985 a; Molina 1985 b) have been observed [i.e. mononuclear (predominantly lymphocytes and plasma cells) and neutrophilic]. In general, mononuclear inflammatory vascular disease is observed within muscle more commonly than neutrophilic vasculitis. The mononuclear cells surround and invade small epi- and endomysial blood vessels and capillaries.

The frequent association of vascular inflammation with myositis in Sjögren's syndrome stands in contrast to the low frequency of vasculitis in poly/and dermatomyositis (Bohan 1977). Vascular lesions, on the other hand, appear to be a feature of the childhood form of myositis (Banker 1975).

The observation that inflammatory vascular disease may involve skeletal muscle in Sjögren's syndrome has several important clinical ramifications. Such vascular and other muscle inflammatory infiltrates may well be related to the common musculoskeletal syndrome (see Chapter II. B. 2.) in which myalgias are a frequent symptom. It is possible that locally synthesized lymphokines, mediators, or antibodies might induce musculoskeletal discomfort and subtly affect neuromuscular conduction without giving rise to sufficient damage of muscle fibers to elevate the muscle enzymes or induce characteristic electromyographic changes.

The detection of inflammatory vascular disease in muscle has another important clinical ramification. We have observed that approximately two-thirds of patients with biopsy documented peripheral inflammatory vascular disease (i.e. involving skin, nerve, or muscle) develop nervous system complications (Molina 1985). The presence of vascular inflammation in muscle, may be indicative of more generalized vascular inflammation. If a patient is suspected of having systemic vasculitis, a diagnostic muscle biopsy may be indicated even in the absence of muscle enzyme elevation or electromyographic changes. If in the process of evaluating a patient for myositis or a myopathy, a muscle biopsy shows inflammatory vascular disease, the patient should be carefully observed and evaluated for possible systemic disease including neurologic complications.

Immunofluorescence studies have been performed on muscle biopsies from 10 patients (Whitaker 1972; Alexander 1982b; Ringel 1982). Direct immunofluorescence showed linear epimysial and connective tissue staining for immunoglobalia most commonly. Mottled or punctate and homogeneous staining of isolated necrotic fibers were also observed. Vascular deposition of IgG, IgM or C_3 was observed in seven of eight patients studied (Whitaker 1972; Alexander 1982b; Ringel 1982).

Electron microscopic studies have been performed in eight patients (Ringel 1982; Alexander 1982b) and showed microvascular changes including endothelial cell swelling and proliferation with prominant micropinocytosis, numerous intracytoplasmic vesicles and inclusions (including tubuloreticular structures), and subendothelial deposits of homogeneous, electron-dense material, with associated basement membrane thickening and disruption.

Systemic

In addition to peripheral inflammatory vascular disease (i.e. involving skin, nerve, or muscle), patients with Sjögren's syndrome can develop vascular inflammation of other organs (i.e. systemic vasculitis). A single or multiple organ systems may be involved. Since the inflammatory vascular disease of Sjögren's syndrome appears to affect predominantly small vessels (see below), the manifestations tend to be subacute, insidious, and slowly progressive over time. It is our experience that under such circumstances, considerable cumulative end-organ damage can occur over time, before the process becomes manifest and is recognized clinically. A subset of patients, however, particularly those with larger vessel involvement indistinguishable from polyarteritis nodosa (Ramage 1956; Alexander 1982a) or severe diffuse small vessel involvement, have a more precipitous onset of the clinical manifestations of their vasculitis and a more aggressive course.

Inflammatory vascular disease in Sjögren's syndrome has been observed to affect the salivary and lacrimal glands, kidneys, lung, gastrointestinal tract (stomach, small bowel, colon) pancreas, liver, spleen, breast, reproductive tract, and peripheral and central nervous systems (Alexander 1982a; Alexander 1983a; Molina 1985a, b, 1986; Molina 1983c; Clinicopathologic conference 1964; Bloch 1965; Peyronnard 1982; Alexander et al, unpublished observations).

A spectrum of clinical presentations associated with vasculitis has been observed. On the one hand, when systemic vascular complications emerge clinically, they can be protean and devastating. For example, we have observed two patients with long standing primary Sjögren's syndrome, cutaneous leukocytoclastic vasculitis, and prominent sero-reactivity who died abruptly of acute central nervous system complications. Post-mortem examination showed extensive diffuse disseminated inflammatory vascular disease involving essentially every organ. In neither case was systemic vasculitis suspected prior to the terminal event. On the other hand, the development of systemic complications may be more subtle. For example, we also have observed patients in whom the antemortem clinical expression of systemic vasculitis, documented by biopsy, was limited to one or two organs (particularly, kidney and lung).

We have been particularly interested in the central nervous complications of primary Sjögren's syndrome, which can occur alone or with other systemic organ involvement. These findings will be discussed in detail in Chapter II. B. 2. Briefly, there is a striking association between the presence of peripheral, particularly cutaneous, biopsy documented vasculitis and concomitant central nervous system disease (Molina 1985a).

Two Histopathologic Types of Inflammatory Vascular Disease

New Observations

In our early work with Sjögren's syndrome, we examined the clinical, hematologic, and serologic associations with the presence of precipitating autoantibodies (determined by gel double immunodiffusion) to Ro (SS-A) and La (SS-B) (Table 2) (Alexander 1982d, 1983a). We demonstrated a striking association of anti-Ro (SS-A) antibodies with purpuric skin lesions ($p = 0.0005$), vasculitis ($p = 0.0005$), seroreactivity for rheumatoid factor ($p = 0.0005$), antinuclear antibodies ($p = 0.0005$), cryoglobulins ($p = 0.001$) and hypocomplementemia ($p = 0.005$). Similar, but less strik-

Table 2. Primary Sjögren's syndrome: cutaneous manifestations/histopathologic correlates (Alexander & Provost 1983)

Histopathology	Clinical features (no. of patients)		
	Purpura	Urticaria	Other
Leukocytoclastic angiitis	6	5	1
Mononuclear vasculitis	2	1	2
Both leukocytoclastic angiitis and mononuclear vasculitis	2	0	0
Perivascular cuffing only	0	1	2
Total patients	10	7	5

ing associations were observed for anti-La (SS-B) antibodies. In this study, we observed that a small subset of patients without precipitating antibodies to Ro (SS-A) or La (SS-B) also had vasculitis. In general, these patients were seronegative and normocomplementemic.

When we reviewed the histopathologic features of the biopsies from Sjögren's patients with and without precipitating autoantibodies to Ro (SS-A) and La (SS-B), we observed striking differences. The patients with precipitating antibodies to Ro (SS-A)/La (SS-B) generally had leukocytoclastic vasculitis characterized by a predominance of polymorphonuclear cells within vascular infiltrates. In contrast, the patients without precipitating antibodies to Ro (SS-A)/La (SS-B) had inflammatory vascular disease which was characterized by the presence of mononuclear cells (predominantly lymphocytes) within the vessel walls.

Based on these preliminary observations, we subsequently described two distinct histopathologic types of inflammatory vascular disease in primary Sjögren's syndrome; neutrophilic inflammatory vascular disease (NIVD) and mononuclear inflammatory vascular disease (MIVD) (Alexander 1983c; Molina 1985b). Neutrophilic inflammatory vascular disease is defined as vascular disease associated with infiltration of the vessel wall by neutrophils (Figure 3A, B). Neutrophils constitute more than 5% of the total of inflammatory cell population within the vessel wall, and at least one of the following features are also present: fibrinoid necrosis, lumen occlusion, leukocytoclysis (nuclear debris or dust), or extravasation of erythrocytes. In neutrophilic inflammatory vascular disease, neutrophils usually comprise between 40 and 80% of the total number of cells within the infiltrates. This type of inflammatory vascular disease is indistinguishable from leukocytoclastic vasculitis (Sams 1976).

Mononuclear inflammatory vascular disease is defined as frank invasion and disruption of mural integrity of the blood vessel by mononuclear cells (lymphocytes, plasma cells and monocytes) with less than 5% neutrophils and at least one other accompanying feature listed above (Figure 4A, B). If present, fibrinoid necrosis tends to be less prominent in this form of inflammatory vascular disease. Patients may have neutrophilic inflammatory vascular disease alone, mononuclear vascular disease alone, or both. Those patients categorized as having mononuclear inflammatory vascular disease are patients with only mononuclear vasculitis, while those characterized as having neutrophilic inflammatory vascular disease have either neutrophilic vasculitis alone or, less commonly, mixed vasculitis (i.e. neutrophilic and mononuclear).

Both histopathologic types of inflammatory vascular disease appear to be able to induce significant vascular injury resulting in end-organ dyfunction. This statement is supported by the observation that both histopathologic types of vascular inflammation can result in identical cutaneous manifestations of vasculitis (Table 2). In addition, it is not possible to predict the histopathologic type of vasculitis by the clinical appearance of the lesions. Furthermore, both histopathologic types of vascular inflammation have been associated with systemic vasculitis and serious end-organ compromise (Molina 1985a, 1986).

Classically, vasculitides are defined, not only by the type of inflammatory cells infiltrating blood vessel walls, but also with respect to the types and sizes of the involved blood vessels. A wide range of blood vessel types are involved in primary

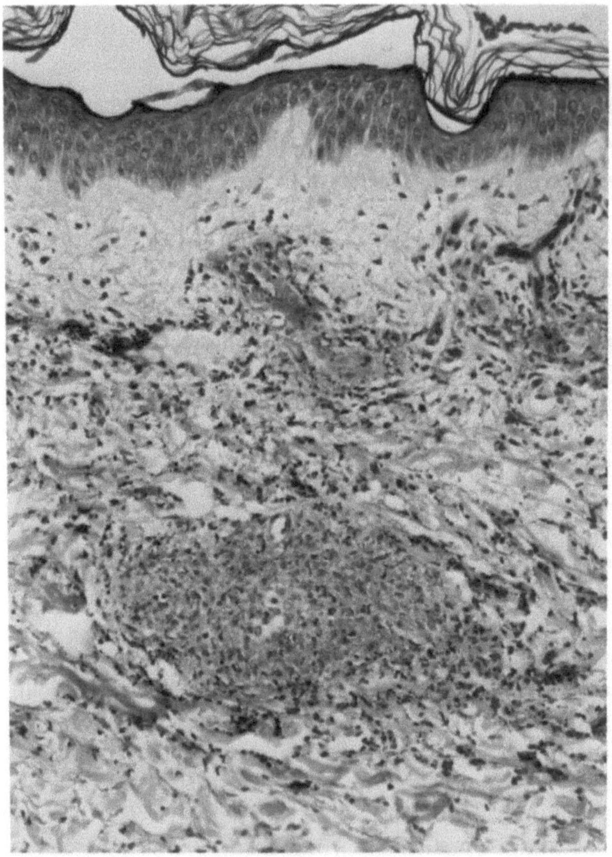

A

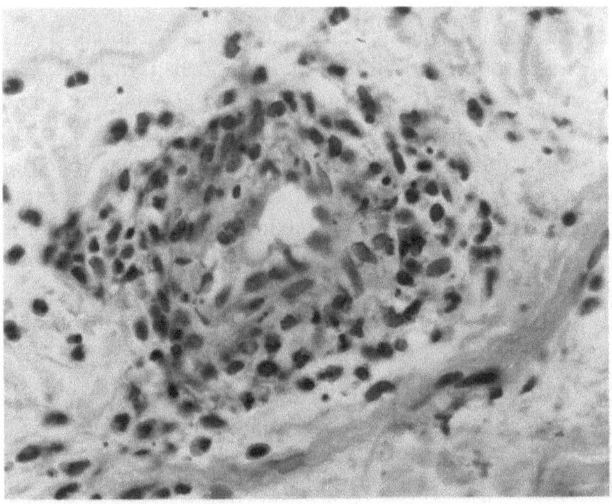

B

Fig. 3. **A** Neutrophilic inflammatory vascular disease (NIVD) in a cutaneous lesion from a "seropositive" patient with primary Sjögren's syndrome. Neutrophilic inflammatory vascular disease involving vessels of superficial and deep dermis. Venules and arterioles are affected, and there is extensive necrosis of vessel walls with fibrin deposition and extravasation of erythrocytes (hematoxylin and eosin stained, original magnification ×180). **B** Early neutrophilic inflammatory vascular disease in a dermal arteriole. Endothelial cells are swollen and distorted, with lumen compromise. The integrity of the vessel wall architecture is disrupted with inflammatory infiltrates containing mononuclear cells and neutrophils. Nuclear dust is present (hematoxylin and eosin stained, original magnification ×800)

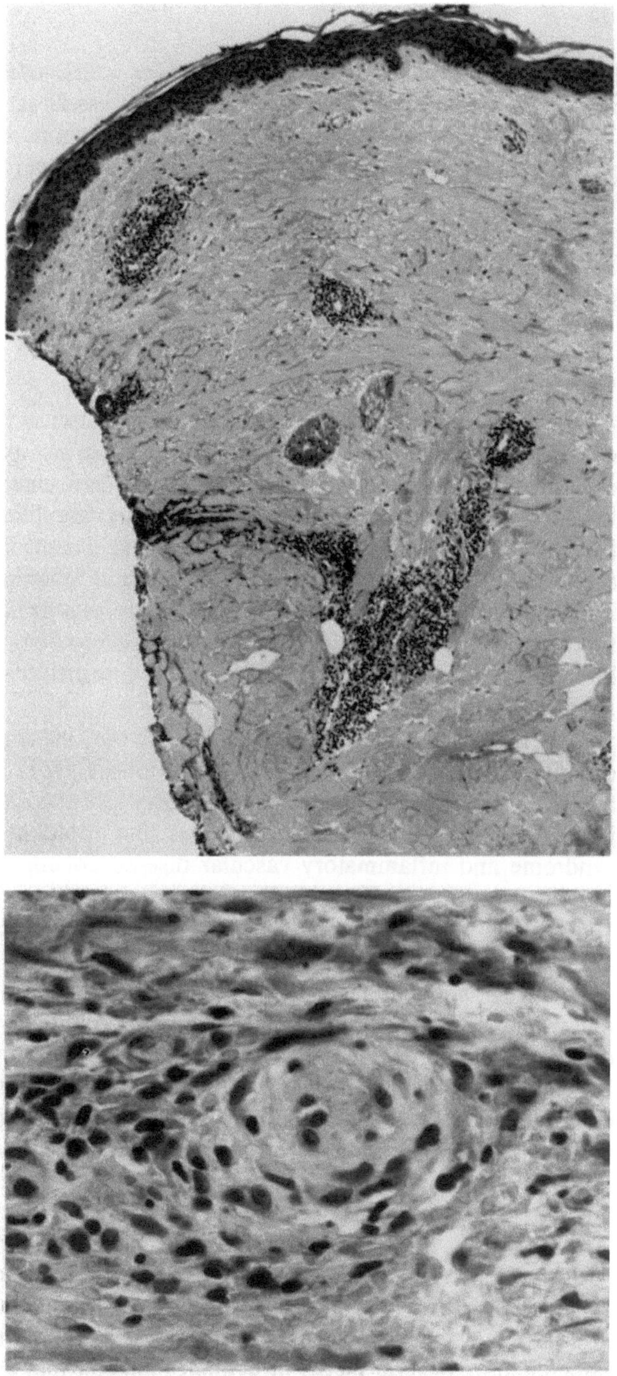

A

B

Fig. 4. A Mononuclear inflammatory vascular disease (MIVD) in a cutaneous lesion from a "sero-negative" patient with primary Sjögren's syndrome. Mononuclear inflammatory vascular disease affecting venules and arterioles within superficial and deep dermis (hematoxylin and eosin stained, original magnification ×57) **B** Mononuclear inflammatory vascular disease involving a small arteriole. Mononuclear cells surround and invade vessel which shows lumen occlusion and erythrocyte extravasation. Lymphocytes and plasma cells are the predominant cell type (hematoxylin and eosin stained, original magnification ×730)

Sjögren's syndrome (i. e. capillaries, venules, veins, arterioles, and arteries). With respect to blood vessel size, however, small vessels are involved predominantly. Medium size muscular arteries are involved less commonly and may cause vascular pathology indistinguishable from polyarteritis nodosa (Ramage 1956). Large vessels are usually spared. We have seen, however, unusual cases in which there was mononuclear inflammation of the vasa vasorum of large arteries. In addition, we have observed small vessel vasculitis accompanied by large vessel disease radiographically indistinguishable from Takayasu's arteritis (Alexander 1983 a).

Historical Perspectives

Although mononuclear inflammatory vascular disease in connective tissue disorders has not been proposed previously as a distinct histopathologic form of vascular injury with the potential for causing systemic involvement, other investigators also have recognized two distinct types of cutaneous vasculitis. Soter et al. described two histopathologic forms of necrotizing arteritis (i. e. neutrophilic and lymphocytic) in a series of fourteen patients, four of whom had Sjögren's syndrome (Soter 1976). Soter has indicated that additional patients in that group probably had Sjögren's syndrome (Soter, personal communication, 1985). Two types of inflammatory cellular infiltrates also have been described in chronic urticarial vasculitis (Provost 1980; Monroe 1981).

The histopathologic characteristics of the inflammatory vascular lesions described by these authors (Soter 1976; Monroe 1981) are indistinguishable from the features of the two types of inflammatory vascular disease described in our patients. A review of the literature indicates that a total of 17 women with Sjögren's syndrome and inflammatory vascular disease documented by biopsy have been described previously (Soter 1976; Kaltreider and Talal 1969; CPC Amer. J. Med 1964; Bloch 1965; Whitehouse 1967; Peyronnard 1982). The clinical, pathologic, and serologic features of these patients, which closely resemble those observed in our patients, are summarized in Table 3. Purpuric skin lesions were the most frequent cutaneous manifestations occurring in 13 patients. Chronic urticaria, the second most common cutaneous manifestation in our group, occurred in one patient. Inflammatory vascular disease was documented histopathologically in skin (6 patients), muscle (9 patients), or other tissue (3 patients). Neutrophilic inflammatory vascular infiltrates occurred in 13 patients and mononuclear infiltrates were observed in 8 (four patients had both types of inflammatory vascular disease). Serious systemic complications were documented in 13 patients.

Classically, it has been postulated that neutrophilic inflammatory vascular disease (i. e. leukocytoclastic vasculitis) is the histopathologic manifestation of the acute insult to the blood vessel wall, while mononuclear inflammatory vascular infiltrates have been considered to represent "chronic" or "healing" vascular inflammation. Several pieces of evidence suggest that a different series of immunopathogenic events might be operative in inflammatory vascular disease of Sjögren's syndrome. The available evidence suggests that, in contrast to the classical concept of the evolution of inflammatory vascular disease, mononuclear inflammatory vascular disease, in some cases, may actually transform into neutrophilic inflammatory vascular disease.

Table 3. Clinical and laboratory features in patients with anti-Ro (SS-A) antibodies

Features	Patients with Anti-Ro (SS-A)		
	Positive (n=33)	Negative (n=42)	p Value
	n	n	
Clinical			
Vasculitis	24	4	0.0005
Salivary gland enlargement	26	15	0.0005
Lymphadenopathy	19	4	0.0005
Purpura	12	1	0.0005
Hematologic*			
Anemia	19	6	0.0005
Leukopenia	14	3	0.001
Thrombocytopenia	7	1	0.025
Serologic**			
Hyperglobulinemia	21	8	0.0005
Rheumatoid factor	29	17	0.0005
Antinuclear antibody	31	10	0.0005
Cryoglobulinemia	7/13	0/22	0.001
Hypocomplementemia	11	2	0.005

* Anemia = hematocrit <35%; leukopenia = <4000 leukocytes/mm^3; thrombocytopenia = <150,000 platelets/mm^3.

** Hyperglobulinemia = serum globulins >4.0 g/dL; rheumatoid factor ≥1:80; antinuclear antibodies ≥1:40; cryocrit ≥2%; total hemolytic complement <25 units

Both types of inflammatory vascular disease have been observed to occur in the same individual, both in our series and in previously recorded cases (Table 3; Reference Kaltreider and Talal 1969). In addition, in a subset of these patients the transition from mononuclear inflammatory vascular disease to neutrophilic inflammatory vascular disease has been documented, not only by our group (Alexander 1983c; Molina 1985b; Alexander et al, personal observations), but also by others (Kaltreider and Talal 1969). Neither we nor Soter, et al. (Soter 1976; Soter NA, personal communication, 1985) have observed a temporal transition from neutrophilic to mononuclear inflammatory vascular disease in Sjögren's patients who have had multiple biopsies over time. Furthermore, mononuclear inflammatory cells always are present in significant numbers (usually aproximately 20 to 60% of total number of cells) in neutrophilic inflammatory vascular disease (Soter 1976; Alexander 1983c; Molina 1985b). This finding has been recognized, but not emphasized, in descriptions of classical leukocytoclastic vasculitis (Sams 1976). *In toto,* these data suggest that there is a subset of patients with mononuclear inflammatory vascular disease whose inflammatory vascular lesions may eventually evolve into a neutrophilic form of inflammatory vascular disease.

Differential Serologic and Complement Associations Between Two Histopathologic Types of Vasculitis

The two histopathologic types of inflammatory vascular disease in Sjögren's syndrome have distinct serologic associations (Molina 1985b) (Table 4). Neutrophilic inflammatory vascular disease is characterized by a striking association with seroreactivity with respect to precipitating antibodies (determined by gel double immunodiffusion) to Ro (SS-A), La (SS-B), rheumatoid factor, and antinuclear antibodies. Cryoglobulins, if present, are seen in these patients. In contrast, mononuclear inflammatory vascular disease occurs in the setting of seronegativity with respect to these autoantibodies.

The most striking serologic correlations with inflammatory vascular disease involve the presence of precipitating antibodies to Ro (SS-A), La (SS-B) and serum rheumatoid factor. Twenty of twenty-seven (74%) patients with neutrophilic inflammatory vascular disease had anti-Ro (SS-A) antibodies in contrast with two (11%) of those with mononuclear inflammatory vascular disease ($p = 0.00006$). A similar but less significant association ($p = 0.036$) was seen between neutrophilic inflammatory vascular disease and the presence of antibodies to La (SS-B). Serum rheumatoid factor was present in 18 (67%) patients with neutrophilic inflammatory vascular disease, but in only 3 (17%) of those with mononuclear inflammatory vascular disease ($p = 0.002$).

When analyzed further, an even stronger association between neutrophilic inflammatory vascular disease and the concomitant presence of both autoantibod-

Table 4. Histopathologic documentation of inflammatory vascular disease in 17 female patients with Sjögren's syndrome

Ref. no.	Age	Race	Skin lesion	Biopsy site	Histopathologic diagnosis	RF
18	46	U	p	Skin	NIVD	ND
18	50	U	p	Skin	NIVD	ND
18	67	U	p	Skin	NIVD	ND
18	37	U	p	Skin	MIVD	ND
22	52	B	p, u	Muscle	MIVD, NIVD+	H
22	49	W	p	Skin	NIVD	L
22	48	W	p	Skin	MIVD	L
22	73	W	–	Muscle	MIVD, NIVD+	H
22	55	W	p	Muscle	MIVD, NIVD	H
22	69	W	–	Muscle	NIVD	H
22	64	W	–	Muscle	MIVD	H
22	52	W	p	Muscle	NIVD	H
22	41	W	p	Muscle	MIVD	L
23	57	W	p	Colon	NIVD	H
24	52	W	–	Parotid, muscle, bowel	NIVD	H
25	54	W	p	Muscle	NIVD	H
26	66	W	p	Gall bladder, spleen	MIVD, NIVD	H

(*RF* rheumatoid factor, *U* unknown, *p* purpura, *NIVD* neutrophilic inflammatory vascular disease, *ND* not done, *MIVD* mononuclear inflammatory vascular disease, *u* urticaria, *H* high-titer RF using bentonite flocculation test or latex agglutination, *L* low-titer RF + Transition from MIVD to NIVD) (Molina 1985a) ies to Ro (SS-A) and rheumatoid factor was demonstrated. Sixteen (59%) of the patients with neutrophilic inflammatory vascular disease had antibodies to both Ro (SS-A) and rheumatoid factor, while no patient with mononuclear inflammatory vascular disease had both of these autoantibodies ($p = 0.00006$). Twenty-two patients (81%) with neutrophilic inflammatory vascular disease had antibodies to Ro (SS-A) or rheumatoid factor (or both), in contrast to only 5 patients (28%) with mononuclear inflammatory vascular disease ($p = 0.0008$). A similar, but less significant, association between neutrophilic inflammatory vascular disease and hyperglobulinemia ($p = 0.01$) and antinuclear antibodies ($p = 0.02$) was observed.

The data described here involved the determination of Ro (SS-A) and La (SS-B) antibodies employing gel double diffusion techniques. More recent quantitative studies performed with a sensitive ELISA using purified antigens indicate that almost all Sjögren's syndrome patients possess abnormal quantities of Ro (SS-A) and La (SS-B) antibodies (Harley 1986). In general, Ro (SS-A) and La (SS-B) antibody detection by gel double diffusion correlates with high titer antibody levels detected by ELISA, whereas a negative gel double diffusion assay for Ro (SS-A) and La (SS-B) antibodies correlates with low titers of Ro (SS-A) and La (SS-B) antibodies. For a more complete discussion see Chapter III. 2.

Previous studies also have linked serologic abnormalities with inflammatory vascular disease in connective tissue disorders. The presence of high titer IgG- and IgM-rheumatoid factor has been associated with vasculitis in rheumatoid arthritis (Theofilopoulos 1974; Scott 1981). Similarly, the presence of rheumatoid factor has been associated with clinical vasculitis in SLE (Zizic 1982). Antibodies to Ro (SS-A) antigen have been observed in necrotizing renal vasculitis in SLE (Maddison 1979). Of the Sjögren's syndrome patients with biopsy-documented vasculitis described in the literature (Table 2), serologic data on rheumatoid factor were available in 13. Nine of 10 patients with neutrophilic inflammatory vascular disease had rheumatoid factor in high titer, in contrast to only one of three patients in the small group of patients with mononuclear vasculitis. Sufficient data were not available on antibodies to Ro (SS-A) in these patients.

There also are differences in serum complement levels between the two groups of inflammatory vascular disease patients. Patients with neutrophilic inflammatory vascular disease had significantly lower mean total hemolytic complement levels (25.2 ± 11.6 units) than did patients with mononuclear inflammatory vascular disease (33.4 ± 10.1 units) ($p = 0.03$). The percentage of neutrophilic inflammatory vascular disease patients with abnormal CH_{50} values (50%) was also higher than that of mononuclear inflammatory vascular disease patients (12.5%) ($p = 0.03$). There were no differences between the 2 groups in the mean C_3 concentrations (NIVD, 110.6 ± 51.6 mg/dl; MIVD, 122.8 ± 49.1 mg/dl) or C_4 concentrations (NIVD, 22.1 ± 15.7 mg/dl; MIVD 23.6 ± 10.2 mg/dl). Nor were there differences between the two groups in the percentage of individuals with abnormal values (C_3 concentrations: NIVD, 26%; MIVD, 9%; C_4 concentrations: NIVD, 53%; MIVD, 35%). Of the 13 patients with decreased CH_{50} levels who also had C_3 and C_4 determinations, however, 11 (85%) had decreased C_4 and 8 (62%) had decreased C_3 concentrations.

Other investigators also have found a difference in serum complement levels between the two histopathologic types of vasculitis. Soter et al. found that hypocomplementemia was more common in the neutrophilic form of vasculitis (Soter et al. 1974a, b, 1976). Hypocomplementemia with an urticaria-like leukocytoclastic vasculitis also has been observed (McDuffie 1973; Soter 1974b; Sanchez 1982).

The two histopathologic types of inflammatory vascular disease also had differences in the quantity of circulating immune complexes. IgG immune complexes as measured by a solid phase anti-C_3 assay were present at higher mean serum concentration in patients with neutrophilic inflammatory vascular disease (4.0 ± 4.4) than in patients with mononuclear inflammatory vascular disease (0.4 ± 1.4) ($p = 0.002$). Sixteen of 25 (64%) patients with neutrophilic inflammatory vascular disease had elevated IgG immune complex levels, while only 6 of 26 (23%) patients with mononuclear inflammatory vascular disease had elevated levels. There was no significant difference between the two groups with respect to immune complexes detected by a solid phase anti-Clq binding assay. Circulating immune complexes have been described in Sjögren's syndrome previously (Lawley 1979; Yoshinoya 1982; Hersey 1983), but their association with vascular inflammation has not been reported.

The differences between the two types of vasculitis with respect to the presence of autoantibodies, immune complexes, and serum complement levels suggest that, if immune complexes and activation of the complement pathway do play a role in the development of vascular inflammation, there may be differences in the immunopathogenesis of the two types of inflammatory vascular lesions. In addition, if there is a transition of mononuclear to neutrophilic vasculitis, these serologic parameters may play a pathogenetic role in the development of leukocytoclastic vasculitis.

Murine Models

In parallel with our work on vasculitis in Sjögren's syndrome patients, we have developed the MRL/Mp mouse as a model for studying the immunopathogenesis of inflammatory vascular disease (Alexander 1983b, 1985; Jabs 1985) in autoimmune disorders. MRL/Mp mice traditionally have been proposed as models of lupus erythematosus or rheumatoid arthritis, but recently they have been recognized as also having features of Sjögren's syndrome (Alexander 1983b, 1985, Jabs 1985, Hoffman 1984). MRL/Mp mice uniformly and spontaneously develop inflammatory vascular disease which is histopathologically indistinguishable from that seen in patients with Sjögren's syndrome. The importance of these mice lies not in their precise identity with a specific established rheumatic disorder, but rather relates to their potential value in dissecting immunopathologic mechanisms of such disorders as vasculitis.

A major cause of morbidity and mortality in MRL/Mp mice is inflammatory vascular disease (Alexander 1985). When MRL/Mp mice are followed until moribund and sacrificed, vascular complications such as hemorrhage or infarct of one or more organs can be documented in most animals. Correlative histopathologic examination of tissues from these mice demonstrates the concomitant presence of inflammatory vascular disease.

Two main histopathologic types of inflammatory vascular disease (i.e. neutrophilic (NIVD) and mononuclear (MIVD) have been observed (Table 5) in both substrains of MRL mice (e.g. MRL/Mp-lpr/lpr and MRL/Mp-+/+). Mononuclear vasculitis always antedates the development of neutrophilic vasculitis. Characteristically, there is a serial transition from mononuclear inflammatory vascular disease to neutrophilic inflammatory vascular disease. In no case has the development of neutrophilic vasculitis been observed to precede the onset of mononuclear vasculitis. The presence of the lpr gene in the homozygous recessive form in MRL/Mp-lpr/lpr mice accelerates the transition from mononuclear to polymorphonuclear inflammatory vascular disease and is associated with decreased survival secondary to vascular complications. Our studies on MRL/Mp-+/+ mice and other strains of mice into which the lpr gene has been introduced, indicate that there is an important contribution of the genetic background to the development of vasculitis (Table 6).

The serologic associations seen in human Sjögren's syndrome patients with the two types of inflammatory vascular disease are paralleled, in part, in the mice. Mice with neutrophilic inflammatory vascular disease are seropositive with respect to serum rheumatoid factor, immune complexes, cryoglobulins, and antinuclear antibodies. MRL/Mp mice of either substrain, however, do not develop anti-Ro (SS-A) or La (SS-B) antibodies. Mice with mononuclear inflammatory vascular disease are seronegative with respect to the autoantibodies outlined above. With the transition from mononuclear to neutrophilic inflammatory vascular disease there is an associated characteristic development of seropositivity for these autoantibodies. MRL/

Table 5. Serologic/histopathologic correlates in inflammatory vascular disease in patients with Sjögren's syndrome*

	ANA	Globulins	Rheumatoid Factor	Anti-Ro (SS-A)	Anti-La (SS-B)
NIVD (n=27)	21 (78)+	14 (52)	18 (67)	20 (74)	12 (44)
MIVD (n=18)	7 (39)	2 (11)	3 (17)	2 (11)	2 (11)
P	0.02	0.01	0.002	0.00006	0.036

* Antibodies to Ro (SS-A) and La (SS-B) determined by gel double-diffusion

Table 6. Cellular infiltrates in inflammatory vascular disease (IVD) in MRL/Mp mice (*NIVD* neutrophilic IVD, *MIVD* mononuclear IVD) (Alexander 1985)

IVD type	No. (Percent)	
	MRL/Mp-lpr/lpr	MRL/Mp-+/+
NIVD alone	9 (31)*	0
MVD alone	3 (10)**	11 (58)**
NIVD and MIVD	17 (59)	8 (42)
Total	29 (100)	19 (100)

* P<0.025.
** P<0.005
(*ANA* antinuclear antibodies on mouse liver substrate >1:40, *Glob.* serum globulin concentrations >4 mg/dl; *RF* rheumatoid factor by latex fixation >1:80, *NIVD* neutrophilic inflammatory vascular disease, *MIVD* mononuclear inflammatory vascular disease. + Numbers in parentheses are percentages) (Molina 1985 a)

Mp mice have been reported to develop hypocomplemententemia (Theofilopoulos 1981), although the temporal association with the development of vascular inflammation has not yet been established.

These observations in MRL/Mp mice establish that mononuclear vasculitis antedates neutrophilic vasculitis and occurs prior to the development of circulating autoantibodies and immune complexes. These data also establish that there is a subsequent transition from mononuclear to neutrophilic vasculitis that is associated with the development of seropositivity. The presence of the lpr gene accelerates the development of this histopathologic transition.

The Immunopathogenesis of Inflammatory Vascular Disease - A Model

An Overview

Our observations on the immunopathogenesis of inflammatory vascular disease in primary Sjögren's syndrome appear to be important for several clinical and basic reasons. From a clinical standpoint, peripheral vasculitis (primarily cutaneous) occurs in approximately 25% of patients with primary Sjögren's syndrome evaluated at our institution. In our experience, subtle clinical manifestations of cutaneous vasculitis are often overlooked in this disorder. In addition, systemic complications in patients with peripheral inflammatory vascular disease may be more common than appreciated previously.

Peripheral inflammatory vascular disease may serve as a marker for those patients at risk for the development of potential systemic complications including central nervous system involvement (see Chapter II. B. 2.). It is equally important to recognize, however, that not all Sjögren's patients with systemic complications or central nervous system disease have evidence of peripheral inflammatory vascular disease. This is becoming increasingly clear with our recent observations of Sjögren's patients with early subtle neurologic disease characterized by psychiatric or cognitive abnormalities which neurodiagnostic studies indicate have an organic etiology (see Chapter III. B. 2). The documentation of peripheral inflammatory vascular disease and associated immunologically mediated autoimmune nervous system disease, unattributable to other etiologies, however, suggests to us that these manifestations and their association are previously under-recognized features of primary Sjögren's syndrome.

The findings regarding the two histopathologic types of inflammatory vascular disease (i. e. mononuclear and neutrophilic) and their distinctive serologic associations also have practical clinical implications. Since both types of inflammatory vascular disease can give rise to a spectrum of identical cutaneous lesions, can cause systemic vascular complications, and are both associated equally with neurologic disease, we reason that mononuclear inflammatory vascular disease, as well as the better recognized leukocytoclastic vasculitis, can cause similar clinically significant blood vessel injury and destruction. We recognize, however, that all neurologic complications of Sjögren's syndrome are not secondary to inflammatory vascular disease (i.e. vasculitis), but may be secondary to other immunologic mechanisms (see Chapter II. B. 2.)

It is also important to realize that not all patients with primary Sjögren's syndrome are seroreactive by standard techniques. A subset of patients with primary Sjögren's syndrome are "seronegative" and a subgroup of these develop mononuclear inflammatory vascular disease. This subgroup of "seronegative", in contrast to "seropositive", patients with primary Sjögren's syndrome, may have, as yet undefined, fundamental immunologic and immunogenetic differences. The uniform presence of anti-Ro (SS-A)/La (SS-B) antibodies detected by ELISA, rather than by gel double diffusion, (Harley 1986) and HLA DRw52 (Wilson 1980; Harley 1986), an immunogenetic marker for Sjögren's syndrome, in these "seronegative" Sjögren's patients, however, indicates to us that they are appropriately categorized as primary Sjögren's syndrome. These observations emphasize that the diagnosis of primary Sjögren's syndrome is not predicated on "seroreactivity" by traditional methods. Furthermore, most importantly, "seronegative" patients may develop the same clinical vasculitic, systemic, and neurologic complications as "seropositive" patients.

Evidence that mononuclear inflammatory vascular disease is important in other clinical settings comes from several sources. Lymphocytic vasculitis, histopathologically indistinguishable from that observed in Sjögren's syndrome, has been observed in other connective tissue disorders and is associated with systemic disease. Mononuclear inflammatory vascular disease has been described in a subset of systemic lupus erythematosous patients (Provost 1980) and in Behcet's syndrome (Lehner 1969; McMenemy 1957). Similarly, mononuclear inflammatory vascular disease has been reported in the setting of infectious diseases and malignancy (Cupps 1981).

Hypothesis

Our studies on the immunopathogenesis of inflammatory vascular disease in Sjögren's syndrome and in autoimmune MRL/Mp mice have provided new, and in some respects unexpected, information about the immunopathogenesis of inflammatory vascular disease. We have established the existence of two distinct histopathologic types of vascular inflammation in man and in the murine model. In Sjögren's syndrome patients we have limited direct evidence that mononuclear inflammatory vascular disease may transformed into neutrophilic vasculitis. In MRL/Mp mice we have presented evidence that this transition is the rule and that it is accelerated by the presence of the lpr gene.

Support for the concept that mononuclear inflammatory vascular disease may be a specific entity and may antedate, rather than follow, the development of neutrophilic vasculitis is provided by unique data from the first prospective clinical, pathologic, and immunologic study of human serum sickness (Lawley 1984). This serendipitous experiment, in which neutropenic patients given horse anti-thymocyte sera to minimize a graft-versus-host reaction following allogeneic bone marrow transplantation developed serum sickness, allows the dissection of the relative and temporal contributions of the two main cellular types of vascular inflammation.

Eight patients with bone marrow failure and severe neutropenia, who were treated with intravenous infusions of horse anti-thymocyte globulin, developed serum sickness and vasculitic cutaneous lesions (chronic urticaria- and erythema multiforme-like lesions) between the 8th and 12th post-treatment days. These cutaneous lesions resembled some of those seen in our Sjögren's patients. Biopsies of the fresh skin lesions (i.e. less than 24 hours old) showed perivascular lymphocytic cuffing and blood vessel wall invasion and damage in the absence of neutrophils (Lawley 1984; Lawley personal communication, 1986). Deposition of horse immunoglobulin or human IgG was not observed, although scattered lesional blood vessels in the superficial dermis had deposition of IgM, IgE, IgA or C_3 in most, but not all, cases. In the only patient with restitution of neutrophils histopathologic features of neutrophilic vasculitis developed (Lawley personal communication, 1986).

These observations indicate that even in putative immune complex mediated disease (i.e. classical serum sickness), mononuclear cells play an important role in vascular inflammation and damage. It is important to note that the mononuclear infiltrate occurred at the height of the suspected immune complex deposition (i.e. days 8-12) and not following the immune complex deposition phase as in the one shot serum sickness model in rabbits. In addition, these findings suggest that immune complex disease can induce vascular injury without the participation of neutrophils. The clinical appearance of the cutaneous lesions caused by lymphocytic inflammatory vascular disease in these patients was indistinguishable from those caused by either type of inflammatory vascular disease in Sjögren's patients. Furthermore, these data suggest that lymphocytic inflammatory vascular disease in humans may antedate, or at least occur simultaneously, with neutrophilic vasculitis and, that under normal circumstances, there probably is not a temporal transition of neutrophilic to mononuclear inflammatory vascular disease, but rather than the converse.

The exact role, of immune complexes in the development of vascular lesions in experimental human serum sickness and in Sjögren's syndrome is unclear. Several pieces of evidence in man and in the murine model, however, would suggest that the passive deposition of circulating serum immune complexes may not necessarily be the initiating event in inflammatory vascular injury. For example, in human experimental serum sickness (Lawley 1984), neither horse immunoglobulin nor human IgG was observed within cutaneous blood vessel walls by immunofluorescence. Not all vessels demonstrated immunoglobulin or complement deposition.

In inflammatory vascular disease accompanying Sjögren's syndrome, circumferential immunoglobulin and complement deposition within cutaneous blood vessel walls has been demonstrated in only a minority of cases by immunofluorescence (Alexander, unpublished observations 1986). What has been observed by immunocytochemical techniques, however, is the presence of focal aggregates of immunoglobulin containing B and plasma cells with adjacent extracellular immunoglobulin deposition. Identical histopathologic findings have been observed in blood vessels in the MRL/Mp murine model of inflammatory vascular disease. These findings suggest that immunoglobulin, rather than or in addition to being passively deposited, may be synthesized locally within the vessel wall and immune complexes deposited *in situ*.

Further support for the suggestion that the passive deposition of circulating immune complexes is not sufficient to induce inflammatory vascular disease comes from genetic studies in autoimmune mice. MRL/Mp mice develop high titers of circulating immune complexes and autoantibodies. The transition of mononuclear to neutrophilic inflammatory vascular disease in MRL/Mp-lpr/lpr mice is associated with the development of circulating immune complexes and autoantibodies. Mice with other genetic backgrounds, into which the lpr gene has been introduced (i.e. C3H/HeJ-lpr/lpr and C57BL/6J-lpr/lpr), also develop very high titers of circulating immune complexes and autoantibodies. They do not develop, however, inflammatory vascular disease. These studies demonstrate that high levels of circulating immune complexes alone do not necessarily result in immune complex mediated vascular damage.

On the basis of these observations we propose a new model of vascular inflammation which is an alternative to the classical model of immune complex mediated vascular damage. We suggest that mononuclear vascular infiltrates may initiate and perpetuate blood vessel injury, and, thus, may exist as a distinct form of inflammatory vascular disease. In the case of neutrophilic vasculitis, we further propose that mononuclear vasculitis may commonly antedate, or at least occur simultaneously with, neutrophilic vascular inflammation. A schematic hypothesis for the development of inflammatory vascular disease is presented in Fig. 5.

We postulate that mononuclear cells (i.e. lymphocytes and perhaps macrophages) may be the first type of inflammatory cell to initiate vascular inflammation.

Mononuclear phase: Lymphocyte adherence to vascular endothelium

↓

Diapedesis through vascular endothelium

↓

Perivascular cuffing
(Accumulation and proliferation of lymphocytes around blood vessels)

↓

Mononuclear inflammatory vascular disease
(Accumulation and proliferation of lymphocytes within blood vessels)

↘ Destructive mononuclear vasculitis
(Invasion and destruction of vessel wall with lumen occlusion, erythrocyte extravasation, fibrinoid degeneration)

↓

Transition phase: Proliferation of cells of B lineage

↓

In situ production of immunoglobulin and/or immune complexes by B lymphocytes or plasma cells

↓

Neutrophilic phase: *In situ* activation of complement pathway

↓

Chemotaxis of polymorphonuclear leukocytes

↓

Neutrophilic inflammatory vascular disease

Fig. 5. Model of inflammatory vascular disease

We suggest that T lymphocytes are probably the first cells to transgress the vessel wall. Cytotoxic T cells or macrophages could damage or kill vascular endothelium and helper T cells could enhance proliferation of infiltrating cells of the B lineage. Continued migration of cells from the vascular compartment and proliferation within the vessel wall would then produce mononuclear vascular inflammation. If vascular damage occurs and repair does not re-establish vascular integrity, mononuclear inflammatory vascular disease would be established and potentially could result in vascular insult and end-organ damage.

The transition of mononuclear to neutrophilic inflammatory vascular disease could be initiated by the migration and proliferation of cells of the B lineage within the vessel walls. B lymphocytes (and plasma cells) stimulated by T helper cells could synthesize immunoglobulins (autoantibodies such as rheumatoid factor, anti Ro (SS-A)/La (SS-B) antibodies, anti-nuclear antibodies or cryoglobulins) within the vessel wall. The local *in situ* deposition of immunoglobulin or immune complexes could activate the complement pathway. Reaction products of the complement pathway are potent chemotactic factors and may cause the additional migration of monocytes and neutrophils into the vessel wall.

In this model of inflammatory vascular disease, we postulate a role for the local production of complement fixing immune complexes in the transition of mononuclear to neutrophilic vasculitis, rather than a primary role for the passive deposition of circulating immune complexes in initiating vascular inflammation. Thus, this model proposes that cell (predominantly lymphocytic) mediated immunologic events are primary in the initiation of vascular inflammation in autoimmune connective tissue disorders. Our laboratory currently is performing studies to test this hypothesis of the immunopathogenesis of inflammatory vascular disease.

Acknowledgements

I would like to express my sincere appreciation to Dr. Thomas T. Provost and my collaborators whose continued support, critical discussions, and enthusiasm have made the continuation of these studies possible, and particularly intellectually rewarding. I would also like to thank Vicky Rogers for her professional clerical assistance.

Figures 1-4 reprinted with permission of the authors and *Arthritis and Rheumatism*.

References

Alexander GE, Provost TT, Stevens MB, Alexander EL (1981 a) Sjögren's syndrome: Central nervous system manifestations. Neurology 31: 1391-1396

Alexander EL, Craft C, Dorsch C, Moser RL, Provost TT, Alexander GE (1982 a) Necrotizing arteritis and spinal subarachnoid hemorrhage in Sjögren's syndrome. Ann Neurol 11: 632-635

Alexander EL, Josifek L, Provost TT, Alexander GE (1982 d) Myositis/vasculitis in primary Sjögren's syndrome (SS). Arthritis Rheum 25: S15

Alexander EL, Provost TT, Stevens MB, Alexander GE (1982 c) Neurologic complications of primary Sjögren's syndrome. Medicine 61: 247-257

Alexander EL, Hirsch TJ, Arnett FC, Provost TT, Stevens MB (1982 b) Ro (SS-A) and La (SS-B) antibodies in the clinical spectrum of Sjögren's syndrome. J. Rheumatol 9: 239-246

Alexander EL, Arnett FC, Provost TT, Stevens MB (1983 a) Sjögren's syndrome: Association of anti-Ro (SS-A) antibodies with vasculitis, hematologic abnormalities, and serologic hyperreactivity. Ann Intern Med 98: 155-159

Alexander EL, Murphy ED, Roths JB, Alexander GE (1983b) Congenic autoimmune murine models of central nervous disease in connective tissue disorders. Ann Neurol 14: 242-248

Alexander EL, Provost TT (1983c) Cutaneous manifestations of primary Sjögren's syndrome: a reflection of vasculitis and association with anti-Ro (SS-A) antibodies. J Invest Dermatol 80: 386-391

Alexander EL, Moyer C, Travlos GS, Roths JB, Murphy ED (1985) Two histopathologic types of inflammatory vascular disease in MRL/Mp autoimmune mice. Arthritis Rheum 28: 1146-1155

Banker BQ (1975) Dermatomyositis of childhood: Ultrastructural alterations of muscle and intramuscular blood vessels. J Neuropathol Exp Neurol 34: 46

Bloch KJ, Buchanan WW, Wohl MJ, Bunim JJ (1965) Sjögren's syndrome: a clinical, pathological, and serological study of sixty-two cases. Medicine (Baltimore) 44: 187-231

Bunim JJ, Talal N (1963) The association of malignant lymphoma with Sjögren's syndrome. Trans Assoc Am Physicians 26: 45-55

Clinicopathologic conference: Sjögren's syndrome (1964) Am J Med 37: 578-591

Cupps TR, Fauci AS (1981) Central nervous system vasculitis. In: Smith LH, Jr (Ed) The Vasculitides, WB Saunders Co., Philadelphia, pp. 127-131

Harley JB, Alexander EL, Bias WB, Fox OF, Provost TT, Reichlin M, Yamagata H, Arnett FC (1986) Anti-Ro (SS-A) and anti-La (SS-B) in patients with Sjögren's syndrome. Arthritis Rheum 29: 196-206

Harrist TJ, Murphy GF, Mihm MC Jr (1982) Lymphomatoid vasculitis: a subset of lymphocytic vasculitis. In: Moschella S (ed) Dermatology Update, pp 115-133

Hersey P, Lawrence S, Prendergast D, Bindon C, Benson W, Valk P (1983) Association of Sjögren's syndrome with C4 deficiency, defective reticuloendothelial function and circulating immune complexes. Clin Exp Immunol 52: 551-560

Hoffman RW, Alspaugh MA, Waggie KS, Durham JB, Waler SE (1984) Sjögren's syndrome in MRL/l and MRL/n mice. Arthritis Rheum 27: 157-165

Jabs D, Alexander EL, Green WR (1985) Ocular inflammation in autoimmune MRL/Mp mice. Invest Ophthalmol Vis Sci 26: 1223-1229

Kahn M et al (1962) Renal concentrating defect in Sjögren's syndrome. Ann Intern Med 56: 883-895

Kaltreider HB, Talal N (1969) The neuropathy of Sjögren's syndrome. Trigeminal nerve involvement. Ann Intern Med 70: 751-762

Kyle RA, Gleich GJ, Bayrd ED, Vaughan JH (1971) Benign hypergammaglobulinemic purpura of Waldenstrom. Medicine (Baltimore) 50: 113-123

Lawley TJ, Moutsopoulos HM, Katz SI, Theofilopoulos AN, Chused TM, Frank MM (1979) Demonstration of circulating immune complexes in Sjögren's syndrome. J Immunol 123: 1382-1386

Lawley TJ, Bielory L, Gascon P, Yancey KB, Young NS, Frank MM (1984) A prospective clinical and immunologic analysis of patients with serum sickness. N Engl J Med 311: 1407-1413

Lehner T (1969) Pathology of recurrent oral ulceration in Behcet's syndrome: Light, electron and fluorescence microscopy. J Pathol 97: 481-494

Maddison PJ, Reichlin M (1979) Deposition of antibodies to a soluble cytoplasmic antigen in the kidneys of patients with systemic lupus erythematosus. Arthritis Rheum 22: 858-863

Malinow KL, Yannakakis GD, Glusman SM, Edlow DR, Griffin J, Pestronk A, Powell DL, Ramsey-Goldman R, Eidelman BH, Medsger TA, Alexander EL (1986) Subacute sensory neuropathy secondary to dorsal root ganglionitis in primary Sjögren's syndrome. Ann Neurol, 20: 535-537

Mason AM, Golding PL (1970) Hyperglobulinaemic renal tubular acidosis: a report of nine cases. Br Med J 1: 143-146

Mason AMS et al (1973) Sjögren's syndrome - a clinical review. Semin Arthritis Rheum 2: 301-331

McCurdy DK et al (1967) Hyperglobulinemic renal tubular acidosis. Ann Intern Med 67: 110-117

McDuffie FC, Sams WM, Moldonado JE, Audreini PH, Conn DL, Samayoa EA (1973) Hypocomplementemia with cutaneous vasculitis and arthritis: possible immune complex syndrome. Mayo Clin Proc 48: 340-348

McMenemey WH, Lawrence BJ (1957) Encephalomyelopathy in Behcet's disease: Report of necropsy findings in two cases. Lancet 2: 353

Molina R, Provost TT, Alexander EL (1985 a) Peripheral inflammatory vascular disease in Sjögren's syndrome: association with nervous system complications. Arthritis Rheum 28: 1341-1347
Molina R, Provost TT, Alexander EL (1985 b) Two histopathologic prototypes of inflammatory vascular disease in Sjögren's syndrome: differential association with seroactivity to rheumatoid factor and antibodies to Ro (SS-A) and with hypocomplementemia. Arthritis Rheum 28: 1251-1258
Molina R, Provost TT, Arnett FC, Bias WB, Hochberg MC, Wilson RW, Alexander EL (1986) Primary Sjögren's syndrome in men - Clinical, serologic, and immunogenetic features. Am J Med 80: 23-31
Monroe EW, Schultz CI, Maize JC, Jordan RE (1981) Vasculitis in chronic urticaria: an immunopathologic study. J Invest Dermatol 76: 103-107
Pasternack A, Linder E (1970) Renal tubular acidosis: an immunopathological study on four patients. Clin Exp Immunol 7: 115-123
Peyronnard JM, Charron L, Beaudet F, Couture F (1982) Vasculitic neuropathy in rheumatoid disease and Sjögren's syndrome. Neurology 32: 839-845
Provost TT, Zone JJ, Synkowski DR, Maddison PJ, Reichlin M (1980) Urticaria-like lesions in SLE, I: Correlation with clinical and serological abnormalities. J Invest Dermatol 75: 495-499
Ramage JH, Kinnear WF (1956) Keratoconjunctivitis sicca and collagen diseases. Brit J Ophthal 40: 416-420
Sams WM, Thorne EG, Small P, Mass MF, McIntosh RM, Stanford RD (1976) Leukocytoclastic vasculitis. Arch Dermatol 112: 219-226
Sanchez NP, Winklemann RR, Schroefer AL, Dicken CH (1982) The clinical and histopathologic spectrums of urticarial vasculitis: study of forty cases. J Am Acad Dermatol 7: 599-604
Scott DG, Bacon PA, Allen C, Elson CJ, Wallington T (1981) IgG rheumatoid factor, complement and immune complexes in rheumatoid synovitis and vasculitis: comparative and serial studies during cytotoxic therapy. Clin Exp Immunol 43: 54-63
Shearn M (1971) Sjögren's syndrome. WB Saunders, Philadelphia
Soter NA (1977) Chronic urticaria as a manifestation of necrotizing venulitis. N Engl J Med 296: 1470
Soter NA, Austen KF, Gigli I (1974) The complement system in necrotizing angiitis of the skin: Analysis of complement component activities in serum of patients with concomitant collagen-vascular disease. J Invest Dermatol 63: 219
Soter NA, Austen KF, Gigli I (1974) Urticaria and arthralgias as manifestations of necrotizing angiitis (vasculitis). J Invest Dermatol 63: 485-490
Soter NA, Mihm MC Jr, Gigli I, Dvorak HF, Austen KF (1976) Two distinct cellular patterns in cutaneous necrotizing angiitis. J Invest Dermatol 66: 344-350
Steinberg AD, Green WT, Talal N (1971) Thrombotic thrombocytopenic purpura complicating Sjögren's syndrome. JAMA 215: 757-761
Strauss WG (1959) Purpura hyperglobulinemia of Waldenstrom. N Engl J Med 260: 857-860
Szanto L, Farkas K, Gyulai E (1957) On Sjögren's disease (1957) Rheumatism 13: 60-63
Talal N (1966) Sjögren's syndrome. Bull Rheum Dis 16: 404-407
Talal N et al (1967) Extrasalivary lymphoid abnormalities in Sjögren's syndrome (reticulum cell sarcoma, "pseudolymphoma," macroglobulinemia). Am J Med 43: 50-65
Talal N et al (1968) Renal tubular acidosis, glomerulonephritis and immunologic facts in Sjögren's syndrome. Arthritis Rheum 6: 774-786
Theofilopoulos AN, Burtonboy G, LoSpalluto JJ, Ziff M (1974) IgM rheumatoid factor and low molecular weight IgM: an association with vasculitis. Arthritis Rheum 17: 272-284
Theofilopoulos AN, Dixon FJ (1981) Etiopathogenesis of murine SLE. Immunologic Review 55: 179-216
Waldenstrom J (1943) Kliniski metooler for pavisande av hyperproteinami och deras praktiska varde for diagnostiken. Nord Med 20: 2288-2292
Waldenstrom J (1952) Abnormal proteins in myeloma. Adv Intern Med 5: 398-440
Whaley K, Webb J, McAvoy BA, Hughes GRV, Lee P, MacSween RNM, Buchanan WW (1973) Sjögren's syndrome. II. Clinical associations and immunological phenomena. Quart J Med 42: 513-548
Whitaker JN, Engel WK (1972) Vascular deposits of immunoglobulin and complement in idiopathic inflammatory myopathy. N Engl J Med 286: 333-338

Whitehouse AC, Buckley CE, Nagaya H, McCarter J (1967) Macroglobulinemia and vasculitis in Sjögren's syndrome. Am J Med 43: 609-619
Wilson R, Provost TT, Bias WB, Alexander EL, Edlow DW, Hochberg MC, Stevens MB, Arnett FC (1984) Sjögren's syndrome: Influence of multiple HLA-D region alloantigens on clinical and serologic expression. Arthritis Rheum 27: 1245-1253
Yoshinoya S, McDuffy S, Alarcon-Segovia D, Pope RM (1982) Detection and partial characterization of immune complexes in patients with rheumatoid arthritis plus Sjögren's syndrome and with Sjögren's syndrome alone. Clin Exp Immunol 48: 339-347
Zizic TM, Klaussen JN, Stevens MB (1982) Acute abdominal complications of systemic lupus erythematosus and polyarteritis nodosa. Am J Med 73: 525-531

C. Lymphoid Malignancy

1. Lymphoid Malignancy and Monoclonal Proteins

A. G. Tzioufas, H. M. Moutsopoulos and N. Talal

Introduction

Bunim and Talal (1963) first reported an increased incidence of non-Hodgkin's lymphoma in patients with SS over two decades ago and suggested that the chronic antigenic stimulation triggered a malignant transformation event. There were three cases of lymphoma and one case of Waldenstrom's macroglobulinemia which developed in 58 patients with SS. Since then, several case reports have suggested an association between SS and frank lymphoma (Talal and Bunim 1964; Hornbaker et al. 1966; Talal et al. 1967) or Waldenstrom's macroglobulinemia (Anderson and Talal 1972; Whitehouse et al. 1967) as well as an aggressive lymphoid infiltrative disorder termed "pseudolymphoma" (Talal et al. 1967). There are now over one hundred examples of this association in the medical literature (Kassan et al. 1978; Schmid et al. 1982).

Stimulated by these reports, Kassan and co-workers (1978) studied the incidence of malignancies in a population consisting of 136 female patients with SS who were diagnosed and followed-up at the NIH.

The average period of follow-up was 8.1 years per patient, covering a total of 1099 person years. In addition, an age, sex, race, and time specific matched control population was used for comparison. The relative risk (RR) was calculated by dividing the number of malignancies observed in SS patients by the number that would have been expected in the control group.

Fifteen cases of cancer (excluding skin cancer) were observed during the follow-up period. These included seven cases of non-Hodgkin's lymphoma and eight cases of other types of malignancies. The number of non-lymphoma malignancies expected, based on the rates in the general population, was 6.6. This was similar to the eight non-lymphoma malignancies observed in the SS population. In contrast, the seven cases of lymphoma were 43.8 times higher than the expected number of 0.16 in the control group. Thus, the risk of lymphoma in the SS population was about 6.4 cases per thousand per year.

The risk of lymphoma was similar for primary and secondary SS in this study, although we believe lymphoma to be more common in primary SS. In addition, the risk of lymphoma was not associated with either age or duration of SS. However, patients with parotid swelling were more prone to develop lymphoma (RR = 66.7) compared with patients without parotid swelling (RR = 12.5). In addition, two other risk factors were identified, lymphadenopathy (RR = 3.7) and splenomegaly (RR = 6.7).

Clinical Picture, Laboratory Findings and Histopathology

The autoimmune disorder may precede the development of lymphoma by intervals as long as 20 years (range 0.5–29 years), so that the natural history of this slowly evolving immunoregulatory disease can be separated into three stages (Fig. 1). Some patients with SS develop a clinical picture suggestive of malignancy which cannot be clearly classified as malignant even after tissue biopsy. Features of autoimmunity are often present. The term "pseudolymphoma" has been applied to such cases (Talal et al. 1967; Anderson and Talal 1971). The course of these patients is quite variable, and many of them respond to corticosteroids or immunosuppressive drugs. Some, however, later develop a frankly malignant lymphoma.

The lymphomas are of two major types: either composed of highly undifferentiated B cells (Zulman et al. 1978) once incorrectly termed reticulum cell sarcoma or histocytic lymphoma, or highly pleomorphic and sometimes associated with monoclonal macroglobulinemia. In the first type, antibodies tend to disappear and hypogammaglobulinemia may develop when the malignancy appears (Talal and Bunim 1964).

SS patients who develop lymphoma usually have several features of systemic extraglandular disease (Talal and Bunim 1964). The lymphoma may involve salivary glands or major parenchymal organs such as lungs, kidney, and gastrointestinal tract. One patient in our initial series died from generalized lymphoma 13 years after the resection of a localized process in the inguinal lymph nodes.

Lymphomatous involvement of the major salivary glands occurs but is infrequent in SS. It should be suspected in a patient who suddenly develops massive, firm or hard salivary gland enlargement. It is difficult to classify male patients who lack features of autoimmunity and therefore do not have an "autoimmune exocrinopa-

Benign ⟵	⟶	Malignant
Autoimmune exocrinopathy →	Pseudolymphoma →	Lymphoma
Clinical:		
Xerostomia Xerophthalmia R. A. (or another systemic rheumatic disease)	Lymphadenopathy Splenomegaly Purpura Pulmonary infiltrates Renal Infiltrates	Massive lymphadenopathy Massive salivary gland enlargement Wasting
Pathology:		
Benign lymphoid infiltrates confined to glandular tissue	Atypical extraglandular lymphoid infiltrates	B Cell Lymphoma
Serology:		
Hypergammaglobulinemia Anti-Ro and La (+)	Hypergammaglobulinemia Anti-Ro and La (+) Monoclonal spike	Hypogammaglobulinemia Loss of autoantibodies

Fig. 1. Pathogenesis of Sjögren's syndrome

thy." Indeed Mikulicz's own case may be such an example. As a rule, males presenting with parotid enlargement in the absence of RA should be evaluated carefully to rule out lymphoma, leukemia, amyloidosis, fatty parotid, alcoholism, or other metabolic/nutritional causes. Moreover, we have recently seen a male patient who showed in the same biopsy specimen lesions of both a benign lymphoproliferative process as well as a true lymphoma.

A recent immunohistologic study suggests that myoepithelial sialadenitis (formerly called the benign lymphoepithelial lesion of SS) with areas of confluent lymphoid proliferation producing mostly monoclonal IgM/kappa represents a "manifest malignant lymphoma" (Schmid et al. 1982). These were all immunocytomas or immunoblastic lymphomas (i.e. all B cell lymphomas). These lesions were considered "early lymphomas", analogous to carcinoma *in situ,* which after a variable latent period, transformed into true lymphomas. There were no cases of germinal center cell lymphoma or Hodgkin's disease.

SS patients who develop lymphoma may lose their autoantibodies and even develop hypogammaglobulinemia with immunodeficiency and lowered resistance to ordinary bacterial infections. Zulman et al. (1978) studied biopsies from SS patients with lymphoma with an immunoperoxidase technique and showed that these lymphomas are primarily of B-cell origin having exclusively IgMk immunoglobulin in their cytoplasm. A sequential progression from Ig-positive to Ig-negative stages could be demonstrated immunohistologically, analogous to the progression from hyper- to hypogammaglobulinemia.

Monoclonal Immunoglobulins in SS Patients

There is evidence to suggest that monoclonal immunoglobulins and RF may be produced very early in the salivary glands in SS (Anderson et al. 1972). Sometimes monoclonal immunoglobulins are part of the pseudolymphoma process, while in other patients they appear to represent a neoplasm from the disease onset. It is often difficult to distinguish between these two possibilities.

Isotype differences have been observed in the monoclonal immunoglobulins found in lymphoma cells or in serum of SS patients from different ethnic groups. North American SS patients with lymphoma have IgMκ cytoplasmic immunoglobulins (Zulman et al. 1978). Another study from Mexico (Diaz-Zuanen 1981) showed that the monoclonal lymphoid cells contain IgMλ monoclonal immunoglobulin. Finally, Japanese patients with SS have a high incidence of IgA or IgG gammopathies II.C.3.

Papadopoulos et al. (1967, 1982) have introduced a new high resolution agarose gel electrophoresis. This method can detect minute amounts of monoclonal immunoglobulins which are undetectable by routine electrophoretic methods. Identification of the monoclonal immunoglobulins is performed by immunofixation using monospecific antisera to human κ, λ light and α, γ and μ chains (Pascali et al. 1982). With this method, Magrath et al. (1983) demonstrated the in vitro production and circulation of a monoclonal IgM in lymphoma patients without SS. This finding and the previous knowledge that SS patients develop B-cell lymphomas prompted a study of the serum and urine of SS patients. It was shown that 67% of 21 American patients with primary SS had monoclonal bands in their serum which, by immunofixation, were identified as λ light chains (Moutsopoulos et al. 1983). The highest proportion of monoclonal light chains was observed in patients with extraglandular features (100%); in contrast, only 22% of patients with sicca complex (glandular SS) had monoclonal light chains.

A second study with Greek patients further substantiated these findings, demonstrating that 70% of SS patients with extraglandular involvement had monoclonal immunoglobulins and/or light chains in their serum (Moutsopoulos et al. 1985). In addition, all patients excreted monoclonal light chains in the urine (Moutsopoulos et al. 1985). Retrospective serial studies on frozen sera from SS patients who developed lymphoma were not possible because the monoclonal immunoglobulins were not detected even after a limited storage at −20 °C.

In agreement with our study (Moutsopoulos et al. 1985), Walters et al. (1986) failed to demonstrate monoclonal light chains in the urine of three primary SS patients without extraglandular manifestations or in patients with probable or secondary SS. However, three patients with SS who developed lymphoma had such monoclonal light chains. Interestingly, in one patient with lymphoma the level of urinary free light chains was monitored and correlated with disease activity.

Patients with primary SS have a high incidence of cryoglobulins in their sera (Tzioufas et al. 1986). The presence of cryoglobulins is associated with higher prevalence of extraglandular disease and autoantibodies to Ro (SS-A) and RF, as compared to patients without cryoglobulins. The type of cryoglobulin was investigated by high resolution agarose gel electrophoresis combined with immunofixation. It was demonstrated that these are mixed cryoglobulins containing an IgMκ monoclonal immunoglobulin.

Furthermore, Fox et al. (1986), using a monoclonal antibody (MoAb 17-109) and immunoblotting, have shown that monoclonal rheumatoid factors in 12 of 15 patients with primary SS contain on their κ chain a cross-reactive idiotype which is shared by the monoclonal rheumatoid factors found in patients with Waldenstrom's macroglobulinemia and lymphoma. This cross-reactive idiotype is also present on cytoplasmic immunoglobulins of B cells from salivary gland biopsies as demonstrated by immunoperoxidase techniques on stained frozen tissue sections. It is of great interest that serial biopsies studied over a 4-year period revealed a progressive increase in the proportion of B cells bearing the cross-reactive idiotype (Fox et al. 1986).

It is primary SS among all autoimmune diseases that frequently exhibits this monoclonal expression. In fact, patients with SLE, RA and scleroderma very rarely display monoclonal light chains and/or immunoglobulins in their serum and urine (Moutsopoulos et al. 1983; Moutsopoulos et al. 1985). In addition, the cryoglobulins of these patients are mixed polyclonal in type (Tzioufas et al. 1986). Finally, B cells in the synovial membrane of patients with classical RA (another tissue which is known as an active site of rheumatoid factor synthesis) do not express the cross-reactive idiotype found in primary SS patients (Fox et al. 1986).

Review of the above data leads to speculation that patients with primary SS often contain a B cell subset producing monoclonal immunoglobulins. Most of these B cells are located in affected salivary glands rather than in the circulation (Fox et al. 1986). These observations complement the histologically demonstrated "in situ"

Table 1. Monoclonality expressed early and is selective

1. Monoclonal Ig and RF produced in salivary gland
2. Monoclonal IgM/kappa in USA
3. Monoclonal IgG and IgA in Japan
4. One particular RF (kappa chain idiotype) expressed in serum and salivary gland
5. Homogeneous light chain bands

lymphoma described by Schmidt et al. (1982). Monoclonality is expressed very early (Table 1), together with polyclonal B cell activation (Tzioufas et al. 1986) and progressively increases (Fox et al. 1986). Serial follow up of these patients should help determine whether monoclonal expression is a marker for lymphoma development in Sjögren's syndrome.

Conclusion

The clinical and laboratory data suggest that SS is a disease of unusually aggressive B-cell activation which begins in the salivary glands and later becomes extraglandular with a strong propensity to malignant transformation at any time in its course (Table 1).The finding of monoclonal immunoglobulins or light chains in many SS patients suggests that a monoclonal process is present very early and coexists with the polyclonal B-cell disorder.

This natural history of lymphoproliferation in SS suggests a multistage process analogous to carcinogenesis. Patients may progress through three stages: 1) *initiation,* in which isolated salivary gland lesions or perhaps only serum autoantibodies may be present in otherwise asymptomatic patients, 2) *promotion* into frank SS, perhaps with pseudolymphoma and monoclonal Ig, 3) *progression* to B cell lymphoma with possible accompanying hypogammaglobulinemia and immunodeficiency (Fig. 2). Careful serial immunohistologic studies (Schmid et al. 1982; Zulman et al. 1978) as well as clinical studies (Talal and Bunim 1964; Talal et al. 1967; Anderson and Talal 1971) support this concept of pathogenesis.

This sequence in SS is analogous to the relationship between benign monoclonal spikes and myeloma/macroglobulinemia, or between ARC (AIDS-Related Com-

Autoimmunity	Initiation Serum autoantibodies (RO:SS-A)	→	Promotion Sjögren's syndrome Pseudolymphoma	→	Progression B cell lymphoma Immunodeficiency
Malignancy		Benign monoclonal Spike		Myeloma Macroglobulinemia	
		AIDS-related Complex		AIDS	

Fig. 2. Autoimmunity and malignancy are multistage processes

Table 2. Similarities between AIDS and Sjögren's syndrome

Polyclonal B cell activation
Immune complexes
Increased serum βeta-2-microglobulin
Acid labile interferon
Decreased autologous mixed lymphocyte response
Decreased interleukin-2
Decreased natural killer cells
Lymphoma development

Table 3. Possible immune mechanisms contributing to lymphoma

1. Polyclonal B cell activation
2. Decreased IL-2 production and T cell effector function
3. Activated T cells (OKT10 and HLA-DR positive)
4. Decreased NK cell activity
5. Absence of Leu-11 cells in salivary gland

plex) and AIDS (Acquired Immunodeficiency Syndrome). Indeed, many immunologic features occur commonly in both SS and AIDS patients (Table 2).

SS is not the only disease in which this progression from an autoimmune process to a lymphoma occurs. A recent study found lymphoproliferative malignancies in 10 of 489 patients (2.2%) (RR = 24.1) with rheumatoid arthritis developing after a mean interval of 11.8 years. As in SS, cytotoxic drugs could not be implicated in pathogenesis and the lymphomas were mostly B cell (non-Hodgkin's) in type (Symmons 1984).

A spectrum of immunopathology combining features of autoimmunity with benign or malignant lymphoproliferation also occurs following experimental chronic graft-vs-host disease (Pal et al. 1985). Moreover, patients with chronic GVH may develop histologic changes in the salivary glands resembling SS (Gratwhol et al. 1977).

There are numerous immune abnormalities in SS patients that may contribute to the transformation from a benign polyclonal reactive response into a malignant proliferation (Table 3). The intense polyclonal B cell activation in SS could be an initiating event setting the stage for the emergence of a malignant B cell clone. Activated B cells are present in the salivary gland lesions (Segerberg-Konttinen et al.). Promoting mechanisms might be intrinsic to B cells (e.g. oncogene activation, viral expression) as well as extrinsic (e.g. immunoregulatory failure to control B cells). There is abundant evidence for such failure in SS including inappropriate activation of B and T cells in the lesions, impaired IL-2 production and NK cell activity (Miyasaka et al. 1983), and the absence of NK cells (Leu-11 positive) in the salivary gland lesions (Fox et al. 1985; Moutsopoulos et al. 1986) where Ig production is so excessive (Talal et al. 1970).

References

Anderson LG, Cummings NA, Asofsky R, Hylton MB, Tarpley TM Jr, Tomasi TB Jr, Wolf RO, Schall GL, Talal N (1972) Salivary gland immunoglobulin and rheumatoid factor synthesis in Sjögren's syndrome. Natural history and response to treatment. Am J Med 53: 456

Anderson LG, Talal N (1972) The spectrum of benign to malignant lymphoproliferation in Sjögren's syndrome. Clin Exp Immunol 9: 199-219

Bunim JJ, Talal N (1963) The association of malignant lymphoma with Sjögren's syndrome. Trans Assoc Am Phys 76: 45-56

Diaz-Zuanen E, Ruiz-Arguelles G, Vega-Ortiz JM, Villareal G, Alarcon-Segovia D (1981) From benign polyclonal to malignant monoclonal lymphoproliferation in a patient with primary Sjögren's syndrome. Arth Rheum 24: 850-853

Fox RI, Chen P, Carson DA, Fong S (1986) Expression of a cross-reactive idiotype on rheumatoid factor in patients with Sjögren's syndrome. J Immunol 136: 477-483

Gratwohl AA, Moutsopoulos HM, Chused TM, Akizuki M, Wolf RO, Sweet JB, Deisseroth AB (1977) Sjögren type syndrome after allogeneic bone marrow transplantation. Ann Intern Med 87: 703-706

Hornbaker JH, Forster EA, Williams GS, Davis JS (1966) Sjögren's syndrome and nodular reticulum cell sarcoma. Arch Intern Med 118: 449-452

Kassan S, Thomas T, Moutsopoulos HM, et al. (1978) Increased risk of lymphoma in sicca syndrome. Ann Intern Med 89: 888-892

Magrath I, Benjamin D, Papadopoulos NM (1983) Serum monoclonal immunoglobulin bands in undifferentiated lymphomas of Burkitt and non-Burkitt types. Blood 61: 26-31

Miyasaka N, Seaman W, Bakshi A, Sauvezie B, Strand V, Pope R, Talal N (1983) Natural killing activity in Sjögren's syndrome: an analysis of defective mechanisms. Arth Rheum 26 (8): 954-960

Moutsopoulos HM, Steinberg AD, Fauci AS, Lane HC, Papadopoulos NM (1983) High incidence of free monoclonal γ light chains in the sera of patients with Sjögren's syndrome. J Immunol 130: 2263-2265

Moutsopoulos HM, Costello R, Drosos AA, Mavridis AK, Papadopoulos NM (1985) Demonstration and identification of monoclonal proteins in the urine of patients with Sjögren's syndrome. Ann Rheum Dis 44: 109-112

Moutsopoulos HM, Hooks JJ, Chan CC, Dalavanga YA, Skopouli FN, Dietrick B (1986). HLA-DR expression by labial minor salivary gland tissues in Sjögren's syndrome. Ann Rheum Dis 45: 677-683

Pals ST, Radaszkiewicz T, Roozendaal L, Gleichmann E (1985) Chronic progressive polyarthritis and other symptoms of collagen vascular disease induced by graft-vs-host reaction. J Immunol 134: 1475-1482

Papadopoulos NM, Kintzios JA (1967) Differentiation of pathological conditions by visual evaluation of serum protein electrophoretic patterns. Proc Soc Exp Biol Med 123: 927-929

Papadopoulos NM, Elin RJ, Wilson DM (1982) Incidence of γ-globulin banding in the healthy population by high resolution electrophoresis. Clin Chem 28: 707-709

Schmid U, Helbron D, Lennert K (1982) Development of malignant lymphoma in myoepithelial sialadenitis (Sjögren's syndrome). Pathol Anat 395: 11-43

Segerberg-Konttinen M, Bergroth V, Jungell P, Malmstrom M, Nordstrom D, Sane J, Immonen I, Konttinen YT (manuscript submitted) Lymphocytes activation in Sjögren's syndrome

Strand V, Talal N (1980) Advances in the diagnosis and concept of Sjögren's syndrome (autoimmune exocrinopathy). Bull Rheum Dis 30: 1046-1052

Sugai S, Konda S, Shirasaka T, Murayama T, Nishikawa T (1980) Non-IgM monoclonal gammopathy in patients with Sjögren's syndrome. Am J Med 68: 861-867

Symmons DPM (1984) Neoplasms of the immune system in rheumatoid arthritis. Am J Med 78: 22-28

Talal N, Bunim JJ (1964) Development of malignant lymphoma in the course of Sjögren's syndrome. Am J Med 36: 529-540

Talal N, Sokoloff L, Barth WF (1967) Extrasalivary lymphoid abnormalities in Sjögren's syndrome (reticulum-cell-sarcoma, "pseudolymphoma", macroglobulinemia). Am J Med 43: 50-65

Talal N, Asofsky R, Lightbody P (1970) Immunoglobulin synthesis by salivary gland lymphoid cells in Sjögren's syndrome. J Clin Invest 49: 49-54

Talal N, Dauphinee MJ, Ahmed SA, Christadoss P (1983) Sex factors in immunity and autoimmunity. In: Progress in Immunology V, Yanamura Y, Tada T (eds) Academic Press, NY, pp 1589–1600

Talal N (in press) The etiology of systemic lupus erythematosus. In: Third Edition of Monograph on Lupus Erythematosus, Dubois E, Wallace D (eds) Lea and Febiger, Philadelphia, PA

Tzioufas AG, Manoussakis MN, Costello R, Silis M, Papadopoulos NM, Moutsopoulos HM (1986) Cryoglobulinemia in autoimmune rheumatic diseases: Evidence of circulating monoclonal cryoglobulins in patients with primary Sjögren's syndrome. Arth Rheum (In press)

Walters MT, Stevenson FK, Herbert A, Cawley MID, Smith JL (1986) Urinary monoclonal free light chains in primary Sjögren's syndrome: an aid to the diagnosis of malignant lymphoma. Ann Rheum Dis 45: 210–219

Whitehouse AC, Burkley CE, Nagaya H, McCarter J (1967) Macroglobulinemia and yasculitis in Sjögren's syndrome. Am J Med 43: 609–619

Zulman J, Jaffe R, Talal N (1978) Evidence that the malignant lymphoma of Sjögren's syndrome is a monoclonal B-cell neoplasm. N Eng J Med 299: 1215–1220

2. Detection of Lymphoma in Sjögren's Syndrome by Analysis of Immunoglobulin Gene Rearrangements*

M. L. CLEARY, N. GALILI, N. LEVY, N. TALAL, and J. SKLAR

The marked predilection for the development of lymphoma in patients with Sjögren's syndrome (SS) has been well-documented in recent years (Talal and Bunim, 1964 ; Talal et al. 1967; Kassan et al. 1978). In view of this fact, biopsy tissues obtained from Sjögren's patients must be carefully scrutinized for atypical lymphoid proliferations that may prompt the diagnosis of lymphoma, sometimes before the lymphoma is clinically manifest. However, using morphologic criteria alone, the diagnosis of lymphoma in tissue sections of biopsy material from Sjögren's patients is often difficult.

In part, the difficulty of diagnosing lymphoma in specimens from SS patients reflects the considerable problems associated with the histologic diagnosis of lymphoma in general. Paramount among these problems is that cytologically, neoplastic lymphocytes may resemble normal lymphocytes under various conditions of activation. Additional difficulty in SS derives from the frequency with which lymphoma in these patients arises in or involves extranodal sites. Lymphoma in these patients may present in lymph nodes, but more often it is found within lymphoid infiltrates present in salivary glands, lungs, kidneys, bone marrow, gastrointestinal tract, and skin (Heckmayr et al. 1976). When lymphoma involves these extranodal sites, some of the observations usually helpful in making the diagnosis of lymphoma are not applicable. For instance, effacement of the normal anatomical architecture of the lymph node, a valuable criterion of lymphoma in the usual intranodal situation, cannot be used. Instead, diagnosis must rely entirely upon atypical cytologic features of lymphocytes and the homogeneous, monomorphic cellular composition of the lymphoid infiltrates that is the consequence of the clonal nature of the lymphomatous proliferation. Assessment of these tissues is further complicated by the frequent necessity of distinguishing small foci of early lymphoma among the numerous reactive lymphocytes within the biopsy tissue (Schmid et al. 1982).

To some degree, immunophenotyping of tissue sections has simplified the task of diagnosing lymphoma in SS, as well as indicating several important points about the biology of these neoplasms. Primarily, the impact of these techniques has been to permit identification of clonal lymphoid proliferations, by determining the presence of lymphocytes containing monotypic cellular immunoglobulins restricted to either the kappa or lambda light chain type (Zulman et al. 1978; Schmid et al. 1982). These techniques have also demonstrated that although the histology of these lesions varies (the majority are diffuse large cell tumors, often showing immunoblastic differentiation, while smaller numbers are low-grade, small cell tumors),

* This work was supported by grants CA38621 and CA34233. MLC is a Lucille P. Markey Scholar.

almost all are B cell neoplasms (Heckmayr et al. 1976; Kassan et al. 1978; Colby and Dorfman 1979; Schmid et al. 1982). Finally, immunophenotyping has highlighted the subtle focal pattern of involvement by early lymphoma frequently encountered in Sjögren's disease (Schmid et al. 1982).

Despite the considerable advance that immunophenotyping has represented for diagnosing lymphoma, both as a whole and specifically in SS, this method has a number of problems associated with it. These have been discussed elsewhere (Cleary et al. 1984a) and mostly relate to obtaining tissue and antibody reagents of high quality, to the reproducible interpretation of the results, and to the diagnosis of lymphomas which fail to express cellular immunoglobulins. An additional problem of special relevance in SS is the possibility of missing a small cluster of neoplastic lymphocytes during sectioning of the biopsy or failure to detect within a section a clonal population of lymphocytes evenly admixed among benign lymphocytes.

Recently the method of immunogenotyping has been introduced to facilitate the diagnosis of lymphoma in cases that appear equivocal by conventional histopathology or immunophenotyping (Cleary et al. 1984a). We have begun to explore the application of this technique to SS and have obtained results that indicate that this method will probably contribute to the evaluation of Sjögren's biopsy specimens for lymphoma in the future.

Immunogenotyping involves analysis of clonal rearrangements of DNA within antigen receptor genes - immunoglobulin and T cell receptor genes - of biopsy specimens (Cleary and Sklar 1985; Sklar et al. 1986). Immunoglobulin genes are analyzed in the diagnosis of B cell processes and T cell receptor genes in T cell processes. Given the B cell derivation of the great majority of lymphomas in SS, analysis of immunoglobulin genes is clearly the most pertinent form of immunogenotyping in the present context. Further discussion will therefore concentrate on these genes.

There are three immunoglobulin genes in the human genome. One of these encodes the heavy chain immunoglobulin gene and the other two encode the light chain genes kappa and lambda, respectively. Prototypic immunoglobulin molecules consist of two identical heavy chain polypeptides and two identical light chain polypeptides. The outstanding biologic feature of these proteins is their specificity for the binding of a wide variety of antigens based on the variation in amino acid sequences from immunoglobulin to immunoglobulin molecule. Studies of the genes for these molecules, using recombinant DNA techniques, have revealed that to a great extent the diversity among immunoglobulin proteins is generated by an unusual structure and physiology of the immunoglobulin genes (in fact, the only other known genes with similar properties are the recently discovered and functionally analogous T cell receptor genes).

In the germline and all non-hematopoietic tissues each of the three immunoglobulin genes is divided into three or four segments (four segments in the heavy chain gene, three segments in the light chain genes). All but one of these segments is represented by at least several related but unique copies of coding sequence spread out along large distances of DNA in each gene. During B cell development a series of recombination events take place first in the DNA of the heavy chain genes and then in the DNA of the light chain genes. In the course of these rearrangements, one copy from each set of segments is brought together to create a contiguous, intact immunoglobulin gene. One or both alleles of each gene may rearrange in this manner, but only one allele is ever functional within a single lymphocyte. Diversity of immunoglobulin protein structure is largely a result of the many different possible combinations with which the individual gene segments from the three or four sets of segments can assemble into a functional immunoglobulin gene. Once immunoglobulin gene rearrangement has occurred, the configuration of DNA in the rearranged locus appears to be fixed. Consequently, this configuration is a marker for the B cell in which it is present and any clonal progeny of that cell.

Analysis of the configuration of DNA in rearranged immunoglobulin genes is carried out by way of the Southern blot hybridization procedure (Southern 1975). In this procedure, DNA is extracted from a biopsy specimen and digested *in vitro* by a bacterial restriction enzyme that cuts the DNA at numerous defined sites specific for each different kind of restriction enzyme. For analysis of immunoglobulin genes, one of several usable enzymes is selected that places cuts on either side of a region of the gene in which recombination takes place during the normal process of gene rearrangement. In unrearranged DNA, cleavage with this restriction enzyme produces a fragment of immunoglobulin DNA which has characteristic and predictable size. However, after rearrangement, the size of this fragment changes because of recombination of DNA within this region. The length of the restriction fragment derived from this region of DNA depends upon how rearrangement has taken place - that is, which gene segments have been substituted in this region. The end effect is that the length of the restriction fragment generated from this region of DNA is a specific marker for the configuration of DNA in this rearranged locus and, in turn, for the individual lymphocyte in which it has occurred (Arnold et al. 1983; Cleary et al. 1984a; Cleary et al. 1984b).

To detect both germline and rearranged fragments, the restriction fragments in a digest of total biopsy DNA are separated by size using agarose gel electrophoresis. After electrophoresis, fragments of different sizes form invisible bands in the gel which are then transferred from the gel onto a membrane to which the DNA fragments stick, forming a replica of the bands as they were situated in the gel prior to transfer. To recognize the immunoglobulin bands from the many thousands of other bands on this membrane, the membrane is hybridized with a radiolabeled fragment of immunoglobulin DNA prepared by molecular cloning techniques. This fragment, referred to as a probe, recognizes and binds only to bands on the membrane that contain homologous DNA sequences. After hybridization, rinsing, and drying of the membrane, autoradiography is performed using a standard X-ray film. The final product of the analysis is an autoradiogram which reveals the positions of bands containing DNA of the particular immunoglobulin gene being tested.

A feature of the Southern blot procedure critical for diagnosing lymphoma is that it detects rearranged bands in autoradiograms only if about 1% or more of the cells within a biopsy specimen contain the same immunoglobulin gene rearrangement (Cleary et al. 1984a). Uniform rearrangements present in clonal populations of cells composing a smaller fraction of the specimen are not generally detectable by this method. In other words, a reactive benign lymphoid proliferation will show only germline bands due to unrearranged immunoglobulin alleles in some portion of the lymphocytes and in all nonlymphoid elements within the biopsy (for example, endothelial cells, fibroblasts, granulocytes, and epithelial cells). Although numerous rearranged immunoglobulin genes lie within the lymphocytes of such tissues, none of the lymphocytes represent clones above the 1% threshold of detection. In analysis of biopsy specimens containing lymphoma, in which the lymphomatous cells exceed a concentration of 1%, the germline bands will still be present, but in addition, one or two rearranged bands will also be visible. These correspond to rearrangement of one or both alleles for the immunoglobulin gene being analyzed, and will have an intensity roughly proportional to the ratio of the lymphoma to other cells within the specimen.

Figure 1 illustrates application of these principles to two cases of lymphoma in SS. Case 1 is a 71-year-old white woman who had a ten-year history of swelling of the submandibular glands eventually leading to bilateral submandibular gland resection in 1977. There was no history of a connective tissue disease, but the patient described symptoms of dry mouth and a sandy sensation in the eyes. Sections of the submandibular gland showed lymphocytic infiltration and islands of myoepithelial proliferation characteristic of Mikulicz's disease. Over the subsequent five years, the patient noted progressive enlargement of both parotid glands. These were biopsied in 1982 and showed reactive lymphoid follicles with germinal centers and interfollicular lymphocytic infiltrates that appeared atypical. However, an unequivocal diagnosis of lymphoma could not be made. Two years later a follow-up biopsy of the right parotid gland was performed and revealed histologic features unchanged from 1982. Studies of cell surface immunoglobulin in this specimen

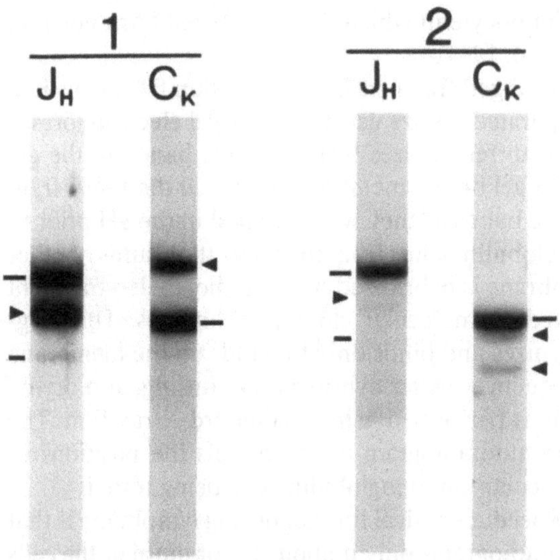

Fig. 1. Autoradiograms showing clonal rearrangements of immunoglobulin genes in biopsy tissues from patients with Sjögren's disease.
Each analysis was performed with 10 μg of DNA digested with Bam HI restriction enzyme and electrophoresed in a 0.8% agarose gel. After transfer to nylon membranes, the DNA was hybridized with a ^{32}P-labeled J_H DNA probe, which detects rearrangements of the heavy chain locus regardless of the class of heavy chain expressed by the lymphocytes, or a C_K probe which detects rearrangements of the kappa light chain locus. The bars indicate germline bands and the arrows indicate clonal rearranged bands

were reported to show a polyclonal pattern. The patient has continued to the present time with findings similar to those described above. The parotids have remained enlarged but there has been no adenopathy or hepatosplenomegaly. The patient has received no form of therapy.

Analysis of immunoglobulin gene rearrangements was performed on one of the parotid biopsy specimens from 1982. Both heavy chain and kappa light chain studies show a single non-germline band consistent with a single clone of neoplastic B lymphocytes in which one rearrangement had occurred in both the heavy chain and kappa light chain loci.

Case 2 is a 55-year-old white woman with a 20 year history of dry mouth and eyes, intermittent parotid swelling, and Raynaud's phenomenon. In 1982, this patient developed a perihilar mass, lung lesions, and multiple erythematous skin plaques. Enlarged soft and mobile lymph nodes were palpated in the cervical and axillary regions but there was no hepatosplenomegaly. Biopsies of the lung and skin showed angiocentric lymphoid infiltrates, some of which were felt to contain atypical lymphocytes. Biopsy specimens of minor salivary glands and the perihilar mass showed only reactive changes. Staining for cellular immunoglobulins in the lung and skin specimens revealed an excess of mu/kappa immunoglobulins suggesting a clonal lymphoproliferative process. The patient was begun on low dose cyclophosphamide and prednisone in 1983 and generally has done well with resolution of skin and lung lesions but persistence of dry eyes and mouth.

The tissue analyzed for immunoglobulin gene rearrangements was a specimen of skin removed prior to the therapy. The results of these analyses show a single rearranged band for the heavy chain gene and two rearranged bands for the kappa light chain gene. This tissue, therefore, probably contained a monoclonal B cell lymphoma in which one heavy chain gene and two kappa light chain genes had rearranged.

The results obtained in these two cases demonstrate a number of advantages intrinsic in the method of immunogenotyping for diagnosing lymphoma. First, the diagnostic data is more objective than that obtained by histopathology or immunophenotyping. A clonal population of B cells is indicated by a simple presence or absence of non-germline bands. Both cases in Figure 1 illustrate this point by showing non-germline bands indicative of a major clonal population of B cells despite morphologic diagnoses of atypia that in neither case could be called definite lymphoma. In case 1, the rearranged bands are intense, suggesting that there was abundant lymphoma in the specimen, although, as mentioned, this could not be determined morphologically.

Another strength of immunogenotyping is that this technique offers the opportunity to independently confirm a diagnosis by separately analyzing two or three immunoglobulin genes, if necessary by utilizing several hybridization probes and a number of different restriction enzymes that are appropriate for each gene. The usefulness of this feature is well illustrated by case 2, in which analysis of heavy chain immunoglobulin rearrangements showed only one light rearranged band. This band may have been overlooked under some circumstances; however, two clear rearranged bands were found in kappa light chain gene analysis in the same tissue, providing an unequivocal diagnosis of a lymphoproliferative process in this specimen.

Sensitivity is another positive attribute of the Southern hybridization procedure. The sensitivity of the procedure for detecting minor clonal constituents in biopsy tissues has already been discussed. The technique is also extremely sensitive with regard to the amount of total material required for each analysis. In practice, each analysis for a single immunoglobulin gene requires a minimum of about 10^6 cells, which is the equivalent of about 1 milligram or 1 cubic millimeter of tissue (Cleary et al. 1984a). This means that biopsy specimens can almost always be divided for simultaneous evaluation by histopathology, immunophenotyping, and immunogenotyping. In addition, immunogenotyping can be satisfactorily performed on specimens of the size obtained by percutaneous thin-needle aspiration (Hu et al. 1986). Such procedures are particularly relevant for SS in which one may wish to avoid excisional biopsy of a parotid gland because of potential damage to the facial nerve.

Fresh or fresh frozen tissue constitutes the best material for immunogenotyping, although even tissue obtained several days after death often gives good results. The tissue used for immunogenotyping must be stored frozen, but it can simply be placed in a tube at −20 °C maintained this way indefinitely. Drying does not affect the reliability of the test.

Besides a number of significant virtues, analysis of immunoglobulin gene rearrangements also carries with it several limitations and the potential for certain kinds of artifacts. The major theoretical limitation of immunogenotyping for diagnosing lymphoma is that a positive result - detection of a non-germline band in Southern blot autoradiograms - is not absolutely specific for lymphoma. Rather, the presence of these bands indicates a clonal proliferation of lymphocytes within the tissue being tested. Fortunately, clonal proliferations of B lymphoid cells appear to be uncommon outside of neoplasia. However, at least one clinical entity exists, namely, benign monoclonal gammopathy, suggesting that benign clonal B lymphoid proliferations do occur on occasion. In this condition, analysis of immunoglobulin gene rearrangements would not distinguish these benign cells from malignant ones. Consequently, immunoglobulin gene rearrangements should always be used in conjunction with histologic and immunophenotypic data whenever possible.

So-called DNA polymorphisms can also represent a problem in immunogenotypic analyses. These inherited, phenotypically silent mutations in the DNA of a given individual may result in germline bands having positions that differ from the positions of these bands in the general population. The possibility exists that such bands may be mistaken for rearranged bands in analyses of tissues that actually lack clonal populations of B cells. This appears to be a rare event since polymorphisms with the enzymes usually used (Bam HI, Eco RI, and Hind III) are either infrequent or are known to occur at specific sites in the DNA, producing an alternative pattern of germline bands which can be easily recognized. If need arises, control tissue from the same patient (e.g., blood) can be used to show the positions of germline bands in normal tissues.

Another type of potential artifact involves incomplete or partial digestion of DNA. Failure to completely digest the DNA prior to gel electrophoresis may lead to spurious rearranged bands within autoradiograms at discrete positions above that of the germline bands because some germline immunoglobulin fragments do not become separated from the DNA of flanking fragments during the digestion. Therefore, care must be taken to be sure that the digest of DNA had proceeded to completion before large bands at certain positions are regarded as indicating clonal rearrangements.

A final limitation of immunoglobulin gene rearrangement analysis is the time and labor required to produce interpretable results. At the present time this is probably the major drawback of immunogenotyping. The technique currently takes about seven days from start to finish in order to obtain diagnostic data. In addition several steps in the procedure require technical skill and close adherence to the Southern blot protocol. However, considerable efforts are now being made to automate the Southern blot hybridization technique and some progress has already been achieved in certain phases of the methodology. Further advances can probably be expected in the near future, and these will undoubtedly expand the role of immunogenotyping in the diagnosis of lymphoma in SS and other clinical settings.

Acknowledgements

The authors wish to thank Dr. Kim Margolin for her cooperation in these studies.

References

Arnold A, Cossman J, Bakhshi A, Jaffe ES, Waldmann TA, Korsmeyer SJ (1983) Immunoglobulin gene rearrangement as unique clonal markers in human lymphoid neoplasms. N Engl J Med 309: 1593-1598

Cleary ML, Chao J, Warnke R, Sklar J (1984a) Immunoglobulin gene rearrangement as a diagnostic criterion of B cell lymphoma. Proc Natl Acad Sci USA 81: 593-597

Cleary ML, Warnke R, Sklar J (1984b) Monoclonality of lymphoproliferative lesions in cardiac-transplant recipients: Clonal analysis based on immunoglobulin-gene rearrangements. N Engl J Med 30: 477-482

Cleary ML, Sklar J (1985) DNA rearrangements in non-Hodgkin's lymphomas. Cancer Surveys 4: 331-348

Colby TV, Dorfman RF (1979) Malignant lymphoma involving salivary glands. Pathol Annu 14: 307-324

Heckmayr M, Seifert G, Donath K (1976) Malignant lymphomas and immunosialadenitis. Laryngol Rhinol Otol (Stultg) 55: 593-607

Hu E, Horning SJ, Flynn S, Brown S, Warnke R, Sklar J (1986) Diagnosis of B cell lymphoma by analysis of immunoglobulin gene rearrangements in biopsy specimens obtained by fine needle aspirations. J Clin Onc 4: 278-283

Kassan SS, Thomas TL, Moutsopolos HM, Hoover R, Kimberly RP, Budman DR, Costa J, Decker IG, Chused TM (1978) Increased risk of lymphoma in Sicca syndrome. Ann Intern Med 89: 888-892

Schmid U, Helbron D, Lennert K (1982) Development of malignant lymphoma in myoepithelial sialadenitis (Sjögren's syndrome). Virchows Arch (Pathol Anat) 395: 11-43

Sklar J, Weiss LM, Cleary ML (1986) The diagnostic molecular biology of non-Hodgkin's lymphoma. In: Berard CW, Dorfman RF (eds) Malignant lymphoma, leukemia, and the immune system: from cacaphony to clarity. Williams and Wilkins, Baltimore. In press.

Southern EM (1975) Detection of specific sequences among DNA fragments separated by gel electrophoresis. J Mol Biol 98: 503-517

Talal N, Bumin JJ (1964) The development of malignant lymphoma in the course of Sjögren's syndrome. Am J Med 36: 529-540

Talal N, Sokoloff L, Barth WF (1967) Extrasalivary lymphoid abnormalities in Sjögren's syndrome (reticulum cell sarcoma, "pseudolymphoma," macroglobulinemia). Am J Med 43: 50-64

Zulman J, Jaffe R, Talal N (1978) Evidence that the malignant lymphoma of Sjögren's syndrome is a monoclonal B-cell neoplasm. N Engl J Med 299: 1215-1220

3. Lymphoproliferative Disorders in Japanese Patients with Sjögren's Syndrome

SUSUMU SUGAI, SHIRO SHIMIZU, SUSUMU KONDA, and NOBUYUKI MIYASAKA

Introduction

Sjögren's syndrome (SS) is characterized by lymphoproliferation in exocrine organs such as the salivary and lacrimal glands, and in various extraglandular sites such as the lymphoid system, the liver, kidneys, muscles and lungs. A high incidence of lymphoproliferative disorders (LPD) has occurred in SS (Talal and Bunim 1964; Talal et al. 1967; Anderson and Talal 1971; Kassan et al. 1978; Zulman et al. 1978). According to Talal (1974), SS can be divided into three stages. The first is benign, localized, and characterized by hypergammaglobulinemia and the presence of multiple autoantibodies; the second is benign, generalized, and associated with generalized lymphoid hyperplasia, pseudolymphoma, and macroglobulinemia; and the third is malignant with lymphoid malignancy, e.g., reticulum cell sarcoma. The association of LPD is described in animal models of autoimmunity such as NZB/W F1 (Talal and Steinberg 1974), MRL/l and BXSB (Andrews et al. 1978) mice. Immunological disorders such as B cell hyperactivity and T cell dysfunction observed in mice and humans are possible factors that link SS to the development of LPD.

In this study we describe some features of Japanese SS patients and LPD such as monoclonal gammopathies and malignant lymphomas, and also discuss some differences between Japanese and non-Japanese SS patients.

Clinical Features

Because of the subtlety of many SS symptoms, its presence was determined through careful questioning for symptoms of xerophthalmia and xerostomia, and parotid pain and swelling. Our diagnoses were based primarily on the criteria of the Japan SS Research Committee (Ofuji 1977). These criteria include patients who have sicca syndrome of unknown etiology and more than one of the following: 1) keratoconjunctivitis sicca (KCS) of unknown etiology (more than +2 abnormal staining with rose bengal dye and positive results from Schirmer's tests or fluorescence staining tests), 2) characteristic histological abnormalities of lacrimal or salivary glands (more than one aggregate around the salivary ducts consisting of more than 50 mononuclear cells in a lobule) and 3) characteristic sialographic abnormalities (diffuse, punctate or spotty opaque shadows of more than 1 mm in diameter). Instead of 3), however, we often substituted the abnormal findings of sequential salivary scintigraphy assessed according to the criteria of Schall et al. (1971). Table 1

Table 1. Symptoms, signs and tests for dry mouth and eyes

	+	Patients	%
Dry mouth and/or eyes	80	92	97.5
Parotid pain and/or swelling	27	92	29.3
Angular cheilitis	20	89	22.5
Abnormalities in			
Schirmer's test	87	92	94.6
Rose bengal staining	52	57	91.7
Salivary flow	85	91	93.4
Scintigraphy	72	74	97.3
Lip biopsy	69	72	95.8

shows the symptoms, signs and abnormal test results of our 92 patients; 97.5% had dry mouth and/or dry eyes; 29.3% had parotid pain and/or swelling and angular cheilitis was found in 22.5% of the patients. A positive Schirmer's test and abnormal staining with rose bengal dye were present in more than 90% of patients. All patients were examined by ophthalmologists and most were diagnosed as having KCS. The salivary flow rate by gum chewing decreased in 93.4%. Sequential salivary scintigraphy using 99mTc-pertechnetate was performed in 74 patients out of whom most showed more than grade 2 abnormality. Histological examination of salivary glands classified 69 out of 72 patients (95.8%) at higher than grade 2 abnormality, according to Tarpley et al. (1974). The results of other studies are shown in Table 2. Elevation of the erythrocyte sedimentation rate (ESR) was found in 89.5%; hypergammaglobulinemia was noted in 76.1%; the IgG level was high in 64.3% of the patients but a high level of IgA and IgM was found in only 27.8% and 13.9%, respectively; a decreased level of IgA or IgM was seen in some patients. The level of C3 and/or C4 was low in 27.1% and 34.9% of the patients.

Various autoantibodies were present; the rheumatoid factor (RF) was positive in 69.9%; anti-nuclear antibody (ANA) in 54.8%; anti-DNA antibody in 27.3%; anti-SSA and -SSB antibody in 42.4% and 18.2%, respectively; and anti-salivary duct antibody in 25.0%. Antibodies against the thyroid gland and microsomal antigens were also positive (41.5 and 46.2%, respectively). Dermal delayed-type hypersensitivity (DTH) was tested in 41 patients and 33 patients showed impaired responses (80.5%); more than 3 antigens such as tuberculin purified protein derivatives (PPD), candida albicans, streptokinase/streptodornase (SK/SD), mumps antigen, streptococcal polysaccharides or phytohemagglutinin (PHA) were tested in 37 patients and 31 patients (83.8%) showed negative or hyporeactions to more than half of the antigens tested. Blastogenic responses to nonspecific mitogens in peripheral blood lymphocytes were studied in 50 patients; decreased responses were obtained against PHA (20.0%), concanavalin A (ConA; 28.6%) and pokeweed mitogen (PWM; 32.7%). The T cell markers of peripheral blood lymphocytes were examined using monoclonal antibodies (OKT series) in 32 patients; the percentage of T cells (OKT3) had decreased in 3 patients and T4 and T8 cells had decreased in 4 and 9 patients, respectively. The ratio of OKT4/T8 was high (>2.5) in only 4, and low (<1.0) in only 3 patients; the majority of our SS patients showed normal OKT4/T8 ratios.

Table 2. Laboratory data

	SS (92)			G1-SS[a] (27)			Exgl-SS[b] (39)			SS/CTD[c] (26)		
	Pt	+	%	Pt	+	%	Pt	+	%	Pt	+	%
ESR high	86	77	89.5	23	14	60.9**	39	39	100.0**	24	24	100.0
Gamma-gl high	88	67	76.1	25	16	64.0	39	32	82.1	24	19	79.2
Gamma-gl low	88	1	1.1	25	0	0	39	1	2.6	24	0	0
IgG high	84	54	64.3	27	14	51.9	37	26	70.3	20	14	70.0
IgG low	84	0	0	27	0		37	0	0	20	0	0
IgA high	79	22	27.8	25	1	4.0**	34	13	38.2**	20	8	40.0
IgA low	79	6	7.6	25	3	12.0	34	3	8.8	20	0	0
IgM high	79	11	13.9	25	2	8.0	34	6	17.6	20	3	15.0
IgM low	79	5	6.3	25	1	4.0	34	2	5.9	20	1	5.0
C3 low	48	13	27.1	12	3	25.0	26	10	38.5*	12	0	0*
C4 low	43	15	34.9	12	3	25.0	20	7	35.0	11	5	45.5
RF	83	58	69.9	23	17	73.9	39	24	61,5	21	17	81.0
Coombs' test	38	5	13.2	3	0	0	22	1	4.5*	13	4	30.8*
ANA	62	34	54.8	20	6	30.0	27	14	51.9**	15	14	93.3**
A-DNA Ab	44	12	27.3	10	0	0*	22	7	31.8*	12	5	41.7
LE test	57	4	7.0	16	0	0	23	1	4.3	18	3	16.7
A-SSA Ab	33	14	42.4	7	4	57.1	17	6	35.3	9	4	44.4
A-SSB Ab	33	6	18.2	7	1	14.3	17	2	11.8	9	3	33.3
A-Salivary Ab	40	10	25.0	8	1	12.5	19	5	26.3	13	4	30.8
A-Thyroid Ab	41	17	41.5	6	2	33.3	25	10	40.0	10	5	50.0
A-Microsome Ab	39	18	46.2	6	1	16.7	23	12	52.1	10	5	50.0
Decreased DTH	41	33	80.5	9	3	33.3**	18	18	100.0**	14	12	85.7
Blastogenic Resp												
PHA low	50	10	20.0	12	2	16.7	24	6	25.0	14	2	14.3
ConA low	49	14	28.6	12	5	41.7	23	7	30.4	14	2	14.3
PWM low	49	16	32.7	12	4	33.3	23	7	30.4	14	5	35.7
OKT3 low (<50%)	32	3	9.4	7	0	0	14	2	14.3	11	1	9.1
T4 high (>50%)	32	3	9.4	7	2	28.6	14	0	0	11	1	9.1
T4 low (<30%)	32	4	12.5	7	2	28.6	14	1	7.1	11	1	9.1
T8 high (>40%)	32	3	9.4	7	0	0	14	2	14.3	11	1	9.1
T8 low (<20%)	32	9	28.1	7	0	0	14	5	35.7	11	4	36.4
T4/8 high (>2.5)	32	4	12.5	7	1	14.3	14	2	14.3	11	1	9.1
T4/8 low (<1.0)	32	3	9.4	7	2	28.6	14	0	0	11	1	9.1

[a] glandular SS
[b] extragrandular SS
[c] SS associated with connective tissue diesases
* $p<0.05$
** $p<0.01$

Among SS associated with other diseases, connective tissue diseases were seen in 26 patients (28.5%); rheumatoid arthritis (RA) in 12 patients, progressive systemic sclerosis (PSS) in 7, mixed connective tissue disease (MCTD) in 5, and systemic lupus erythematosus (SLE) in 2. There were 71 autoimmune diseases or related disorders such as hypergammaglobulinemic purpura (HPG; 9 patients), chronic thyroiditis (ChTD; 8), interstitial pneumonitis (5), renal tubular acidosis (RTA; 4), hyperviscosity syndrome (HVS; 3), autoimmune hemolytic anemia (AIHA; 1), primary biliary cirrhosis (PBC; 1) and peripheral neuropathy (3). Raynaud's phenomenon was seen in 19 patients. Monoclonal gammopathy in 6 patients (one IgG, 2 IgA and 3 IgM), B cell malignant lymphomas (4), pseudolymphoma (PL; 1) and gastric carcinoma (1) were observed. Subclinical RTA, studied by ammonium chloride loading, was found in 7 out of 11 patients (63.6%).

Table 3. IL-2 production in patients with Sjögren's syndrome

	No.	KMUH[a] IL-2 Activity (unit) (Mean ± SD)	No.	TMDUH[b] IL-2 Activity (unit) (Mean ± SE)
Normal	20	0.82 ± 0.46	14	0.89 ± 0.06
SS	16	0.19 ± 0.14**	32	0.57 ± 0.06**
Primary SS				
G1-SS[c]	7	0.22 ± 0.19*	17	0.62 ± 0.06**
Exgl-SS[d]	4	0.21 ± 0.07*	6	0.57 ± 0.05**
Secondary SS	5	0.11 ± 0.09*	9	0.47 ± 0.06**

[a] KMHU, Kanazawa Medical University hospital
[b] TMDUH, Tokyo Medical and Dental University hospital
[c] glandular SS
[d] extraglandular SS
* $p < 0.01$-0.002
** $p < 0.001$

Laboratory data according to the subgroups of SS is shown in Table 2; there were 66 primary SS patients, including 27 glandular SS (Gl-SS), 39 extraglandular SS patients (Exgl-SS) and 26 secondary SS patients (SS/CTD). There were significant differences ($p < 0.05$ or 0.01) in the rates of high ESR, high IgA, positive anti-DNA-antibody, and decreased DTH between patients with Gl-SS and with Exgl-SS; the low titer of C3 positive Coombs' tests and ANA were significantly higher in patients with SS/CTD than in those with Exgl-SS.

We examined IL-1 production by peripheral blood monocytes in 17 patients but the data showed no differences between SS patients and normal controls. IL-2 production by peripheral blood mononuclear cells was examined by stimulation with PHA in 16 (Kanazawa Medical University) and 32 SS patients (Tokyo Medical and Dental University). Table 3 shows that there was a significant decrease in the IL-2 production of SS patients ($p < 0.01$ to 0.001) in both groups, especially in patients with Exgl-SS and SS/CTD.

Monoclonal Gammopathy

Serum electrophoresis on cellulose acetate membranes and agar gel was performed to detect electrophoretically homogeneous bands. M proteins were assessed by immunoelectrophoresis (Sugai 1972). Preparative agar gel electrophoresis, Sephadex column chromatography and sucrose density gradient ultracentrifugation techniques were used to obtain M proteins. For purification of M proteins with RF activity, affinity column chromatography using Sepharose 4B coupled with human IgG was done. Because some M proteins showed rather broad patterns on electrophoresis, especially in cases of M proteins with RF activity, polyclonal and monoclonal anti-idiotypic (Id) antisera against M proteins were prepared to obtain additional evidence of the monoclonality of electrophoretically homogeneous proteins

(Sugai et al. 1985). Polyclonal anti-Id antisera were raised in rabbits and $F(ab')_2$ fractions were used. The specificity of the antisera were examined by immunofluorescence tests and enzyme-linked immunosorbent assay (ELISA).

We studied 14 sera of SS patients with monoclonal gammopathy; among these patients, we encountered 3 patients, 3 additional patients were sent to our hospital and 8 sera were submitted to us by other doctors. Serum electrophoretic patterns on agar gel and cellulose acetate membranes are shown in Fig. 1. The IgG class of monoclonal gammopathy was found in 3 patients, IgA in 6 patients, IgM in 3, and 2 M proteins (IgM/IgG and IgA/IgG) were observed in 2 patients. The M proteins in patients 7, 13, 14 (IgA) and 19 (IgM) showed RF activity. Hyperviscosity was seen in the serum of patients 7, 8, 11 and 13 resulting in broad electrophoretic patterns on the M proteins.

Polyclonal anti-Id antisera were produced in 11 out of 14 patients (patients 4, 6-8, 13-14, 19-20, and 27-28); each anti-Id antiserum reacted only against autologous M protein except for patients 27 and 28 who had 2 M proteins. In these patients, 2 anti-Id antisera were prepared against 2 M proteins; in patient 27, IgMK and IgGK M proteins turned out to belong idiotypically to 2 different clones (Sugai et al. 1985), whereas IgGK and IgAK M proteins in patient 28 were idiotypically shown to belong to one clone by ELISA. The relationship between the activity of monoclonal RF and the Id determinant was studied with polyclonal and monoclonal anti-Id antisera. Anti-Id antisera against monoclonal RF inhibited only the autologous RF activity in 4 patients. Fig. 2 shows the inhibition curves of RF activity by polyclonal anti-Id antisera in these patients. Cross-reactive Id was studied among RF-positive sera. We previously reported that 2 polyclonal anti-Id antisera

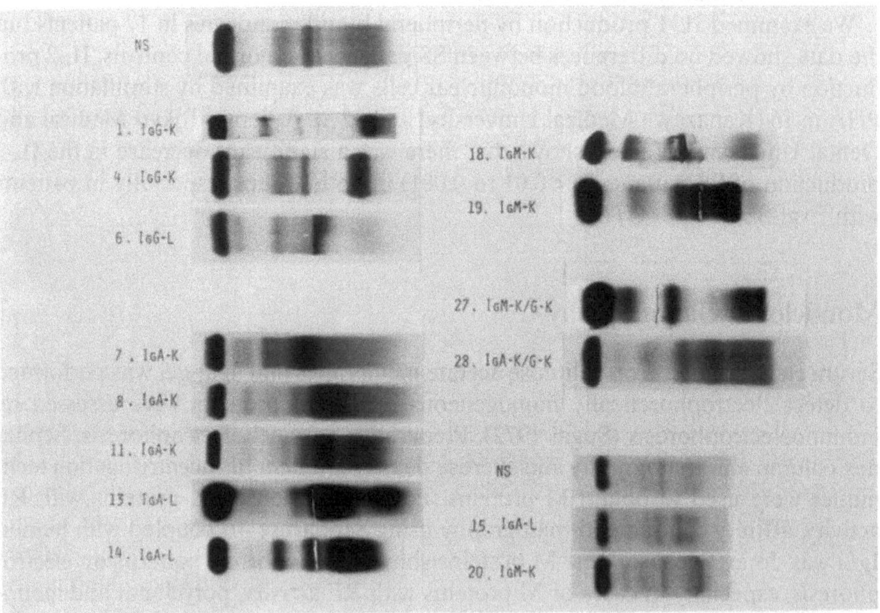

Fig. 1. Serum electrophoretic patterns on agar gel or cellulose acetate membranes in 14 SS patients

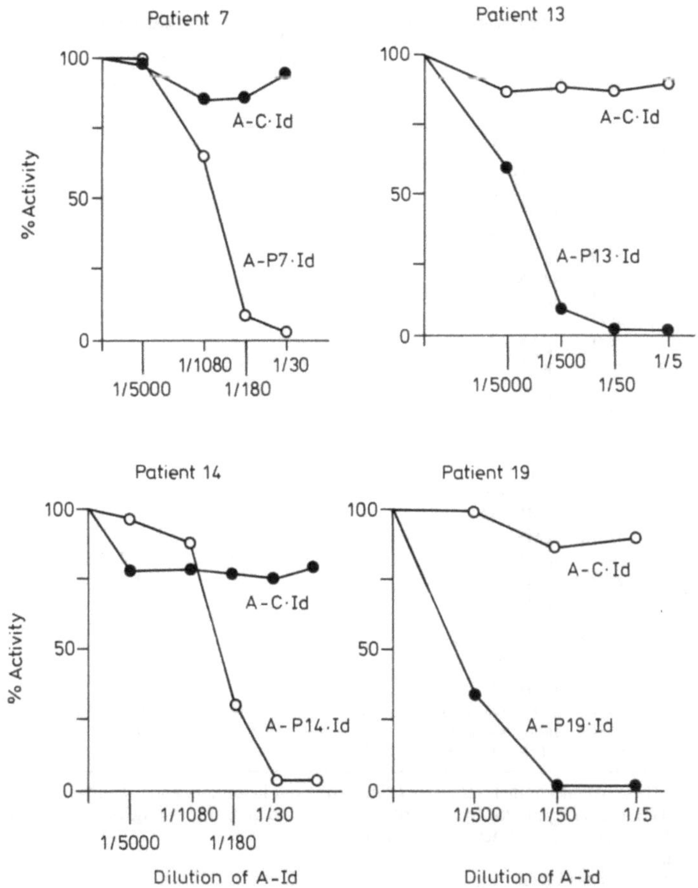

Fig. 2. Inhibition of RF activity by polyclonal anti-Id antisera. RF activity of patients 7, 13, 14 (IgA) and 19 (IgM) was inhibited only by anti-Id antisera against autologous monoclonal RFs, but not by anti-Id antisera against other control monoclonal RFs (A-C · Id)

(patients 13 and 19) reacted with 4 different sera out of 85 RF-positive sera (Sugai et al. 1980; Sugai et al. 1985). One monoclonal A-Id antiserum (patient 7) showed cross-reactivity with 3 out of 106 RF-positive sera that differed with previous ones. This antiserum additionally reacted with the nuclear antigens of only proliferating cells (T and B cells) and saline extracts of rabbit calf thymus.

A review of the Japanese literature and records of academic meetings on SS patients with monoclonal gammopathy disclosed 15 such patients; 3 patients were of IgG class, 5 of IgA class, 6 of IgM class and one case of Bence Jones protein. The clinical and serological features of all Japanese SS patients with monoclonal gammopathy, including our 14 patients, are listed in Table 4. There were 5 males and 24 females; the mean age of the patients was 53.9 years. The average duration of SS before the diagnosis of monoclonal gammopathy was 4.5 years. KCS was present in 21 out of 25 patients and objective salivary dysfunction assessed by sialography and/or scintigraphy was present in 17 out of 18 patients. Histologic abnormalities

Table 4. Japanese patients with Sjögren's syndrome who developed monoclonal gammopathies

Case No	Age/ Sex	M Protein (g/dl)	SS (yrs)	KCS	Decreased Salivary Flow	Histologic Abnormalities	RF	Coombs' Test	DTH[a] (+/Ag)
1#	54/F	IgGK (2.0)[b]	4	+	+	+4	+	U[c]	0/1
2	65/F	IgGK 2.9	1	+	–	U	+	U	1/2
3	61/F	IgGK 3.7 + BJP[d]	3	–	U	+	+	U	1/4
4#	/F	IgGK 6.0	1	+	+	–	–	U	U
5	54/F	IgGL 2.1	4	+	+	+	+	U	U
6#	55/F	IgGL 2.8	6	U	U	+	U	U	U
7#	61/F	IgAK 2.7	0	+	U	U	+(MP)	–	U
8#	27/F	IgAK 5.8	0	+	U	+2	+	–	0/2
9	45/F	IgAK 5.5	10	+	+	U	–	–	2/4
10	74/F	IgAK 2.1	2	+	+	+3	+	+	1/1
11#	42/M	IgAK 2.2	2	+	+	+3	+	–	U
12	72/F	IgAK 3.1	5	U	+	+	U	U	U
13#	49/F	IgAL 1.8	2	+	+	+3	+(MP)	–	0/4
14#	53/F	IgAL 0.8	27	+	+	+	+(MP)	+	U
15#	51/F	IgAL 1.5	8	+	+	+3	–	–	2/4
16	36/F	IgAL U	U	U	U	U	U	U	U
17	68/F	IgA + BJP	3	+	+	+3	+(MP)	U	U
18#	66/M	IgMK (4.5)	1	+	+	U	+	+	0/1
19#	31/M	IgMK 2.3	2	+	+	+3	+(MP)	–	0/1
20#	64/F	IgMK 0.5	1	+	+	+2	–	+	U
21	28/F	IgMK 0.8	5	–	U	+4	+	–	U
22	55/F	IgMK 4.0	0	–	U	+	U	U	U
23	49/M	IgMK 1.0	0	U	U	U	U	U	U
24	63/M	IgMK 3.3 + BJP	U	+	U	–	U	U	U
25	48/F	IgMK 2.4	0	+	U	U	+	–	U
26	66/F	IgML 4.0	U	–	U	U	U	U	U
27#	46/F	IgMK 0.5/IgGK 3.3	2	+	+	U	–	U	0/2
28#	56/F	IgGK 4.4/IgAK 0.9	25	+	+	+	–	–	U
29	69/F	BJPK 1.6 (Ur[e])	2	+	+	+	+	U	U

\# These patients or their sera were examined in our laboratory and are shown in Fig. 1
[a] DTH, skin delayed-type hypersensitivity reaction to antigens; +/Ag, positive reactions/tested antigens
[b] the gamma globulin fraction in parenthesis
[c] unknown
[d] Bence Jones protein
[e] urine

were documented in 18 out of 20 patients. RF was present in 16 out of 22 and 5 of these were monoclonal in nature (4 IgA and one IgM). Coombs' tests were positive in 4 out of 14 patients. DTH was impaired in 10 out of 11 patients.

We reviewed the literature on monoclonal gammopathy in non-Japanese SS patients and found 26 such patients (including 8 whites and one black). Five were men and 20 were women; their age ranged from 46 to 85 years (average, 62.6 years). Of these M proteins, 19 were of IgM class, 4 were of IgG class, 2 of IgA class and one was of Bence Jones protein. The average duration of SS was 5.9 years. Histologic abnormalities were documented in most of these patients. RF was present in 10 out of 16 patients, one of which was monoclonal (IgAK) (Aizawa et al. 1979). Table 5 shows a comparison of the Ig class between Japanese and non-Japanese SS patients. The IgM class is dominant in non-Japanese patients (73.1%), whereas in Japanese, the IgG and IgA classes were predominant (58.6%). The difference was statistically significant ($p < 0.01$).

The association of other diseases was studied in these 29 Japanese and 26 non-Japanese patients. Among associated connective tissue diseses, RA was recognized

Table 5. Monoclonal gammopathies in patients with Sjögren's syndrome

Class	Japanese (%)	Non-Japanese (%)
IgM	9 (31.0)	19 (73.1)
IgG	6 (20.7)	4 (15.4)
IgA	11 (37.9)	2 (7.7)
IgM/IgG	1 (3.4)	0
IgG/IgA	1 (3.4)	0
Bence Jones Protein	1 (3.4)	1 (3.8)
Total	29	26

in 3 Japanese and 2 non-Japanese patients; both groups had one patient each with scleroderma and SLE. The association of connective tissue diseases was 30.2% in our 86 SS patients without monoclonal gammopathy, 42.7% out of the 239 SS patients studied by the Japan SS research Committee (Ofuji et al. 1978), and in Bloch's (Bloch et al. 1965) and Mason's patients (Mason et al. 1973), 62.9% and 52.9% respectively. The difference in the association of connective tissue diseases between SS with and without monoclonal gammopathy was significant ($p < 0.01$). Other associated diseases of both Japanese and non-Japanese patients (55 patients) were non-thrombocytopenic purpura (8), HVS (6), interstitial pneumonitis (4) and nephritis (3), vasculitis (3), ChTD (3), AIHA (2), amyloidosis (2), myositis (1), PBC (1) and pancytopenia (1). There were also LPD such as pseudolymphoma (3), thymoma (2) and immunoblastic sarcoma (IBS; 1), and cancer (1).

Malignant Lymphoma and Related Disorders

Between 1974 and 1985, we encountered 4 SS patients with malignant lymphomas and one with pseudolymphoma. Summaries of these patients are shown in Table 6, and Fig. 3 shows the histologic pictures of these lymphomas.

Patient 1 was a 67-year-old woman with B cell lymphoma in SS associated with PSS (Sugai et al. 1985). She had the onset of Raynaud's phenomenon and symptoms of xeropthalmia and xerostomia in 1971. The diagnosis of SS and PSS was established in our hospital in 1976. In 1982, generalized lymphadenopathy and a mediastinal mass developed. A lymph node biopsy revealed non-Hodgkin's lymphoma, stage 3A, of the diffuse, medium-sized cell type according to the classification of the Japan Lymphoma Study Group (LSG) (Suchi 1981), and the B cell nature of the lymphoma was identified by positive surface membrane IgMK (SmIgMK) and negative cytoplasmic Ig (CIg). The patient was treated with a COPP regimen (cyclophosphamide, vincristine, procarbazine and prednisolone), but she died of interstitial pneumonitis in 1983. Postmortem examination revealed malignant lymphoma and fibrosis of the skin, lungs, esophagus and heart.

Patient 2 is a 77-year-old woman with B cell lymphoma in SS associated with RA. Polyarthritis, Raynaud's phenomenon and xerostomia developed 20 years ago,

Table 6. Summary of patients with malignant lymphoma and pseudolymphoma in Sjögren's syndrome

Case No	1	2	3	4	5
Age/Sex	67/F	77/F	70/F	56/F	63/F
Lymphoma[a]	NHL (B)	NHL (B)	NHL (B)	NHL (B)	PL
SmIg/CIg	IgMK/-	nd/IgML	nd/IgGL	IgML/IgML	Polyclonal
Histology[b]	DM	DL	DL	FMix	Hyperplasia
Autoimmune Dis.	SS/PSS	RA/SS	SS	SS	SS
Duration (Yrs)	11/11	30/1	4	2	0
Steroid Therapy	nd	nd	nd	nd	nd
Autopsy	yes	alive	yes	alive	alive
ESR (mm/hr)	*32/91**	*43/21**	52	24	106
LDH (IU/L)	196/340	211/279	1074	475	379
TP (g/dl)	8.1/6.3	6.4/6.5	5.4	5.4	8.5
gamma-gl (g/dl)	2.0/0.9	0.9/1.0	1.6	0.9	4.1
IgG (mg/dl)	2488/1145	980/1110	1720	1091	5110
IgA (mg/dl)	390/236	144/159	30	436	138
IgM (mg/dl)	162/138	451/430	311	33	142
C3 (mg/dl)	61/80	nd/62	84	66	60
C4 (mg/dl)	34/32	nd/16	nd	18	6
ANA	+/−	nd/+	−	−	+
A-DNA	−/−	−/−	−	−	+
LE Test	+/−	nd/−	−	−	−
RF	+/−	+/+	−	−	−
Thyroid Test	−/−	nd/−	−	−	+
RBC ($\times 10^{12}$/L)	3. 98/3.65	3.35/4.00	4.19	2.49	3.45
WBC ($\times 10^{9}$/L)	3.8/5.7	7.3/4.8	8.1	38.9	5.8
Lymph ($\times 10^{9}$/L)	1.4/1.1	1.2/0.86	0.57	33.4	0.55
E-RFC (%)	53/55	nd/53	nd	48	45
EAC-RFC (%)	10/1	nd/3	nd	2	1
Platelet ($\times 10^{9}$/L)	180/246	228/194	73	81	180
Blst. Resp.[c]	N. N. N/D. N. N	nd	nd	D. D. D	N. N. N
DTH[d]	N. N. D/D. N. D	nd/D	nd	D. D. D	D. D. D.
KCS	+/+	+/+	+	+	+
Abnormality in					
Salivary Scan	+3	+2	nd	+	+3
Salivary Histol.	+2	+3	+3	+3	+3
Pulmonary Fb/IP[e]	+	+	−	−	−

[a] *NHL* non-Hodgkin's lymphoma; *PL* pseudolymphoma
[b] *DM* and *DL* diffuse medium-sized and large cell type; *FMix* follicular mixed cell type
[c] *Blst. Resp.* blastogenic responses of peripheral blood lymphocytes to PHA, ConA and PWM; *N* normal; *D* decreased; *nd* not done
[d] *DTH* skin delayed-type hypersensitivity reactions to one to 3 antigens
[e] *Fb* fibrosis; *IP* interstitial pneumonitis
* one to 8 years before the diagnosis of malignant lymphoma
** at the time of the diagnosis of malignant lymphoma

after a hospital diagnosis of RA. In 1982, she exhibited deformed polyarthritis, dry mouth and dry eyes, and the diagnosis of SS was established by laboratory and histological studies. In 1983, she noticed an elastic, firm, subcutaneous mass in the left pretibial region. A biopsy of the mass and laboratory examination revealed non-Hodgkin's lymphoma, stage 1E, of the diffuse, large cell type of B cell origin

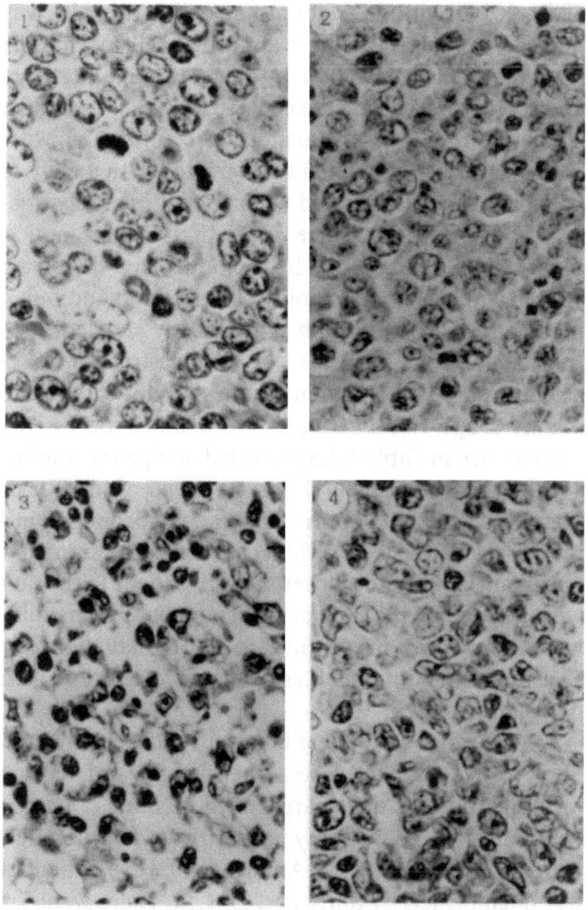

Fig. 3. Histologic pictures of malignant lymphomas in patients 1, 2, 3 and 4. Pictures 1, 3 and 4 are lymph nodes and 2 is a subcutaneous mass

(CIgML). The treatment consisted of local irradiation followed by a mild COP regimen and the patient is now doing well.

Patient 3 was a 70-year-old woman with B cell lymphoma in SS. The patient first noticed dry mouth with parotid pain and swelling in 1971. In 1975, the patient was admitted to our hospital because of tarry stool and weight loss. Malignant change in the transverse and descending colon was disclosed by barium enema examination. She died of massive rectal bleeding in December, 1975. Postmortem examination revealed malignant lymphoma, diffuse, large cell type of B cell origin (CIgGL), involving the colon, stomach, pancreas, mediastinum, heart and lungs. Salivary glands showed marked mononuclear cell infiltration with acinar cell destruction but without any malignant cell involvement.

Patient 4 is a 56-year-old woman with B cell lymphoma in SS. The patient first noticed parotid pain and swelling 10 years ago. Two years ago she noticed symptoms of dry mouth and eyes. In 1984, she was admitted to our hospital for generalized lymphadenopathy and hepatosplenomegaly with ascites. Leukocytosis of

$38.9 \times 10^9/L$ with 85% abnormal lymphoid cells was present. Bone marrow was massively involved by these abnormal cells (94.0%). A lymph node biopsy showed malignant lymphoma of the follicular, mixed-cell type of B cell origin (SmIgML and CIgML). The diagnosis of SS was established by laboratory and histological studies. Minor salivary glands were infiltrated with mononuclear cells but not malignant cells. The patient was treated with a COP regimen and is doing well.

Patient 5 is a 63-year-old woman with pseudolymphoma in SS. She had had Raynaud's phenomenon since 1977. In 1985, she noticed dry mouth and eyes with parotid pain and swelling for 2 months, and then lymph node swelling (1.0×1.0 to 10×15 cm) developed rapidly in the submandibular, both cervical, axillary and inguinal regions. A lymph node biopsy showed nonspecific, marked hyperplasia (polyclonal T and B cells) without destruction of the lymph node architecture. These marked lymphadenopathies disappeared in only 2 months by anti-inflamatory drugs without steroids or immunosuppressives.

As shown in Table 6, SS preceded malignant lymphomas by one to 11 years in our 4 patients and these lymphomas were all of the B cell type with SmIg and/or CIg. Steroids or immunosuppressives had not been used in any of these patients. In laboratory studies, the level of IgG decreased and autoantibodies became negative when malignant lymphoma developed in patient 1. In patients 3 and 4, autoantibodies were negative at the time of malignant lymphoma diagnosis, whereas ANA and RF were still positive in patient 2, in whom malignant lymphoma was in the 1E stage. The T cell functions such as blastogenic responses and DTH were impaired in the patients examined.

A review of the Japanese literature and academic records on LPD associated with SS revealed 22 such cases. The clinical and serological features of 27 patients, including our 5 patients, are shown in Table 7. There were 5 patients with pseudolymphoma (PL); 2 with thymoma; 18 with non-Hodgkin's lymphoma (NHL) and 2 with plasmacytoma (PC). Among 18 NHL, 9 patients were of the B cell type which was documented by SmIg and/or CIg. There were 3 males and 24 females; the patients ranged from 22 to 77 years of age (average 53.3 years). The average interval between the onset of SS and the diagnosis of LPD was 3.6 years. Previous treatment with immunosuppressive drugs other than steroids was not described in any of these patients. KCS was present in 20 out of 21 patients. Objective signs of xerostomia were present in all 19 examined patients. Histologic salivary gland abnormalities were documented in each of the 19 examined patients; in 3, the salivary glands were invaded by malignant cells (patients 9, 11 and 25). RF was present in 16 out of 22 patients; positive Coombs' tests were found in 3 out of 12 patients. Hypergammaglobulinemia was observed in 13 out of 22 patients; hypogammaglobulinemia in 2 patients. A marked increase in gammaglobulin was seen in patients with pseudolymphoma and thymoma. As the thymomas were histologically benign in the latter patients (patients 6 and 7) and thymectomies did not affect hyperviscosity syndrome or the clinical pictures in either patient (Yoshida et al. 1980; Muto et al. 1984), it is probable that these patients could belong to the pseudolymphoma group. DTH tests performed on 11 patients all showed negative or decreased responses to one to 3 antigens. Among associated diseases, 4 patients were associated with connective tissue diseases (2 RA and 2 PSS). Among other diseases, monoclonal gammopathy (3 IgA), HVS (2), cryoglobulinemia (2), ChTD (3) and PBC (1) were found.

Table 7. Lymphoproliferative disorders in Japanese patients with Sjögren's Syndrome

Case No	Age/ Sex	LPD (Histol)	SS (yr)	KCS	Decreased Salivary Flow	Histologic Abnormality Salivary gl	RF	Coombs' Test	Gamma-gl (g/dl)	DTH (+/AG)	Associated Diseases[d]
1	70F	PL[a]	3	+	+	+3	+	+	9.1		
2	28F	PL	1	+	+	+	+	+	3.4	0/3	ChTD, cryoglobulin
3	67F	PL	5			+					
4 #	63F	PL	0	+	+	+	–	–	4.1	0/3	
5	42M	PL	2	+	+	+3	+	–	4.6		M-IgAK
6	27F	Thymoma	0	+		+2	+	–	6.7	0/2	HVS, M-IgAK
7	36F	Thymoma	1	+	+	+	+	–	7.0	0/1	HVS, M-IgAL
8	42F	NHL[b]	0						2.1		
9	44F	NHL	4	+	+	+*	+		0.9		
10	54F	NHL	8	+	+	+3	+	–	1.5	0/3	vasculitis, cryoglobulin
11	76M	NHL	10	+	+	+3*	+	+	3.1		Mikulicz's synd., neuropathy
12	55F	NHL-DS (B)	4		+		+		low	0/1	
13		NHL					+				
14	53F	NHL-FMix	1	+	+	+	+	–	2.1		PSS
15	65F	NHL-FL (B)	1	+	+				normal		
16 #	67F	NHL-DM (B)	11	+	+	+2	–		0.9	0/3	PSS
17	45F	NHL-FM	1	+	+		+		high		RA
18	49F	NHL-DL (B)	10	+	+	+	–		0.5		epilepsy
19	54F	NHL-DM/L (B)									Banti's syndrome
20	62F	NHL-D	1	+			+				
21 #	70F	NHL-DL (B)	4	+		+	–	–	1.6		
22 #	77F	NHL-DL (B)	1	+	+	+3	+	–	1.0	0/3	RA
23 #	56F	NHL-FM (B)	0	–	+	+	–	–	0.9	0/3	
24	52F	NHL-DL (B)	10	+	+						
25	58F	NHL-DL	3	U	U	+3*	+	–	2.0		ChTD
26	22M	PC[c]	4	+	+	+	+		1.1	0/1	
27	53F	PC	6	+	+	+	–		normal	0/3	ChTD, PBC

\# These patients were examined in our section
[a] *PL* pseudolymphoma
[b] *NHL* non-Hodgkin's lymphoma; *DS, DM* and *DL* diffuse small, medium-sized and large cell type; *FM, FL* and *FMix* follicular medium-sized, large and mixed cell type
[c] plasmacytoma
[d] *ChTD* chronic thyroiditis; *HVS* hyperviscosity syndrome; *PBC* primary biliary cirrhosis
* invaded by lymphoma cells

Table 8. Lymphoproliferative disorders in patients with Sjögren's syndrome

Report No.	Japanese (26)					Non-Japanese (65)				
	Cases	M	F	SmIg	CIg	Cases	M	F (W/B)[h]	CIg	T cell
PL[a]	5	1	4			20		17 (9/0)		
IBL[b]	0					5	2	2		
NHL[c]	18	1	17	M2	M5G2[g]	58	9	40 (7/1)	M7G1A1L1Ig1	1
Hodgkin's LM[d]	0					3	1	1		
Plasmacytoma	2	1	1		M1	0				
Thymoma	2	0	2			5				
Lennert's LM[e]	0					2	0	2		
Undeterm LPD[f]	0					8	1	3 (2/0)		
Total	27	3	24	M2	M6G2	101	13	65 (18/1)	M7G1A1L1Ig1	1

[a] pseudolymphoma
[b] immunoblastic lymphadenopathy
[c] non-Hodgkin's lymphoma
[d] Hodgkin's lymphoma
[e] Lennert's lymphoma
[f] undetermined lymphoproliferative disorders
[g] M, G, A and L; IgM, IgG, IgA and light-chain, respectively
[h] W white; B black

We reviewed the literature on LPD in non-Japanese SS patients and found 101 such patients (Table 8). There were 13 males and 65 females. There were 58 NHL (11 B cell type and one T cell type), 20 pseudolymphomas, 5 thymomas, 2 Lennert's lymphomas, one immunoblastic lymphadenopathy (IBL) and 8 undetermined LPD.

Discussion

A high incidence of monoclonal gammopathies and malignant lymphomas has been suggested to occur in SS (Talal and Bunim 1964; Talal et al. 1967; Anderson and Talal 1971; Kassan et al 1978; Zulman et al. 1978) at a higher incidence than in other autoimmune diseases such as RA or SLE (Isomaki et al. 1982; Green et al. 1978). Zulman et al. (1978) reported that some malignant lymphomas associated with SS produce monoclonal IgMK in their neoplastic cells. They suggested a dynamic spectrum of lymphoproliferative lesions in SS ranging from benign polyclonal plasma cell infiltrates to pseudolymphoma, progressing to malignant lymphomas with monoclonal B cell characteristics and finally to dedifferentiated lymphomas with little or no Ig.

Monoclonal gammopathy develops in various immunological disorders such as immunodeficiency (Danon and Seligmann 1973), autoimmune diseases (Zawadzki and Edwards 1978) and lymphoid malignancies such as malignant lymphomas (Alexanian 1975) and adult T cell leukemia (Matsuzaki et al. 1985) suggesting that disorders not only of B cell lineage but also of regulatory T cells play an important role in the development of monoclonal gammopathy as reported by Radle (Radle 1979). We reported the development of macroglobulinemia in aged NZB/NZW F1 mice (Sugai et al. 1973; Sugai et al. 1974) which have been suggested as suitable models for human autoimmune diseases such as SLE and SS. Talal (1974) discussed the similarity of autoimmunity, macroglobulinemia and lymphoid malignancy between SS and New Zealand mice.

Connective tissue diseases such as RA, PSS or SLE are frequently associated with both Japanese and non-Japanese SS patients and these patients comprise the secondary SS group. It is interesting that among 29 Japanese and 26 non-Japanese SS patients with monoclonal gammopathies, there were only 5 patients with RA, 2 with SLE and 2 with PSS. This indicates that monoclonal gammopathy develops at a higher incidence in primary than in secondary SS patients. According to Moutsopoulos et al. (1979), primary SS is different from SS with RA; recurrent parotid gland enlargement, lymphadenopathy, purpura, Raynauds's phenomenon, renal involvement and myositis occur more often in primary than secondary SS. Anti-Ha and anti-SSA antibodies tend to be found in the former. A difference between the two groups is also evident with respect to HLA allo-antigens such as HLA-B8 and DRW3. Monoclonal gammopathy may be another feature of primary SS.

In 29 Japanese SS patients with monoclonal gammopathies, the IgG and IgA classes predominated (58.6%, Table 5), while in non-Japanese SS patients, monoclonal gammopathies were usually confined to the IgM class (73.1%). During B cell differentiation, a clone of antibody-producing cells switches the expression of the Ig heavy-chain from IgM to IgG, IgE or IgA while maintaining its V-region specificity. This process involves T cells via B cell interaction (Isakson et al. 1982; Mayer et al. 1985). The development of IgM class monoclonal gammopathy in SS suggests that a defect on the regulatory T cells which aid the switch from IgM to IgG or IgA at the time of their differentiation may be one of the mechanisms, and the disordered mechanism in B cell differentiation in SS might vary between Japanese and non-Japanese patients.

Rheumatoid factor is one of the most common autoantibodies in patients with SS; this was also the case in Japanese SS patients with LPD such as monoclonal gammopathies and malignant lymphomas (Tables 4 and 7) and in non-Japanese SS patients with monoclonal gammopathies (Sugai et al. 1985). Five Japanese patients manifested monoclonal RF (4 IgA and one IgM) and one IgA monoclonal RF was reported in a Caucasian patient (Aizawa et al. 1979). The occurrence of monoclonal RF in SS is interesting because the autoimmune antigen-antibody reaction which takes place in the salivary gland is thought to stimulate the production of polyclonal RF in situ (Talal et al. 1970) and chronic stimulation would select monoclonal among polyclonal RF (Krause 1970). In two of our patients (Nos. 13 and 27), the polyclonal phase of hypergammaglobulinemia was evidenced before the monoclonal phase by serum electrophoresis. Patient 13 had been followed up for 5 years for polyclonal hypergammaglobulinemia and then IgAL monoclonal RF developed (Murayama et al. 1978). In patient 27, the polyclonal phase of hypergammaglobulinemia was observed for 6 months, then monoclonal IgGK developed, and 5 years later, monoclonal IgMK appeared in the serum (Yamano et al. 1976).

The Id characteristics of 4 monoclonal RFs were examined by ELISA using polyclonal and monoclonal anti-Id antisera. The inhibition test showed that Id determinant was present at the combining site of RF in our 4 patients. Since the report of Kunkel et al. (1973), the Id cross-specificity of RF was studied extensively using monoclonal anti-Id antisera. Major common Id of RF were demonstrated (Chen et al. 1984) and the existence of a family of closely related RF genes was suggested. We found Id cross-specificity between monoclonal RFs (patients 13 and 19) and "non-monoclonal" RFs from patients with other diseases such as RA or connective tissue disease. This suggests that there is a restriction of heterogeneity in some "non-monoclonal" RFs, notwithstanding the fact that usual serum analysis does not reveal monoclonality. It is not known whether these cross-reactive monoclonal RFs were detected as the early stage of distinct monoclonal RFs or whether a small amount of monoclonal RFs are controlled by some mechanisms such as the Id-anti-Id regulatory mechanism. It is interesting that one of the monoclonal A-Id antisera (patient 7) reacted with nuclear antigens of proliferating cells (Shimizu et al. 1986). Analyses of the antigenic determinant between RF Id and the nuclear antigen are now in progress.

Talal and Bunim (1964) described 3 cases of malignant lymphoma and one case of Waldenström's macroglobulinemia among 58 SS patients. Since that report, many reports have supported the association of SS with LPD such as malignant lymphoma, Waldenström's macroglobulinemia and pseudolymphoma. Kassan et al. (1978) reported that patients with SS have an increased risk of non-Hodgkin's lymphoma that is 43.8 times higher than the control group and also a probable high risk of Waldenström's macroglobulinemia. They pointed out that the risk of lymphoma is related to extensive lymphoproliferation such as parotid swelling, splenomegaly and lymphadenopathy.

In this report on LPD in SS patients, non-Hodgkin's lymphoma was most frequent in both Japanese and non-Japanese groups (Table 8). In our 4 patients, lymphomas were of B cell origin; B cell lymphomas were found in 9 Japanese and 11 non-Japanese SS patients. It appears that the incidence of B cell lymphoma in SS is increasing recently, although a case of T cell lymphoma was also reported (Wilke et al. 1984). It is notable that the IgG level declined and autoantibodies such as ANA, an LE test result and RF disappeared in patient 1, and such autoantibodies were negative in patients 3 and 4 at the time of the diagnosis of malignant lymphomas. It was pointed out by Talal and Bunim (1964) that the early decline in gammaglobulin might be the first manifestation of neoplasm which was not yet clinically detectable. Four patients with malignant lymphomas in our study were associated with SS alone or with connective tissue diseases such as PSS or RA, and SS preceded the development of lymphomas. Kassan et al. (1978) and Moutsopoulos et al. (1980) reported that no significant differences were found in the incidence of malignant lymphomas or Waldenström's macroglobulinemia between patients with SS alone and patients with SS and RA. RA, PSS and ChTD were included among the associated diseases in Japanese SS patients. RA, SLE and ChTD are known to be associated with lymphoid malignancy and the association is considered to be significant (Isomaki et al. 1982; Green et al. 1978; Holm et al. 1985).

In our review of the literature on LPD in patients with RA, PSS and SLE, we found 273 LPD in RA (126 NHL, 39 Hodgkin's lymphomas, 46 multiple myelomas and others), 23 LPD in PSS (5 NHL, 5 Hodgkin's lymphomas, 5 multiple myelomas and 4 other monoclonal gammopathies and others), and 73 LPD in SLE (34 NHL, 15 Hodgkin's lymphomas, one multiple myeloma and 9 other monoclonal gammopathies and others). The high rates of PL, monoclonal gammopathies and B cell lymphomas in patients with SS, the high rate of multiple myeloma in RA and the low rate of multiple myeloma or Waldenström's macroglobulinemia and the relatively high rate of Hodgkin's lymphomas in SLE vary considerably. In the case of PSS, it is notable that very few PSS patients with associated Hodgkin's or non-Hodgkin's lymphomas have been reported (to our knowledge, only 7 in non-Japanese and 3 in Japanese patients), although alveolar cell carcinomas are highly associated with PSS. Holm et al. (1985) recently reported that the patients with ChTD had an increased risk of myeloid and lymphoproliferative neoplasms in addition to the high risk of malignant thyroid lymphomas. These facts might indicate that the differences among immunological disorders in these connective tissue diseases have some relation to differences in the kind and the developmental rate of LPD found with autoimmune diseases.

There is evidence in both animals and humans that increased suppressor cell activity is associated with the development or enhancement of certain cancers (Broder and Waldmann 1978). According to Moutsopoulos and Fauci (1980), a spectrum of disorders of immunoregulation in SS ranges from restricted hyperactivity of the B cell function and reversible abnormalities of immunoregulatory T cells to a more broadly expressed B cell hyperactivity and irreversible abnormalities in immunoregulatory T cells that are usually seen in SLE. The proper function of the immune system depends upon appropriate regulation of suppression as well as effector T and B lymphocytes. Autoimmune disorders may disturb this regulatory function resulting in an inability to suppress emerging malignant cell growth.

Acknowledgments

We thank Drs. Y. Yamazaki (Fukui Prefectural Hospital), T. Murayama (Johoku Hospital, Ishikawa), and T. Tohyama (Takaoka City Hospital, Toyama) for referring patients to us, and Drs. S. Kumagai (Kyoto University Hospital), K. Yamauchi (Shimane Medical University Hospital), H. Yamano (Akashi City Hospital, Hyogo), T. Uchida (Fukushima Medical College), T. Tsuchimochi (Saitama Cancer Center), and S. Kamihira (Nagasaki City Hospital), for sending patient sera.

References

1. Aizawa Y, Zawadzki ZA, Micolonghi TS, McDowell JW, Neiman RS (1979) Vasculitis and Sjögren's syndrome with IgA-IgG cryoglobulinemia terminating in immunoblastic sarcoma. Amer J Med 67: 160-166
2. Alexanian R (1975) Monoclonal gammopathy in lymphoma. Arch Intern Med 135: 62-66
3. Anderson LG, Talal N (1972) The spectrum of benign to malignant lymphoproliferation in Sjögren's syndrome. Clin Exp Immunol 10: 199-221
4. Andrews BS, Eisenberg RA, Theofilopoulos AN, Izui S, Wilson CB, McConahey PJ, Murphy ED, Roths JB, Dixon FJ (1978) Spontaneous murine lupus-like syndromes. Clinical and immunopathological manifestation in several strains. J Exp Med 148: 1198-1215
5. Bloch KJ, Buchanan WW, Wohl MJ, Bunim JJ (1965) Sjögren's syndrome. A clinical, pathological and serological study of sixty-two cases. Medicine 44: 187-231
6. Broder S, Waldmann TA (1978) The suppressor-cell network in cancer. N Eng J Med 299: 1281-1284
7. Chen PP, Fong S, Normansell D, Hoghten RA, Karras JG, Vaughan JH, Carson DA (1984) Delineation of a cross-reactive idiotype on human autoantibodies with antibody against a synthetic peptide. J Exp Med 159: 1502-1511

8. Danon F, Seligmann N (1973) Serum monoclonal immunoglobulins in childhood. Arch Dis Childh 48: 207-211
9. Green JA, Dawson AA, Walker W (1978) Systemic lupus erythematosus and lymphoma. Lancct 2: 753-755
10. Holm L-E, Blomgren H, Löwhagen T (1985) Cancer risks in patients with chronic lymphocytic thyroiditis. N Engl J Med 312: 601-604
11. Isakson PC, Pure E, Vitetta ES, Krammer PH (1982) T cell-derived B cell differentiation factor(s). Effect on the isotype switch of murine B cells. J Exp Med 155: 734-748
12. Isomaki HA, Hakulinen T, Joutsenlahti U (1982) Exess risk of lymphomas, leukaemia and myeloma in patients with rheumatoid arthritis. Ann Rheum Dis 41 (Suppl): 34-36
13. Kassan SS, Thomas TL, Moutsopoulos HM, Hoover R, Kimberly RP, Budman DR, Costa J, Decker JL, Chused TM (1978) Increased risk of lymphoma in sicca syndrome. Ann Inter Med 89: 888-892
14. Krause RM (1970) The search for antibodies with molecular uniformity. Adv Immunol 12: 1-56
15. Kunkel HG, Agnello V, Joslin FG, Winchester RJ, Capra JD (1973) Cross-idiotypic specificity among monoclonal IgM anti-γ-globulin activity. J Exp Med 137: 331-342
16. Mason AMS, Gumpel JM, Golding PL (1973) Sjögren's syndrome - A clinical review. Seminar Arth Rheum 2: 301-331
17. Matsuzaki H, Yamaguchi K, Kagimoto T, Nakai R, Takatsuki K, Ogawa W (1985) Monoclonal gammopathies in adult T-cell leukemia. Cancer 56: 1380-1383
18. Mayer L, Posnett DN, Kunkel HG (1985) Human malignant T cells capable of inducing an immunoglobulin class switch. J Exp Med 161: 134-144
19. Miyasaka N, Yamada T, Sato K, Murata H, Nishido T, Yata J, Okuda M (1986) Decreased IL-2 production by peripheral blood lymphocytes in patients with Sjögren's syndrome. Analysis of defective mechanisms. Jap J Rheumatol (in press)
20. Murayama T, Shirasaki Y, Sugai S, Konda S (1978) A case of Sjögren's syndrome with monoclonal IgA rheumatoid factor - Hyperviscosity syndrome and hypergammaglobulinemic purpura. Saishin Igaku 33: 1668-1674 (in Japanese)
21. Muto S, Honma S, Takayasu T, Takazawa K, Ishibashi A, Tsuchiya M, Shiina A, Asanao Y, Hosoda S, Ninomura N (1984) A case of Sjögren's syndrome associated with pulmonary embolism, monoclonal hypergammaglobulinemia, and thymoma. Jap J Intern Med 73: 1001-1008 (in Japanese)
22. Moutsopoulos HM, Fauci AS (1980) Immunoregulation in Sjögren's syndrome: Influence of serum factors on T-cell subpopulations. J Clin Invest 65: 519-528
23. Moutsopoulos HM, Webber BL, Vlagopoulos TP, Chused TM, Decker JL (1979) Difference in the clinical manifestations of sicca syndrome in the presence and absence of rheumatoid arthritis. Amer J Med 66: 733-736
24. Moutsopoulos HM, Chused TM, Mann DL, Klippel JH, Fauci AS, Frank MM, Lawley TJ, Hamburger MI (1980) Sjögren's syndrome (sicca syndrome): Current issues. Ann Intern Med 92: 212-226
25. Ofuji T (1977) Summary of the studies on Sjögren's disease in 1977. Annual Report of the Ministry of Health and Welfare, Sjögren's Disease Research Comittee, p 3-6 (in Japanese)
26. Ofuji T, Miyawaki S, Kageyama K, Azukizawa H (1978) Epideminologic study of Sjögren's disease (Summary of the patients collected from the members of the committee). Annual Report of the Ministry of Health and Welfare, Sjögren's Disease Research Committee p 11-18 (in Japanese)
27. Radle J (1979) Idiopathic paraproteinemia - a consequence of an age-related deficiency in the T immune system. Three-stage development - a hypothesis. Clin Immunol Immunopathol 14: 251-255
28. Schall GL, Anderson LG, Wolf RO, Herdt JR, Tarpley TM, Cummings NA, Zeiger LS, Talal N (1971) Xerostomia in Sjögren's syndrome. Evaluation by sequential salivary scintigraphy. JAMA 216: 2109-2116
29. Shimizu S, Sugai S, Imaoka T, Sawada M, Konda S (1986) Monoclonal anti-idiotypic antibodies against monoclonal rheumatoid factors derived from patients with Sjögren's syndrome. Scand J Rheumatol (in press)
30. Suchi T (1981) A new pathological classification of non-Hodgkin's lymphoma. In: Kojima M, Iijima S, Hanaoka M, Suchi T (eds) Atlas of Malignant Lymphoma by the New Classification, pp 27-40. Bunkodo, Tokyo (in Japanese)

31. Sugai S (1972) IgA pyroglobulin, hyperviscosity syndrome and coagulation abnormality in a patient with multiple myeloma. Blood 39: 224-237
32. Sugai S, Pillarisetty RJ, Talal N (1973) Monoclonal macroglobulinemia in NZB/NZW F1 mice. J Exp Med 138: 989-1002
33. Sugai S, Palmer DW, Talal N, Witz IP (1974) Protective and cellular immune responses to idiotypic determinants on cells from a spontaneous lymphoma of NZB/NZW F1 mice. J Exp Med 140: 1547-1558
34. Sugai S, Konda S, Shirasaki Y, Murayama T, Nishikawa T (1980) Non-IgM monoclonal gammopathy in patients with Sjögren's syndrome. Amer J Med 68: 861-866
35. Sugai S, Shimizu S, Hirose Y, Konda S, Yamano H (1985) Monoclonal gammopathies in Japanese patients with Sjögren's syndrome. J Clin Immunol 5: 90-101
36. Sugai S, Takiguchi T, Hirose Y, Shimizu S, Tachibana J, Konda S, Konishi F (1985) B cell malignant lymphoma in a patient with progressive systemic sclerosis and Sjögren's syndrome. Jap J Med 24: 155-163
37. Talal N (1974) Autoimmunity and lymphoid malignancy in New Zealand black mice. Prog Clin Immunol 2: 101-120
38. Talal N, Bunim JJ (1964) The development of malignant lymphoma in the course of Sjögren's syndrome. Amer J Med 36: 529-540
39. Talal N, Steinberg AD (1974) The pathogenesis of autoimmunity in New Zealand black mice. Curr Topics Microbiol Immunol 64: 79-103
40. Talal N, Sokoloff L, Barth WF (1967) Extrasalivary lymphoid abnormalities in Sjögren's syndrome (reticulum cell sarcoma, "pseudolymphoma", macroglobulinemia). Amer J Med 43: 50-65
41. Talal N, Asofsky R, Lightbody P (1970) Immunoglobulin synthesis by salivary gland lymphoid cells in Sjögren's syndrome. J Clin Invest 49: 49-54
42. Tarpley TM Jr, Anderson LG, White CL (1974) Minor salivary gland involvement in Sjögren's syndrome. Oral Surg 37: 64-74
43. Wilke WS, Tubbs RR, Bukowski RM, Currie TE, Calabrese LH, Weiss RA, Savage RA, Sebek BA (1984) T cell lymphoma occurring in Sjögren's syndrome. Arth Rheum 27: 951-955
44. Yamano H, Noguchi K, Kazuki A, Kitani T, Irie H, Tsuji K, Sugishima S, Ijichi H (1976) A case of Sjögren's syndrome who developed biclonal gammopathy from polyclonal hypergammaglobulinemia. Jap J Clin Hematol 69: 109 (abstr; in Japanese)
45. Yoshida H, Matsuda S, Abe R, Kimura H, Shichishima T, Tanaka T, Akizuki T, Uchida T, Kariyone S (1980) Sjögren's syndrome associated with a benign thymic tumor; Report of a case with wide spectrum of clinical feature. Acta Haematol Jpn 43: 834-841 (in Japanese)
46. Zawadzki ZA, Edwards GA (1978) Nonmyelomatous monoclonal immunoglobulinemia. Prog Clin Immunol 1: 105-156, 1972
47. Zulman J, Jaffe R, Talal N (1978) Evidence that the malignant lymphoma of Sjögren's syndrome is a monoclonal B-cell neoplasm. N Engl J Med 299: 1215-1220

D. Relationship to Other Autoimmune Diseases

1. The Relationship of Sjögren's Syndrome to Rheumatoid Arthritis

R. N. Maini

Introduction

The co-existence of dry eyes, a dry mouth and rheumatoid arthritis, the original components of Sjögren's syndrome, was conceived as a distinct clinical entity (Sjögren 1933, and Sjögren 1951) almost a century after Garrod (1859) proposed the name rheumatoid arthritis for a condition which he perceived as requiring distinction from gout, rheumatic fever, and rheumatism. The expediency and utility of the recognition of conditions such as Sjögren's syndrome and rheumatoid arthritis based on clinical description has undoubtedly stood the test of time and is a part of current rheumatological parlance. Viewed historically, the subsequent emergence of a taxonomy of connective tissue diseases, and criteria for diagnosis of other distinct syndromes, has led to the appreciation that some patients with Sjögren's syndrome have co-existent features of disease classifiable as SLE, scleroderma, polymyositis, polyarteritis nodosa, primary biliary cirrhosis, and fibrosing alveolitis (Bloch und Bunim 1963; Bloch et al. 1965; Mason et al. 1973). At the working level this has been comfortably accommodated by extending the definition of Sjögren's syndrome to include such conditions. However, since the aetiology of all these conditions remains obscure, the basic reason for the co-existence of features remain unexplained, although many theories involving auto-immunity have been advanced. In this chapter the relationship of rheumatoid arthritis to Sjögren's syndrome is examined.

The Clinical Spectrum and Nomenclature of Joint Disease Associated with Sjögren's Syndrome

It is generally accepted that the components of the triad xerophthalmia, xerostomia, and rheumatoid arthritis that constitute Sjögren's syndrome may be expressed singly in individual patients, or in varying combinations, although their precise prevalence in populations is a matter of conjecture since acceptable epidemiological information is only available for definite rheumatoid arthritis, which in Great Britain is estimated to affect 1% of the population (Wood 1978). However, the simplified view that xerophthalmia and xerostomia occurring together as 'sicca syndrome' constitute a single disorder which may be complicated by rheumatoid arthritis in a proportion of patients, and that rheumatoid arthritis is itself a distinct condition which may be associated with sicca syndrome is borne out by clinical observation. Thus, patients with Sjögren's syndrome tend to present in one of the following clinical settings:

1. Complaining of ocular and oral symptoms typical of keratoconjunctivitis sicca and a dry mouth, sometimes associated with episodic parotid swelling. Since the majority of such patients with sicca syndrome continue to suffer from a condition localized to exocrine secretory tissue, the term 'primary' Sjögren's syndrome has been used to describe such patients (Moutsopoulos et al. 1979a). A proportion of such patients may develop intermittent or chronic symptoms compatible with a diagnosis of rheumatoid arthritis, whilst others suffer from arthralgias or, especially in the elderly age group, associated symptoms from coincidental (and aetiopathologically distinct) osteoarthritis.
2. In a proportion of patients suffering from rheumatoid arthritis for some years, there is insidious development of dry eyes and/or a dry mouth compatible with sicca syndrome. According to the suggestion of Moutsopoulos et al. (1979a), such patients are termed as having 'secondary' Sjögren's syndrome.

The 'polar' forms of sicca syndrome and rheumatoid arthritis occurring alone on the one hand, and the 'overlap' form with features of both are best depicted in the form of a Venn diagram (Fig. 1).

This model leads to the hypothesis that patients with sicca syndrome who develop rheumatoid arthritis are clinically indistinguishable from patients with rheumatoid arthritis who develop sicca syndrome, a condition best termed 'RA/SS overlap'. Although there are some grounds for believing this to be true, in reality the position is complex since not only are the antecedent and dominant clinical symptoms (in the individual case) typical of either sicca syndrome or rheumatoid arthritis, but there are other apparent differences; for example, in the severity of the joint disease, in the associated clinical features, specificity of antinuclear antibodies and the HLA phenotypes (discussed later) which suggest an alternative model represented by a different diagram (Fig. 2). This alternative model raises a second

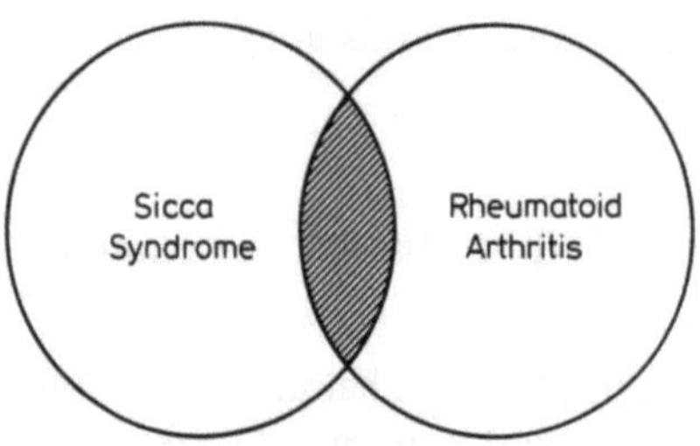

Fig. 1. The 'polar' forms of sicca syndrome and rheumatoid arthritis with co-existing features of both (sicca/rheumatoid 'overlap') represented by shaded area

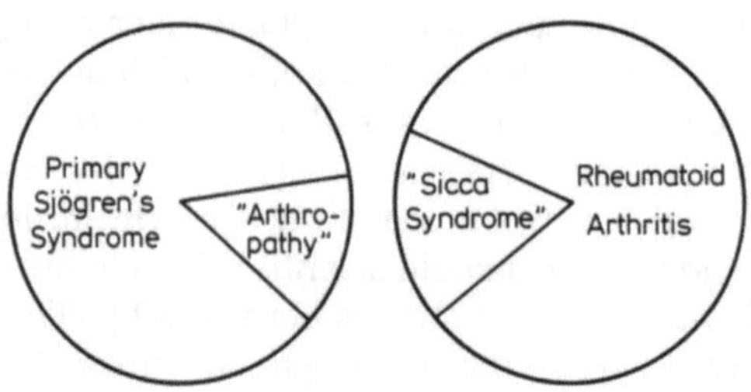

Fig. 2. Primary Sjögren's syndrome and its arthropathy and rheumatoid arthritis associated with sicca syndrome are distinct disorders

hypothesis which suggests the possibility that the arthropathy seen in the context of primary Sjögren's syndrome may in fact be distinct from the usual (or 'classical') form of rheumatoid arthritis; the same theoretical argument of course holds for two forms of 'sicca syndrome' occurring in the distinct settings of rheumatoid arthritis and Primary Sjögren's syndrome.

The problem of nomenclature and classification is further complicated (as we shall see when we examine the details later) by the fact that some patients with the clinical presentation of 'sicca syndrome' may develop features of multi-system disease, especially leukopenia, purpura, panniculitis, nodular vasculitis, Raynaud's phenomenon, and renal disease. The term 'primary Sjögren's syndrome with extraglandular disease' has been used to describe such patients, although it is obvious that many such patients could be classified as 'overlap' syndromes with components of sicca syndrome and SLE. Where the multi-system features of SLE, or another distinct form of connective tissue disease are dominant, the joint symptoms and features are characteristic of that disorder.

In the absence of specific aetiological agents which may clarify the confusion in this area, a situation remniscent of the plethora of syndromes thought to be distinct diseases which in subsequent history were shown to be caused by a single microbial agent, the nomenclature of Sjögren's syndrome remains unsatisfactory and reflects the evolving concepts of this and related diseases.

To summarize, in the context of the relationship of joint disease to Sjögren's syndrome, the following nomenclature based on current usage is recommended:

1. Arthropathy associated with sicca syndrome (primary Sjögren's syndrome): A spectrum of joint symptoms and signs may be observed including arthralgias, myalgias, morning stiffness of joints, intermittent synovitis, and chronic polyarthritis, clinically and histologically indistinguishable from recognized mild forms of rheumatoid arthritis. Components of sicca syndrome are prominent, and often the presenting part of the clinical picture. Leukopenia, purpura, Raynaud's phenomenon, and renal tubular disease may occur in such patients.

2. Rheumatoid arthritis associated with sicca syndrome (secondary Sjögren's syndrome): Patients with established chronic rheumatoid arthritis causing erosive and destructive joint disease may insidiously develop (or be shown on special examination to possess) features of sicca syndrome. Other extra-articular disease features, especially subcutaneous or pulmonary nodules, vasculitis, neuropathy, fibrosing alveolitis, scleritis, pericarditis, and pleural effusions, may occur in such patients. Logically this group could be termed 'primary rheumatoid disease with sicca syndrome'.

3. Arthropathy of other autoimmune diseases associated with sicca syndrome: Patients with SLE, scleroderma, polyarteritis nodosa, idiopathic fibrosing alveolitis and primary biliary cirrhosis, all conditions recognized as associated with articular symptoms and arthropathies, may develop sicca syndrome. Again, although part of the spectrum of secondary Sjögren's syndrome, the logical descriptive terminology should specify the primary disorder.

Other autoimmune diseases	Primary Sjögren's syndrome	Rheumatoid arthritis
sicca syndrome	sicca syndrome	sicca syndrome
arthropathy	arthropathy	destructive/erosive arthritis
multi-system disease	extra-glandular disease	extra-articular disease

Fig. 3. Joint disease, sicca syndrome, and multi-system features may all occur in the context of primary Sjögren's syndrome, rheumatoid arthritis, and other autoimmune diseases

Although the distinct sequence and detailed pattern of clinical features usually permit assignment of patients with joint disease into one of the above categories, Fig. 3 emphasizes the trend for patients with multi-system features to converge towards a clinical picture which may appear the same. Analysis of specificities of autoantibodies and HLA phenotype may assist in their classification. Whether the problem of classification created by the genuine coincidental development of sicca syndrome and destructive chronic rheumatoid arthritis depicted in Figure 1 deserves a separate category - possibly termed 'Sjögren's/RA overlap' - has not been adequately addressed to date.

Joint Disease and Sicca Syndrome: Clinical Features and Differential Diagnosis

As previously noted, the lack of properly conducted epidemiological studies and diagnostic criteria does not permit evaluation of the precise prevalence or nature of the arthropathy associated with sicca syndrome (primary Sjögren's syndrome) and its relationship to rheumatoid arthritis. In patients selected ophthalmologically, presumably indicating severity of ocular symptoms, rheumatoid arthritis was diagnosed in 45-62% of patients (Sjögren 1951; Mason et al. 1973), although in these studies no attempt was made to distinguish primary from secondary forms of Sjögren's syndrome. Bloch and Bunim (1963), reporting on 57 patients with Sjögren's syndrome at the National Institutes of Health, presumably a highly selected group, were able to identify 30 patients with definite or classical rheumatoid arthritis according to the criteria of the Arthritis and Rheumatism Association, and 2 patients with possible rheumatoid arthritis, representing an overall 58% prevalence; in this study 18 patients (35%) had sicca syndrome alone. It is of interest to note that the authors of this study claimed that (although no quantitative differences in biopsies of parotid and submandibular glands were apparent between subgroups) patients with sicca syndrome alone had more severe mouth ulcers and recurrent parotid swelling compared to patients with associated rheumatoid disease. In a subsequent study from the same centre (Bloch et al. 1965) no apparent difference in severity, outcome, or radiological features was found in patients with rheumatoid arthritis with sicca syndrome (who would fulfill criteria for secondary Sjögren's syndrome) compared with rheumatoid arthritis unaccompanied by the sicca complex, though nodules occurred more frequently, and the authors concluded that sicca syndrome suggested an association with the more fully expressed rheumatoid disease. In agreement with the NIH studies (Moutsopoulos et al. 1979b), we find that in patients with sicca syndrome associated with rheumatoid arthritis the chronic joint symptoms antedate the sicca symptoms by several years. In a minority, sicca symptoms occur before or simultaneously with the onset of rheumatoid arthritis and may give rise to an initial categorization of primary Sjögren's syndrome.

Joint symptoms suggestive of rheumatoid arthritis undoubtedly also occur in patients who are categorized as having sicca syndrome alone or primary Sjögren's syndrome. For example, in the study of Bloch et al. (1965), nine of twenty-three patients (40%) gave a history of such symptoms, four of whom could have qualified for consideration of a diagnosis of rheumatoid arthritis in the past. In a study on 31 patients with primary Sjögren's syndrome in which patients with destructive/erosive arthritis were excluded (Castro-Poltroniers and Segovia 1983), polyarticular joint symptoms not ascribable to a known alternative condition (and therefore claimed to be part of the syndrome) occurred in 26 patients. Transient synovitis was present in the majority, complaints of morning stiffness were recorded in six, and chronic continuous polyarticular symptoms were present in five. In none was erosive disease present on x-ray. It will be readily appreciated that such patients with sicca syndrome may be incorrectly labelled as having rheumatoid arthritis, especially since their blood usually contains rheumatoid factor in a high titre (see below) and because in a minority the joint symptoms may precede ocular and oral symptoms. The intermittent nature of the joint symptoms (resembling that observed in palindromic rheumatism), lack of progressive severe destructive joint disease, a positive Schirmer test and Rose Bengal staining (in spite of lack of ocular symptoms), the presence of antinuclear antibody with a speckled pattern, hyperglobulinaemia, and antibodies to SS-A(Ro) or SS-B(La) should alert the clinician to the correct diagnosis.

The clinical pattern of extra-articular disease in rheumatoid arthritis (whether associated with sicca syndrome or not) differs in important respects from the extraglandular features of primary Sjögren's syndrome (Table 1). Nodules are seen in rheumatoid patients but not in patients with primary Sjögren's syndrome; Raynaud's phenomenon is rare in rheumatoid disease and seen in a third of patients with primary Sjögren's syndrome; lower limb purpura (non-palpable, non-thrombocytopenic) is well recognized in primary Sjögren's syndrome and rare in rheumatoid; also commoner in primary Sjögren's syndrome compared to rheumatoid are lymphadenopathy, splenomegaly, renal tubular acidosis, nodular vasculitis (panniculitis), and leukopenia; commoner in rheumatoid disease are digital infarcts, subcutaneous ulcers, mononeuritis multiplex, fibrosing alveolitis, scleritis, pericarditis, pericardial effusions, Felty's syndrome, and amyloidosis.

Table 1. The differences in systemic features of primary Sjögren's syndrome and rheumatoid arthritis. (− indicates not recognized; ± indicates recognized but rare; + to + + + indicates a range of 10% to > 50%)

	Primary Sjögren's syndrome with extra-glandular disease	Rheumatoid Arthritis with extra-articular disease
Nodules	−	+ + +
Raynaud's	+ +	±
Purpura	+ +	±
Lymphadenopathy	+ +	+
Splenomegaly	+	+ (Felty's)
Renal tubular acidosis	+ +	−
Nodular vasculitis	+	−
Digital infarcts	−	+ +
Subcutaneous ulcers	−	+ +
Scleritis	±	+
Mononeuritis multiplex	+	+ +
Fibrosing alveolitis	±	+ +
Pericarditis	−	+
Pleural effusion	−	+
Amyloidosis	−	+ +
Leukopenia	+ +	± (unless Felty's)

Antinuclear Antibodies in the Immunotaxonomy of Sjögren's Syndrome

The concept has been advanced that the specificity and amount of autoantibodies that are found in the blood of patients may form the basis of a taxonomy of the autoimmune diseases (Maini et al. 1985). Unfortunately much controversy has been generated by this approach, largely attributable to poorly reproducible methodology, lack of application of suitable antibody standards, lack of use of purified antigens of known epitope specificity, and biased patient selection. Thus a reliable estimate of the sensitivity and specificity of such tests remains problematical in general. Nevertheless there are grounds for believing that tests for antinuclear antibodies aid in the differential diagnosis of joint disease in relation to Sjögren's syndrome (Alspaugh et al. 1976).

Patients with primary Sjögren's syndrome frequently show the presence in their blood of antinuclear antibodies (ANA), usually with a speckled or nucleolar pattern of staining. In our patients ANA is found in 79% and antibody specificity seen in these patients is anti-SS-A(Ro) in 85%, anti-SS-B(La) in 48%, anti-DNA-protein in 38%, and anti-SS-DNA in 25% (Maini et al. 1985). Clearly many sera contain autoantibodies of multiple specificity, and in particular, anti-SS-B antibodies are invariably found with anti-SS-A. Although anti-SS-A is a sensitive test for primary Sjögren's syndrome, it lacks the diagnostic specificity of anti-SS-B (Venables et al. 1983 and 1986). Thus anti-SS-A also occurs in 45% of our SLE patients (without Sjögren's syndrome); in contrast, anti-SS-B activity by an immunodiffusion assay was detected in 12/200 patients with SLE, and of these 10 had associated sicca syndrome and the remaining 2 had evidence of subclinical sicca syndrome. Thus anti-SS-B and anti-SS-A may be markers of sicca syndrome alone or in association with SLE, although anti-SS-A has been detected in almost half our SLE patients who have not developed sicca syndrome at up to five years of follow-up.

The presence of anti-SS-B, in our experience, practically rules out diagnosis of the usual form of rheumatoid arthritis, with or without sicca syndrome (Venables 1986) and we very rarely detect anti-SS-A in these patients (1 out of 100). It is of interest to reflect that in the study of Bloch et al. (1965) precipitins to SjD and SjT antigens also clearly distinguished patients with rheumatoid arthritis with sicca syndrome from patients with sicca syndrome alone; Tan (1982) has suggested that SjD and SjT antigens were respectively SS-A (RO) and SS-B (La). Although antibodies to SS-A and SS-B are very infrequent in rheumatoid arthritis, we found precipitins to undefined (non-SS-A/B) extractable nuclear antigens (ENA) in a third of 27 patients with extra-articular disease, and most of these showed vasculitis and cryoglobulinaemia (Venables et al. 1980); in this group, the prevalence of sicca syndrome was not increased when compared with a similar number of chronic rheumatoid patients without anti-ENA. We have also published evidence of detectable anti-ds-DNA binding in a minority (3/14) of patients with Sjögren's syndrome associated with rheumatoid arthritis (Holian et al. 1975; Maini and Holborow 1977). The proposal that antibodies to RANA (Alspaugh et 1979), may be specific for rheumatoid arthritis, or rheumatoid associated with sicca syndrome, was not borne out in our studies, since over 50% of normal adults had low titres of anti-RANA antibody; however, there was a trend towards higher anti-RANA titres in rheumatoid patients with a positive Schirmer test (Venables et al. 1981).

Rheumatoid Factors, Immune Complexes, and Complement

Polyclonal rise of IgG, IgA, and IgM occurs with greater frequency in patients with primary Sjögren's syndrome than in rheumatoid patients; in some individuals a rise in monoclonal IgM is present (Gumpel and Hobbs 1970; Anderson and Talal 1972). Rheumatoid factors demonstrated by agglutination of human IgG-coated latex particles or sensitized sheep erythrocytes are present in 96% and 74% respectively (Bloch et al. 1965), a frequency that exceeds that seen in rheumatoid arthritis alone and is equal to that in patients with RA and sicca syndrome. Rheumatoid factor interactions have been implicated in hyperviscosity syndrome. It is claimed that the epitopes on the Fc region of heavy chains of IgG recognized by rheumatoid factors in patients with sicca syndrome and RA include the 'Gm site' more frequently than those detected in patients with sicca syndrome alone (Bunim et al. 1964).

An increased frequency of circulating immune complexes has been reported in patients with all categories of Sjögren's syndrome and rheumatoid arthritis. In patients with definite and classical rheumatoid arthritis, we found no difference in the levels of Clq-binding complexes or of cryoglobulinaemia in patients with or without Sjögren's syndrome (Erhardt et al. 1979); however, cryoglobulinaemia correlated well with the presence of extra-articular disease, suggesting that this parameter correlated with systemic features other than sicca syndrome. In primary Sjögren's syndrome with features such as vasculitis and nephritis, defects of clearance associated with circulating immune complexes have been implicated in pathogenesis (Wilson et al. 1977; Hamburger et al. 1979). Complement components C3 and C4 tend to show no significant differences in sicca syndrome and rheumatoid disease, being slightly raised in both conditions (Moutsopoulos et al. 1979).

Aetiopathogenetic Considerations

Genetic

There is compelling evidence for the involvement of genetic factors and environmental influences in the aetiology of both rheumatoid arthritis and sicca syndrome. In a paradigm which appears to be applicable to autoimmune diseases in general, it is envisaged that one or more genes in the major histocompatibility complex region of the 6th chromosome in man increase susceptibility to autoimmunity, although it seems likely that other gene families (on other chromosomes) may also make a contribution. The gene products that have been consistently implicated in RA and SS thus far are the HLA antigens, especially the HLA-DR antigens, which show restricted expression on B cells, macrophages, and dendritic cells. The concept put forward by Moutsopoulos et al. (1979b) that the dichotomy between rheumatoid arthritis and sicca syndrome has a genetic counterpart in the alleles of the HLA-DR locus. Thus there is an increased prevalence of HLA-DR-4 in rheumatoid arthritis and of HLA-DR-3 in sicca syndrome. Sicca syndrome is also related to the expression of HLA-B-8, the coding gene of which is known to be in linkage disequilibrium with HLA-DR-3, thus confirming the suscipicion that one susceptibility gene is located on the DNA in or around these alleles.

The concept that the arthropathy and systemic features seen in some patients with sicca syndrome (primary Sjögren's syndrome with extra-glandular features) are distinct from sicca syndrome and rheumatoid arthritis is supported by their distinct HLA phenotypic profiles. Thus, in our clinic, for patients with primary Sjögren's syndrome, some of whom have chronic polyarthritis and systemic disease, and the majority of whom show anti-SS-A and/or anti-SS-B antibodies (Venables et al. 1983), the usual HLA phenotype is HLA-B8-DR-3.

In contrast, in an analysis of 79 patients with definite or classical rheumatoid arthritis, the frequency of HLA-DR-4 was 73.6% (controls 36%) and rose to 92% in seropositive patients with extra-articular disease characterized by nodules, vasculitis, fibrosing alveolitis, neuropathy and scleritis (Ollier et al. 1984). This study also provided evidence that when sicca syndrome occurred in the context of rheumatoid arthritis, the frequency of HLA DR-4 was relatively lower (63%) and that of HLA-DW-4 markedly lower (36.8%) than seen in patients with other extra-articular manifestations (Table 2). The apparently slightly different genetic make-up of these sicca syndrome patients was also reflected in the markedly lower frequency of HLA-DR-7 in these patients; HLA-DR-2 on the other hand occurred relatively more frequently than in patients with other extra-articular disease (Table 2). Aside from defining susceptibility factors, these data suggested that the presence of HLA-DR-7 may be a protective factor in the development of sicca syndrome in patients with rheumatoid disease. The possibility that sicca syndrome of primary and sec-

Table 2. The frequencies of HLA antigens in sicca syndrome and other extra-articular disease features in rheumatoid arthritis (Based on Ollier et al. 1984)

	DR-4	DW-4	DR-2	DR-7
All RA (n=77)	73.6	59.4	12.5	8.3
RA with extraarticular disease (n=277)	76.0	62.5	16.0	4.0
RA with sicca (n=23)	63.3	36.8	21.0	0.5
Controls	36.0	26.6	31.1	30.2

ondary varieties may occur in association with a common supratypic HLA antigen was raised by the findings of Moutsopoulos et al. (1979), who found that an antiserum (Ia-172) identified 100% and 82% respectively of patients with primary and secondary Sjögren's syndrome and only 37% of controls.

Viral induction

There is as yet no conclusive evidence that viruses are implicated in aetiology of sicca syndrome and rheumatoid arthritis, although many viruses persist in the salivary glands (Wolf et al. 1984). Sero-epidemiological surveys have raised the possibility that the Epstein-Barr virus (EBV) may be implicated in the aetiology of rheumatoid arthritis (Alspaugh et al., 1981) and claims exist that the titres of IgG and IgM antibodies to the cytomegalovirus (CMV) antigen are raised in primary Sjögren's syndrome (Shillitoe et al. 1982). However, in our survey, rise in anti-CMV antibodies could be ascribed to the amplification of the antibody detecting system by coincident rheumatoid factors, and no differences in antibody titres to EBV or CMV could be discerned in either rheumatoid arthritis or sicca syndrome (Venables et al. 1985). As far as rheumatoid arthritis is concerned, we find that although anti-EBV-VCA titres in the expected range of seroconversion are seen in patients of all ages, antibodies to the EBV-induced nuclear RANA antigen are distinctly elevated in rheumatoid patients who are EBV-antibody positive (Venables et al. 1982). However, classical rheumatoid arthritis occurs in some children and adults who have apparently never been infected by EBV (Gear et al. 1985) and it seems possible that the higher anti-RANA titres in EBV-infected rheumatoid patients could simply reflect an increased virus load due to secondary defects in cellular regulatory mechanisms, or due to the presence of cross-reactive antinuclear antibodies (Venables et al. 1981 and 1984). In either case doubts are raised about adducing an aetiological role for EBV on current evidence.

Pathogenetic mechanisms

The parallelism in the elements of aetiological factors involved in sicca syndrome and rheumatoid arthritis is further demonstrated in the elucidation of pathogenetic mechanisms. Both conditions may be viewed as arising from the ectopic localization and perpetuation of an immune response at abnormal sites - exocrine tissue in the former and synovial membrane in the latter. In both instances the histological features suggest aggregation and organization of immune cells engaged in an antigen-specific response with a predominance of T cells, some of which are activated (Van Boxel and Paget 1975; Talal et al. 1974; Kontrinen et al. 1981; Adamson et al. 1983; Young et al. 1984). Widespread expression of HLA class II antigens (Janossy et al. 1981; Klareskog 1971) including their appearance on epithelial cells of duct tissue in the case of sicca syndrome (Lindahl et al. 1985) suggests that HLA-restricted antigen presentation to T cells may be occurring at these sites. Furthermore, plasma cells are prominent and there is evidence that rheumatoid factors are being locally synthesized in the exocrine tissue in sicca syndrome and in the synovial membrane of rheumatoid patients (Smiley et al. 1968; Anderson et al. 1972). It seems probable that the local immune response is associated with the production of immune complexes which fix complement and mediate local inflammation and tissue damage. It could be suggested that the 'extra-vascular' immune complex disease localized to these tissues spreads to the intravascular compartment and leads to systemic features, and that the pattern of disease and differences in groups reflects the quantity and quality of immune complexes and other host factors; there is some evidence in rheumatoid patients to support this notion (Erhardt et al. 1979; Bourke et al. 1982; Melson et al. 1984). The sequence of events and evolution of disease is diagrammatically shown in Fig. 4.

An intriguing relationship between primary Sjögren's syndrome and the development of lymphoreticular proliferative disorders has previously been noted (Anderson and Talal 1972), suggesting a possible aetiological link between this form of auto-immunity and malignancy. The recent discovery of an increased subpopulation of B cells within the normal number of total circulating B cells in rheumatoid arthritis, with the surface phenotype IgM/D positive and T-1 (CD-5 antigen) positive, resembling the usual type of B cell leukemic cell (Plater-Zyberk et al. 1985),

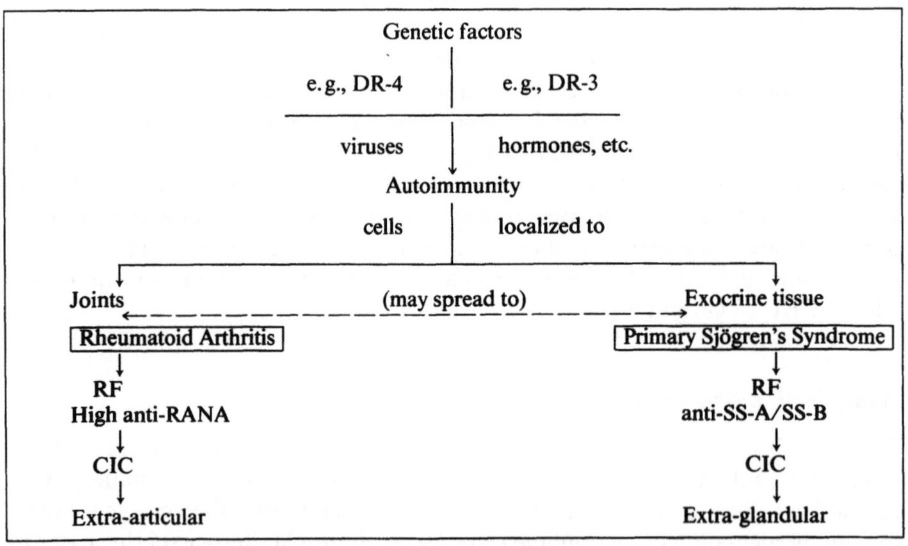

Fig. 4. The dichotomy of aetiopathogenesis of rheumatoid arthritis

extends the concept of the spectrum of benign to malignant proliferation to rheumatoid arthritis. The regulation of the expression of oncogenes and their relationship to virus infection may provide important clues to the aetiology of these conditions and their relationship to each other in the future.

Acknowledgement

I would like to thank Mrs. M. James for her invaluable assistance in the preparation of the manuscript and Dr. Patrick Venables for helpful discussion.

References

Adamson TC, Fox RI, Frisman DM, Howell FV (1983) Immunohistologic analysis of lymphoid infiltrates in primary Sjögren's syndrome using monoclonal antibodies. J Immunol 130: 203-208

Alspaugh MA, Talal N, Tan EM (1976) Differentiation and characterization of autoantibodies and their antigens in Sjögren's syndrome. Arthr Rheum 19: 216-222

Alspaugh MA, Jensen FC, Rabin H, Tan EM (1979) Lymphocytes transformed by EB virus: induction of nuclear antigen reactive with antibody in rheumatoid arthritis. J Exp Med 147: 1018-1027

Alspaugh MA, Henle G, Lennette ET Henle W (1981) Elevated levels of antibodies to Epstein-Barr virus antigens in patients with rheumatoid arthritis. J Clin Invest 67: 1134-1140

Anderson LG, Talal N (1972) The spectrum of benign to malignant lymphoproliferation in Sjögren's syndrome. Clin Exp Immunol 10: 199-211

Anderson LG, Cummings NA, Asofsky R, Hylton MB, Tarpley TM, Tosami TS, Wolf RO, Schall GA, Talal N (1972) Salivary gland immunoglobulin and rheumatoid factor synthesis in Sjögren's syndrome: natural history and response to treatment. Amer J Med 53: 456-463

Bloch KJ, Bunim JJ (1963) Sjögren's syndrome and its relation to connective tissue diseases. J Chron Dis 16: 915-927

Bloch KH, Buchanan WW, Wohl MJ, Bunim JJ (1965) Sjögren's syndrome: a clinical, pathological and serological study of sixty-two cases. Medicine (Balt) 44: 187-231

Bourke BE, Moss IK, Mumford P, Horsfall A, Maini RN (1982) The complement fixing ability of putative circulating immune complexes in rheumatoid arthritis and its relationship to extra-articular disease. Clin Exp Immunol 48: 726-732

Bunim JJ, Buchanan WW, Wertlake DT, Sokoloff L, Bloch KJ, Beck JS, Alepa FB (1964) Clinical, pathologic, and serological studies in Sjögren's syndrome. Ann Intern Med 61: 509-520

Castro-Poltronieri A, Alarcon-Segovia D (1983) Articular Manifestations of primary Sjögren's syndrome. J Rheumatol 10: 485-488

Erhardt CC, Mumford PA, Maini RN (1979) Association of cryoglobulinaemia with nodules, vasculitis and fibrosing alveolitis in rheumatoid arthritis and their relationship to serum Clq-binding activity and rheumatoid factor. Clin Exp Immunol 38: 405-413

Garrod AB (1859) Nature and treatment of gout and rheumatic gout. Walton and Maberly, London

Gear AJ, Venables PJW, Edwards JMB, Maini RN, Ansell BM (1986) Rheumatoid arthritis, juvenile arthritis, iridocyclitis and Epstein-Barr virus. Ann Rheum Dis 45: 6-8

Gumpel JM, Hobbs JR (1970) Serum immune globulin in Sjögren's syndrome. Ann Rheum Dis 29: 681-683

Hamburger MI, Moutsopoulos HM, Lawley TJ, Frank MM (1979) Sjögren's syndrome: a defect in reticuloendothelial system Fc-receptor specific clearance. Ann Intern Med 91: 534-538

Holian J, Griffiths ID, Glass DN, Maini RN, Scott JT (1975) Human anti-DNA antibody reference standards for diagnosis and management of SLE. Ann Rheum Dis 34: 438-443

Janossy G, Duke O, Pulter LW, Panayi G, Bofill M, Goldstein G (1981) Rheumatoid arthritis: a disease of T lymphocyte - macrophage immunoregulation. Lancet 2: 839-842

Klareskog L, Forsum U, Tjernlund UM, Kabelitz D, Wigren A (1981) Appearance of anti-HLA-DR-reactive cells in normal and rheumatoid synovial tissue. Scand J Immunol 14: 183-192

Lindahl G, Hedfors E, Klareskog L, Forsum U (1985) Epithelial HLA-DR expression and T lymphocyte subsets in salivary glands in Sjögren's syndrome. Clin exp Immunol 61: 475-482
Maini RN, Charles PJ, Venables PJW (1985) Antinuclear antibodies in the immunotaxonomy of connective tissue diseases. Scnad J Rheumatol suppl 56: 49-57
Maini RN, Holborow EJ (eds) (1977) Detection and measurement of circulating soluble antigen-antibody complexes and anti-DNA antibodies. Ann Rheum Dis 36, suppl 1
Mason AMS, Gumpel JM, Golding PL (1973) Semin Arthr Rheum 2: 301-331
Melsom RD, Smith PR, Maini RN (1984) Analysis of circulating immune complexes isolated by affinity chromatography from the sera of rheumatoid arthritis patients. Ann Rheum Dis 43: 116-117
Moutsopoulos HM, Webber BL, Vlagopoulous TP, Chused TM, Decker JL (1979a) Differences in the clinical manifestations of sicca syndrome in the presence and absence of rheumatoid arthritis. Am J Med 66: 733-736
Moutsopoulos HM, Mann DL, Johnson AH, Chused TM (1979b) Genetic differences between primary and secondary sicca syndrome. N Engl J Med 301: 761-763
Ollier W, Venables PJW, Mumford PJW, Maini RN, Awad J, Jaraquemada D, D'Amaro J, Festenstein H (1984) HLA antigen associations with extra-articular rheumatoid arthritis. Tussie Antigens 24: 279-291
Plater-Zyberk C, Maini RN, Lam K, Kennedy TD, Janossy G (1985) A rheumatoid arthritis B cell subset expresses a phenotype similar to that in chronic lymphatic leukemia. Arthr Rheum 28: 971-976
Shillitoe EJ, Daniels TE, Whitcher JP, Strand DV, Talal N, Greenspan JS (1982) Antibody to cytomegalovirus in patients with Sjögren's syndrome as detected by enzyme-linked immunosorbend assay. Arthr Rheum 25: 260-265
Sjögren H (1933) Zur Kenntnis der Keratoconjunctivitis sicca (keratitis filiformis bei Hypunfunktion der Tränendrüsen). Acta Ophthal 11: 1-15
Sjögren H (1951) Some problemes concerning keratoconjunctivitis sicca and sicca syndrome. Acta Ophthal (Kbh) 29: 33-39
Smiley JD, Sachs C, Ziff M (1968) In vitro synthesis of immunoglobulins by rheumatoid synovial membrane. J Clin Invest 47: 624-632
Tan EM (1982) Autoantibodies to nuclear antigens (ANA): their immunobiology and medicine. Adv Immunol 33: 167-240
Talal N, Sylvester RA, Daniels TE, Greenspan JS, Williams RC (Jr) (1974) T and B lymphocytes in the peripheral blood and tissue lesions in Sjögren's syndrome. J Clin Invest 53: 180-189
Van Boxel JA, Paget SA (1975) Predominantly T-cell infiltrate in rheumatoid synovial membranes. N Engl J Med 293: 517-520
Venables PJW (1986) Antibodies to nucleic acid binding proteins: their clinical and aetiological significance. MD Thesis, University of Cambridge
Venables PJW, Erhardt CC, Maini RN (1980) Antibodies to extractable nuclear antigens in rheumatoid arthritis: relationship to vasculiis and circulating immune complexes. Clin Exp Immunol 39: 146-153
Venables PJW, Roffe LM, Erhardt CC, Maini RN, Edwards JMB, Porter AD (1981) Titers of antibodies to RANA in rheumatoid arthritis and normal sera. Arthr Rheum 24: 1459-1464
Venables JPJ, Charles PJ, Buchanan RC, Tung Yi, Mumford PA, Schrieber L, Room GRW, Maini RN (1983) Quantitation and detection of isotypes of anti-SS-B antibodies by ELISA and Farr assays using affinity purified antigens. Arthr Rheum 26: 146-155
Venables PJW, Smith PR, Maini RN (1984) Rheumatoid arthritis nuclear antigen and Epstein-Barr virus. Arthr Rheum 27: 476-477
Venables PJW, Ross MGR, Charles PJ, Melsom RD, Griffiths PD, Maini RN (1985) A seroepidemiological study of cytomegalovirus and Epstein-Barr virus in rheumatoid arthritis and sicca syndrome. Ann Rheum Diss 44: 742-746
Wilson MR, Arroyave CM, Miles L, Tan (1977) Immune reactants in cryoproteins, relationship to complement activation. Ann Rheum Dis 36: 540-549
Wolf H, Haus M, Wilmes E (1984) Persistence of Epstein-Barr virus in the parotid gland. J Virol 51: 795-798
Wood PHN (1978) Epidemiology of rheumatic disorders. In: Scott JT (ed) Copeman's Textbook of the Rheumatic Diseases. Churchill Livingstone, Edinburgh London New York, pp 25-61

2. Sjögren's Syndrome with Systemic Lupus Erythematosus/Mixed Connective Tissue Disease

S. S. KASSAN and N. TALAL

Introduction

The co-existence of Sjögren's syndrome (SS) with systemic lupus erythematosus (SLE) has been alluded to since 1959 (Heaton 1959). Since that report, numerous studies on comparing and contrasting these two diseases have been reported (Bencze 1970; Heaton 1959; Kassan 1977; Moutsopoulos 1980a; Moutsopoulos 1980b; Steinberg 1971). Many of the clinical, serological and immunogenetic features of SS and SLE often make precise diagnosis difficult and suggest similar (Moutsopoulos 1980a, 1980b), possible common pathophysiologic features.

In 1959, Heaton reviewed the pathologic and clinical features of SS and SLE and came to the conclusion that SS was a benign form of SLE. This was on the basis of many overlapping systemic symptoms and the presence, grossly, of similar pathologic findings in the two diseases ("oedema, early destruction of the elastic tissue, hyalinization, infiltration with lymphocytes and plasma cells, fibroblastic proliferation, and thickening of blood-vessel walls with hyaline tissue") (Heaton 1959). Since that time, more precise data based on better clinical definitions, serologic and immunologic methods have allowed for critical descriptions of similarities and differences between primary SS, secondary SS with SLE/mixed connective tissue disease (MCTD) and SLE alone.

Incidence

Primary SS evaluated retrospectively (Pavlidis 1982) had an average age at onset of 44 years (± 15 years) as contrasted to 29.3 years (range 2–76 years) (Dubois 1964) for SLE alone. The incidence for the development of SLE following an initial diagnosis of primary SS is between 1% and 9% (Alarcon-Segovia 1974; Moutsopoulos 1980a; Sharp 1975; Shearn 1952).

In contrast, features of SS in SLE (secondary SS) are found more frequently with an incidence varying from 6% (Grennan 1977b; Steinberg 1971) to 90% (Alarcon-Segovia 1974b). This enormous variation is explained by the lack of standardized criteria for the diagnosis of SS. In our experience using recommended criteria outlined in chapter II.E.1, the true incidence probably is around 25%.

The presence of SS in MCTD has been found to vary from 7% (in one multicenter study) (Sharp 1975) to approximately 50% in one clinic (Alarcon-Segovia 1974a) of 25 patients with MCTD. The latter study found symptomatic xerostomia and/or ocular symptoms of keratoconjunctivitis sicca in 12 of 25 patients where confirmation of these findings was accomplished by objective methods.

Clinical Studies

Patients with primary SS and those with SLE may have similar disease manifestations including features of arthritis (usually nonerosive and nondeforming), rash, vasculitis, central nervous system involvement and glomerulonephritis (Moutsopoulos 1980a). A report by Heaton in 1959 postulated on purely clinical grounds that SS may be a milder form of SLE. Clinical experience over the last 25 years suggests that SS and SLE are different diseases although precise diagnosis on clinical grounds alone can be difficult in certain rare patients. Features of lymphadenopathy, hepatosplenomegaly, interstitial renal disease, pulmonary involvement, cutaneous and peripheral nerve vasculitis appear with greater frequency and severity in primary SS than in SLE (Alexander 1983a, 1983b; Bloch 1965; Moutsopoulos 1980a).

The clinical manifestations of SS in SLE patients are often mildly symptomatic or subclinical (Alarcon-Segovia 1974b). Lip biopsy is positive for SS in 50% (Moutsopoulos 1980b) to 94% (Alarcon-Segovia 1974b) of SLE patients in two studies reported. In these same groups, parotid scans were abnormal in 58% (Moutsopoulos 1980b) and 90% (Alarcon-Segovia 1974b) yet clinical symptoms were present in only 30% (Moutsopoulos 1980b) and 42% (Alarcon-Segovia 1974b) respectively.

Grennan et al. (1977a) reported a higher incidence of SS in a group described as overlapping SLE and rheumatoid arthritis (RA) with erosive polyarthritis where an 83% incidence (five of six patients) of SS was found. This was compared with a 13% and a 24% incidence of SS in subsets of patients with SLE/scleroderma and typical SLE respectively. No differences in the incidence of clinical renal disease was noted among the "typical" SLE patients with SS (50%) and those without SS (45%).

Clinical reports of MCTD with SS (Alarcon-Segovia 1974a; Sharp 1975) are limited. Symptomatic SS was found in 50% of 25 patients in one study (Alarcon-Segovia 1974a) where it was postulated that subclinical SS in this disease may be more prevalent as noted in SLE (Alarcon-Segovia 1974b) and scleroderma (Alarcon-Segovia 1976). Overall, the clinical features of MCTD patients with secondary SS did not differ from those with MCTD alone. Symptomatic SS was found to be the presenting symptom in two of twelve patients who later developed other clinical features of MCTD. This is not often seen in other forms of secondard SS (Moutsopoulos 1980a; Moutsopoulos 1979b).

Three cases of childhood MCTD (Fraga 1978) were noted to be associated with secondary SS. Parotid enlargement was also reported in one other case of childhood MCTD (Sanders 1973) and has been seen in one other case by one of the authors (Kassan SS, unpublished data). This is quite significant owing to the fact that both childhood MCTD and childhood SS are both relatively infrequent disorders (Fauci 1980).

Serologic Studies

Patients with primary SS, secondary SS with SLE, and secondary SS with RA all manifest features of B-cell hyper-reactivity as evidenced by the findings of polyclonal hypergammaglobulinemia, non-organ specific autoantibodies, (i.e. rheumatoid factor) and antibodies to extractable nuclear antigens (Alspaugh 1976; Kassan 1977). In primary SS, unlike SLE patients, there is not an increased number of circulating B-cells spontaneously secreting polyclonal antibody.

Comparisons of peripheral B-cell and T-cell markers, by monoclonal antibodies, has demonstrated a relationship between primary SS and active SLE (Morimoto 1982). Specifically, in 71 percent of primary SS patients and in 100% of active SLE patients, there was a decrease in total numbers of T-cells as well as a selective decrease in the T8 suppressor subset in both groups.

Patients with primary SS develop antibodies to the extractable nuclear antigens Ro and La to a high degree (Moutsopoulos 1980b). However, these antibodies are often also present in SLE, although anti-La tends to be more common in primary SS or in SS associated with SLE.

Antibodies to intermediate filaments in the cytoplasmic cytoskeleton have been demonstrated in various connective tissue diseases (Kurki 1983). Antibodies to vimentin filament of the IgG and IgA class were found only in primary SS and the highest prevalence in cytokeratin filament antibodies was found in primary SS (64%) and secondary SS with SLE (57%). The significance of these antibodies is unclear. They have also been found in patients with "autoimmune hepatitis" (Kurki 1981) where the sicca syndrome is also common (Golding 1973). It is possible that the stimulus for the formation of these vimentin and cytokeratin filament antibodies may be a result of breakdown or destruction of cells containing such filaments as synovial lining cells (Osunj 1982), lymphocytes (Linder 1979), hepatocytes and epithelial cells of exocrine glands (Franke 1979).

Genetic Studies

Patients with primary SS have an increased association with HLA-B8 antigen (Fye 1976). Further reports (Chused 1977; Moutsopoulos 1979a) have extended this observation whereby HLA-B8 and HLA-DW3 was noted to be associated with primary SS and not with secondary SS with RA. This data established the genetic differences between primary and secondary SS. B-cell antigen typing showed increased reaction frequencies of individual antisera Ia-172 and Ia-350 in both primary SS and secondary SS with SLE as compared with normals (Moutsopoulos 1979a). Because these B-cell antigens, in the case of secondary SS with SLE, are thought to detect additional B-cell antigens controlled by a gene locus or loci other than the DR-locus, these findings may in some way link primary and secondary SS by a common genetic component and suggests that an immune response gene may contribute to the pathogenesis of the disease (Mann 1980). In contrast, patients with SLE have increased frequencies of HLA-B8, HLA-DRw2, HLA-DRw3 and B-lymphocyte alloantigen Ia-715 (Reinertson 1978). Primary SS patients have similarly increased frequencies of HLA-B8, HLA-DRw3, and B-lymphocyte alloantigens Ia-35, Ia-172, Ia-350 and Ia-715 (Moutsopoulos 1978 κ 1979a). Secondary SS with RA patients do not share any HLA-A or B specificities and have an increased incidence of HLA-DRw4 and B-lymphocyte alloantigens Ia-172 and Ia-350 and not HLA-DRw2, HLA-DRw3, Ia-35 or Ia-715 (Moutsopoulos 1979a). Thus, the various genetic similarities and differences between primary SS, secondary SS with SLE, secondary SS with RA and SLE suggest a possibly greater relationship between primary SS and SLE and enhance the hypothesis that they may share a common pathophysiology different from patients with RA, leading to the development of a sicca syndrome.

References

1. Alarcon-Segovia D (1976) Symptomatic Sjögren's Syndrome in mixed connective tissue disease. J Rheum 3 (2): 191-195
2. Alarcon-Segovia D, Ibanez G, Hermandez-Ortiz J, Velasquez-Forero F, Gonzalez-Jimenez Y (1974a) Sjögren's Syndrome in progressive systemic sclerosis (scleroderma). Am J Med 57: 78-85
3. Alarcon-Segovia D, Ibanez G, Velazguez-Forero F, Hernandez-Ortiz J, Gonzalez-Jiminez Y (1974b) Sjögren's Syndrome in systemic lupus erythematosus; clinical and subclinical manifestations. Ann Intern Med 81: 577-583
4. Alexander EL, Arnett FC, Provost TT, Stevens MB (1983a) Sjögren's Syndrome: association of anti-Ro (SSA) antibodies with vasculitis, hematologic abnormalities and serologic hyper-reactivity. Ann Intern Med 98: 155-159
5. Alexander EL, Provost TT (1983b) Cutaneous manifestations of primary Sjögren's Syndrome: a reflection of vasculitis and association with anti-Ro (SSA) antibodies. J Invest Derm 80: 386-391
6. Alspaugh MA, Talal N, Tan EM (1976) Differentiation and characterization of autoantibodies and their antigens in Sjögren's Syndrome. Arthritis Rheum 19: 216-222
7. Bencze G (1970) Relationship of systemic lupus erythematosus to rheumatoid arthritis, discoid lupus erythematosus and Sjögren's Syndrome; a clinical study. Acta Rheum Scand 16: 191-196
8. Bloch KJ, Buchanan WW, Wohl JJ, Bunim JJ (1965) Sjögren's syndrome: a clinical pathological and serological study of sixty-two cases. Medicine (Baltimore) 44: 187-231
9. Chused TM, Kassan SS, Moutsopoulos HM, Terasaki PI (1977) Sjögren's syndrome associated with HLA-Dw3. New Eng J Med 296: 895-897
10. Dubois EL, Tufanelli D (1964) Clinical manifestations of systemic lupus erythematosus
11. Fauci AS (1980) Immunoregulation in Sjögren's Syndrome In: Moutsopoulos HM (moderator) Sjögren's Syndrome (sicca syndrome): current issues Ann Intern Med 92 (1): 219-220
12. Fraga A, Judino J, Ramos-Niembro F, Alarcon-Segovia D (1978) Mixed connective tissue disease in childhood: relationship with Sjögren's Syndrome. Ann J Dis Child 132: 263-265
13. Franke WW, Appelhans B, Schmid E, et al. (1979) Identification and characterization of peithelial cells in mammalian tissues by immunofluorescence microscopy using antibodies to prekeratin. Differentiation 15: 7-25
14. Fye KH, Teresaki PI, Moutsopoulos HM, Daniels TE, Michalski JP, Talal N (1976) Association of Sjögren's Syndrome with HLA-B8. Arthritis Rheum 19: 883-886
15. Golding PL, Smith M, Williams R (1973) Multisystem involvement is chronic liver disease. Ann J Med 55: 772-782
16. Grennan DM, Ferguson M, Ghobarey AE, Williamson J, Dick WC, Buchanan WW (1977a) Sjögren's Syndrome in SLE: Part 2, an examination of the clinical significance of Sjögren's Syndrome by comparison of its frequency in typical and atypical forms of SLE, overlap syndromes and scleroderma. NZ Med J 86: 376-379
17. Grennan DM, Ferguson M, Williamson J, Mavrikakis M, Dick WC, Buchanan WW (1977b) Sjögren's syndrome in systemic lupus erythematosus: I, The frequency of the clinical and subclinical features of Sjögren's Syndrome in patients with systemic lupus erythematosus. N Z Med J 86: 374-6
18. Heaton JM (1959) Sjögren's Syndrome and systemic lupus erythematosus. Brit Med J 1: 466-469
19. Kassan SS, Akizuki M, Steinberg AD, Reddick RL, Chused TM (1977) Antibody to a soluble acidic nuclear antigen in Sjögren's Syndrome. Am J Med 63: 328-335
20. Kurki P, Helve T, Virtanen I (1983) Antibodies to cytoplasmic intermediate filaments in rheumatic diseases. J Rheum 10 (4) 558-562

21. Kurki P, Miettinen A, Pikkarainen P, et al. (1981) Cytoskeleton antibodies in liver diseases. 16th meeting of the European association for the study of liver. Lisbon, September 3-5, 1981
22. Linder E, Kurki P, Andersson LC (1979) Autoantibody to "intermediate filaments" in infectious mononucleosus. Clin Immunol Immunopathol 14: 411-417
23. Mann DL (1980) HLA-alloantigens in primary and secondary Sjögren's Syndrome. In: Moutsopoulos HM (moderator) Sjögren's Syndrome (sicca syndrome): current issues, Ann Intern Med 92 (1): 215-216
24. Morimoto C, Reinherz EL, Nadler LM, Disfaso JA, Steinberg AD, Schlossman SF (1982) Comparison in T- and B-cell markers in Sjögren's Syndrome and systemic lupus erythematosus. Clin Immunol Immunopathol 22: 270-278
25. Moutsopoulos HM, Chused TM, Mann DL, Klippel JH, Fauci AS, Frank MM, Lawley TJ, Hamburger MI (1980a) Sjögren's Syndrome (sicca syndrome): current issues, Ann Intern Med 92 (Part 1): 212-226
26. Moutsopoulos HM, Klippel JH, Pavlidis N, Wolf RO, Sweet JB, Steinberg AD, Chu FC, Turpley TM (1980b) Correlative histologic and serologic findings of sicca syndrome in patients with systemic lupus erythematosus. Arthritis Rheum 23: 36-40
27. Moutsopoulos HM, Mann DL, Johnson AH, Chused TM (1979a) Genetic differences between primary and secondary sicca syndrome. N Eng J Med 301: 761-763
28. Moutsopoulos HM, Webber BL, Vlajopoulos TP, Chused TM, Deeker JL (1979b) Difference in the clinical manifestations of sicca syndrome in the presence and absence of theumatoid arthritis. Ann I Med 66: 733-736
29. Moutsopoulos HM, Chused TM, Johnson AH, Knudsen B, Mann DL (1978) B-lymphocyte antigens in sicca syndrome. Science 199: 1441-1442
30. Osunj OA, Chandra M, Holborow EJ (1982) Intermediate filaments in synovial lining cells in rheumatoid arthritis and other arthritides are of vimentin type. Ann Rheum Dis 41: 74-77
31. Pavlidis NA, Karsh J, Moutsopoulos H (1982) The clinical picture of primary Sjögren's Syndrome: a retrospective study. J Rheum
32. Reinertson JL, Klippel JH, Johnson AK, Steinberg AD, Decker JL, Mann DL (1978) B-lymphocyte alloantigens associated with systemic lupus erythematosus. N Eng J Med 299: 515-518
33. Sanders DY, Huntley CC, Sharp GE (1973) Mixed connective tissue disease in a child. J Pediatric 83: 642-643
34. Sharp GC (1975) Mixed connective tissue disease. Bull Rheum Dis 25: 828-831
35. Shearn MA, Profsky B (1952) Disseminated lupus erythematosus: an analysis of 34 cases. Arch Intern Med 90: 790-807
36. Steinberg AD, Talal N (1971) The coexistence of Sjögren's Syndrome and systemic lupus erythematosus. Ann Intern Med 74: 55-61

3. Sjögren's Syndrome and Systemic Sclerosis (Scleroderma)

TH. A. MEDSGER, JR.

Historical Background

The occurrence of Sjögren's syndrome in a patient with systemic sclerosis (scleroderma) was first convincingly described by Leriche in 1947 [1]. During the next decade, numerous individual case reports of this association were published [2-9], including one by Sjögren himself [4]. Some of these cases are not well documented, and in fact, appear to be instances of primary Sjögren's syndrome with purpura of the lower extremities resulting in hyperpigmentation of the legs mimicking scleroderma [2, 3]. Beginning with the two patients described by Shearn in 1960 [10], the relationship between Sjögren's syndrome and systemic sclerosis became widely appreciated.

Frequency

Systemic sclerosis in Sjögren's syndrome. In 5 large series of patients with Sjögren's syndrome, including a total of over 400 patients [11-15], the proportion having systemic sclerosis is consistently small (3-6%).

Sjögren's syndrome in systemic sclerosis. Several comprehensive reviews of scleroderma prior to 1955 [16, 17] include no reference to Sjögren's syndrome, and in two subsequent series, this condition was noted only rarely (1-2%) [18, 19]. More recently, there has been increased sensitivity to this relationship and a plethora of new objective methods to detect lacrimal and salivary gland dysfunction (see Chapters II, A.1. and II, A.2.). Consequently, series of systemic sclerosis patients have included increasing proportions of individuals with documented Sjögren's syndrome.

Cipoletti et al. [20] found histologic evidence of Sjögren's syndrome in 6 of 35 (17%) consecutive systemic sclerosis patients, and in an extension of that study [21] the frequency was 17 of 58 (29%). Using similar criteria for minor salivary gland lymphocytic infiltration (2+ or greater, Tarpley grading system) Alarcon-Segovia et al. [22] reported 7 of 20 (35%) with typical Sjögren's syndrome. If other objective clinical features of Sjögren's syndrome are also allowed to contribute as criteria, a considerably higher proportion of patients are found to have one or more abnormality of lacrimal or salivary gland function.

Setting

The systemic sclerosis patient most likely to have associated Sjögren's syndrome is female and older (over age 40), as one might expect considering the demographic features of primary Sjögren's syndrome. These individuals tend to have a prolonged duration of scleroderma and to be classified as having the CREST syndrome variant [20, 23]. One instance of familial CREST syndrome and Sjögren's syndrome (mother and daughter) has been described [24].

Clinical Features

Ocular. The ophthalmologic features of Sjögren's syndrome in patients with systemic sclerosis are essentially the same as those in primary Sjögren's. The complaint of dryness or a "gritty" or "sandy" sensation has been found in 35-70% of patients [20-22], with objective documentation by an abnormal Schirmer's test or rose bengal dye staining in approximately three fourths of these symptomatic cases (Table 1). The complication of corneal ulceration is probably rare but has been described [14]. Another potential contribution in systemic sclerosis is severe facial skin thickening, which may lead to retraction of the lower eyelid and a degree of ectropion.

Oral. Salivary insufficiency is characterized by the complaint of dry mouth and a variety of other symptoms previously described (see Chapter II, A. 1.). Dry mouth is frequent in systemic sclerosis patients (40-80%). There is some discrepancy of opinion regarding enlargement of one or more salivary glands, a physical finding which is reported to occur as seldom as 15% and as often as 80% (Table 1). No simple explanation accounts for these differences, although the reports emanate from different countries. The use of sialography, scintiscans and radionuclide excretion rates appear to be sensitive measures of major salivary gland structure and function. One or more of these evaluations was noted to be abnormal in 75-90% of cases [22].

Table 1. Sicca symptoms, physical examination and laboratory findings in patients with systemic sclerosis

	Cipoletti et al. [20]	Osial et al. [21]	Alarcon-Segovia et al. [22]
Ocular			
Dry eyes	12/35 (34%)	20/53 (38%)	18/25 (72%)
Schirmer test abnormal	9/32 (28%)	14/41 (34%)	10/25 (40%)
Rose bengal staining	3/29 (10%)		11/20 (55%)
Oral			
Dry mouth	15/35 (43%)	17/53 (32%)	21/25 (84%)
Salivary gland enlargement	4/35 (11%)	2/54 (4%)	21/25 (84%)
Lip biopsy abnormal			
inflammation 2+ or greater	6/35 (17%)	17/58 (29%)	7/20 (35%)
fibrosis 2+ or greater	21/35 (60%)	19/58 (33%)	9/20 (45%)

Although one must consider the non-specificity of these tests, results suggest that the great majority of systemic sclerosis patients have subtle, often subclinical, evidence of salivary gland dysfunction.

Laboratory Abnormalities

Serum rheumatoid factor, frequently present in primary Sjögren's syndrome, is also found commonly in the secondary Sjögren's syndrome of systemic sclerosis. Rheumatoid factor is associated with prominent lymphocytic infiltration of the minor salivary glands. Osial et al. noted IgM rheumatoid factor in 8 of 16 (50%) of the latter group compared with only 4 of 34 (12%) in patients whose biopsies showed no significant lymphocytic collections [21]. Antinuclear antibodies are also more frequent in patients with minor salivary gland lymphocytic infiltration [21]. A variety of other serum autoantibodies may be detected, but they are rarely present in more than 10-15% of patients; they include antibodies directed against cell nuclei (anti-DNA, anti-RNP, anti-Sm), cells (direct Coombs), tissue (anti-mitochondrial, anti-smooth muscle, anti-microsomal) and other proteins (anti-thyroglobulin) [20]. Mean serum IgG and IgM levels are significantly higher in patients with anti-SSA, rheumatoid factor and lymphocytic glandular infiltration [21]. Serum immune complexes, in contrast, are found in a majority of patients regardless of other laboratory abnormalities [21].

Other serum autoantibodies more pertinent to Sjögren's syndrome also have been studied. Anti-salivary gland antibody was detected in 12 of 28 (43%) patients in one series [20]. Anti-SSA and/or anti-SSB are often present when the lip biopsy shows lymphocytic infiltration (9/17 or 53%) but seldom in its absence (1/41 or 2%) [25, 26]. Rheumatoid arthritis precipitin (RAP), found in patients with rheumatoid arthritis and rheumatoid arthritis with secondary Sjögren's syndrome, is rare in systemic sclerosis, with or without Sjögren's syndrome [21].

HLA-B8, the tissue typing antigen recognized to be associated with primary Sjögren's syndrome [27], has not been convincingly linked to the secondary Sjögren's syndrome of systemic sclerosis [21]. The MT2 locus appears to be the strongest major histocompatibility complex determinant of both primary and secondary Sjögren's syndrome [28], but HLA-DR3 and DR2 are felt to mediate anti-SSA and anti-SSB responses. These antigens are not increased in systemic sclerosis patients with Sjögren's syndrome.

Pathologic Features

The classic major and minor salivary gland lesions of primary Sjögren's syndrome have been extensively described (see Chapter II, A.4.). Significant glandular and periglandular lymphocytic infiltration is encountered in 20-30% of unselected patients with systemic sclerosis [20-22]. It should be emphasized that false negative biopsies, due to sampling error, must be frequent considering the higher proportion of patients with other objective evidence of salivary gland dysfunction. Immunofluorescent staining has identified IgM as the dominant salivary and tissue immunoglobulin [29].

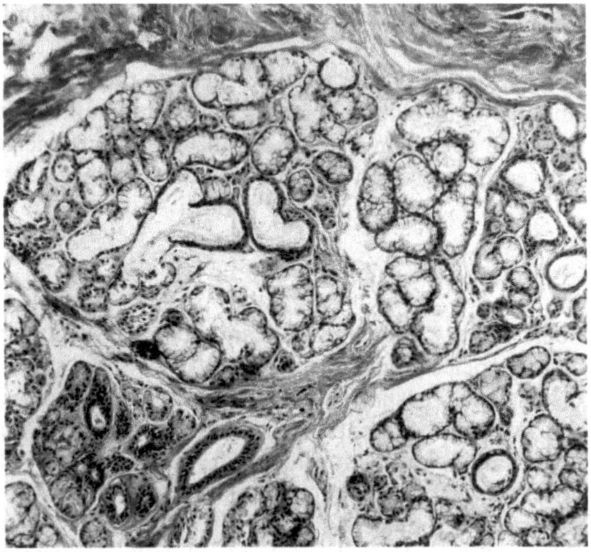

Fig. 1. Photomicrograph of a lip biopsy from a 44-year old woman with systemic sclerosis with limited cutaneous involvement (CREST syndrome) and xerostomia. Note the extensive periglandular (top) and interlobular (center) fibrosis without significant lymphocytic infiltration (magnification ×33)

Table 2. Clinical and laboratory associations in patients with systemic sclerosis according to lip biopsy histologic classification

Lymphocytic Infiltration	*Fibrosis*	*Normal Gland*
older		younger
female		
longer disease duration		
CREST syndrome	diffuse scleroderma	
sicca symptoms	renal involvement	
Schirmer test +		
increased serum IgG		
antinuclear antibody	increased mortality	
rheumatoid factor		
anti-SSA/SSB		

A larger proportion of systemic sclerosis patients (45–60%) have moderate to extensive periglandular and intraglandular fibrosis, as illustrated in Fig. 1 [10, 20]. There appears to be no definite relationship between the degree or extent of cellular infiltration and fibrosis. Most investigators consider that this glandular fibrotic response is integral to systemic sclerosis rather than representing a part of the spectrum of Sjögren's syndrome. Similar fibrosis is found in the thyroid gland [30] and Brunner's glands of the duodenum [31] in patients with systemic sclerosis. Nasal mucosal biopsies have also shown fibrosis surrounding mucous-secreting glands [32].

There may be some utility in dividing patients according to the histopathologic findings on lip biopsy. The important demographic, clinical and laboratory associations are shown in Table 2. Serial biopsy specimens have not been obtained to answer the question whether or not the histologic features change over time.

Associated Conditions

Some of the extraglandular manifestations of Sjögren's syndrome are considered commonplace in scleroderma, such as Raynaud's phenomenon, inflammatory joint disease and bibasilar pulmonary interstitial fibrosis with restrictive lung disease. In contrast, purpura, lymphadenopathy, hepatomegaly, splenomegaly, and renal tubular defects are distinctly unusual in systemic sclerosis. If they occur in a patient with systemic sclerosis, these manifestations should raise the question of associated but unappreciated Sjögren's syndrome. Esophageal dysmotility has been described in primary Sjögren's syndrome but tends to be proximal rather than distal [33]; the latter would be expected in typical systemic sclerosis.

Vasculitis is a frequent finding in primary Sjögren's syndrome but is unusual in typical systemic sclerosis. However, a subgroup of patients with secondary Sjögren's syndrome who also have serum anti-SSA antibodies appear particularly susceptible to developing vasculitis [34]. In our experience, the systemic sclerosis patients at risk to vasculitis have the CREST syndrome variant, ulcerating cutaneous lesions, mononeuritis multiplex and a variety of more severe visceral ischemic events, leukocytoclastic and lymphocytic blood vessel wall infiltration, anti-SSA antibodies, rheumatoid factor, and serum C4 levels disproportionately low compared with C3 [35].

Based on compilation of small series [36-39] and single case reports [40-42] chronic inflammatory (autoimmune) hepatic disease occurs more often in systemic sclerosis patients with Sjögren's syndrome than in those without Sjögren's. The most frequent histologic and immunologic association is with primary biliary cirrhosis, and the majority of reported patients have CREST syndrome.

Autoimmune (Hashimoto's) thyroiditis [43, 44], pernicious anemia [44], thrombocytopenia [45, 46], pulmonary hypertension [46, 47], lymphocytic interstitial pneumonitis [48] and pancreatic exocrine dysfunction [49] have all been noted in patients with systemic sclerosis. Trigeminal neuropathy, which occurs in less than 5% of systemic sclerosis patients, is more frequent when Sjögren's syndrome is also present [50].

An interesting circumstance which highlights the close relationship between the immune system, systemic sclerosis and Sjögren's syndrome is the occurrence of the latter two conditions in patients who develop chronic graft-versus-host disease after allogeneic bone marrow transplantation [51]. Sjögren's syndrome has been noted in four cases of scleroderma following cosmetic breast augmentation [43, 52-54] and in a patient who had received busulfan [55], an agent recognized to precipitate Raynaud's phenomenon and sclerodermatous skin changes [56].

Natural History

The prognosis for survival in Sjögren's syndrome patients with systemic sclerosis is primarily determined by those factors influencing outcome in scleroderma. Poor prognostic features include male sex, older age, classification as the diffuse scleroderma variant, and involvement of the kidney, heart, or lung [57]. The reduced survival reported for patients with minor salivary glandular fibrosis is most likely attributable to the association of this histologic lesion with diffuse scleroderma [20]. We have followed two patients, both with CREST syndrome, in whom Sjögren's syndrome was present for 10-15 years before the development of lymphosarcoma. Although the independent contribution of Sjögren's syndrome to survival has not been determined, extraglandular involvement such as systemic vasculitis and lymphoproliferative malignancy place these patients at high risk.

Therapy

The therapeutic approach to Sjögren's syndrome in patients with scleroderma is symptomatic and similar to that described in Chapter IV. In addition to accelerated dental caries, reduced oral aperture due to facial and perioral skin and subcutaneous thickening may make dental prophylaxis more difficult. Regular visits to the dentist, as often as every 3-4 months, and scrupulous attention to proper oral hygiene are necessary. Since glandular fibrosis is frequent in systemic sclerosis with diffuse scleroderma, one might not expect these patients to respond to antiinflammatory or lympholytic agents such as corticosteroids and immunosuppressive drugs.

References

1. Leriche R (1947) Traitement chirurgical du syndrome de Sjögren (oeil sec et bouche seche), resultat au bout de vingthuit mais d'une double section du nerf vertebral; nature de la maladie. Presse Med 55: 77-78
2. Sheldon JH (1938-39) Sjögren's syndrome associated with pigmentation and scleroderma of the legs. Proc Roy Soc Med 32: 255-256
3. Harrington AB, Dewar HA (1951) A case of Sjögren's disease with scleroderma. Brit Med J 1: 1302-1303
4. Sjögren H (1948) Keratoconjunctivitis sicca and chronic polyarthritis. Acta Med Scand 130: 484-488
5. Holm S (1949) Keratoconjunctivitis sicca and the sicca syndrome. Acta Ophthalmol (Suppl) 33: 1-230
5. Ramage JH, Kinnear WF (1956) Kerato-conjunctivitis sicca and the collagen diseases. Brit J Ophthalmol 40: 416-420
7. Piazzesi W (1956) Su di un caso di sclerodermia con diplegia faciale e sindrome di Sjögren. Riv Pat Nerv Ment 77: 584-592
8. Stava Z (1958) Diffuse scleroderma: a clinical study of 65 cases. Dermatologica 117: 135-147
9. Bertram U (1967) Xerostomia. Clinical aspects, pathology and pathogenesis. Acta Odont Scand 25, Suppl 49: 1-126
10. Shearn MA (1960) Sjögren's syndrome in association with scleroderma. Ann Intern Med 52: 1352-1362
11. Denko CW, Old JW (1969) Myopathy in the sicca syndrome (Sjögren's syndrome). Amer J Clin Path 51: 631-637

12. Vanselow NA, Dodson VN, Angeli DC et al. (1963) A clinical study of Sjögren's syndrome. Ann Intern Med 58: 124-135
13. Bloch KJ, Buchanan WW, Wohl MJ et al. (1965) Sjögren's syndrome: a clinical, pathological, and serological study of sixty-two cases. Medicine 44: 187-231
14. Shearn MA (1971) Sjögren's Syndrome. In: Smith LH Jr (ed) Major Problems in Internal Medicine. WB Saunders Company, Philadelphia
15. Stolze CA, Hanlon DG, Pease GL, et al. (1960) Keratoconjunctivitis sicca and Sjögren's syndrome. Systemic manifestations and hematologic and protein abnormalities. Arch Intern Med 106: 513-522
16. Leinwand I, Duryee AW, Richter MN (1954) Scleroderma. Based on a study of over 150 cases. Ann Intern Med 41: 1003-1041
17. Beigelman PM, Goldman F Jr, Bayles TB (1953) Progressive systemic sclerosis (Scleroderma). N Engl J Med 249: 45-58
18. Rodnan GP (1963) The natural history of progressive systemic sclerosis (diffuse scleroderma). Bull Rheum Dis 13: 301-304
19. Tuffanelli DL, Winkelmann RK (1962) Scleroderma and its relationship to the "collagenoses": Dermatomyositis, lupus erythematosus, rheumatoid arthritis and Sjögren's syndrome. Amer J Med Sci 243: 133-146
20. Cipoletti JF, Buckingham RB, Barnes EL, Peel RL, Mahmood K, Cignetti FE, Pierce JM, Rabin BS, Rodnan GP (1977) Sjögren's syndrome in progressive systemic sclerosis. Ann Intern Med 87: 535-541
21. Osial TA, Whiteside TL, Buckingham RB, Singh G, Barnes EL, Pierce JM, Rodnan GP (1983) Clinical and serologic study of Sjögren's syndrome in patients with progressive systemic sclerosis 26: 500-508
22. Alarcon-Segovia D, Ibanez G, Hernandez-Ortiz J et al. (1974) Sjögren's syndrome in progressive systemic sclerosis (scleroderma) Amer J Med 57: 78-85
23. Medsger TA Jr (1985) Systemic Sclerosis (Scleroderma), Eosinophilic Fasciitis, and Calcinosis. In: McCarty DJ (ed) Arthritis and Allied Conditions, 10th edition. Lea & Febiger, Philadelphia, pp 994-1036
24. Frayha RA, Tabbara KF, Geha RS (1977) Familial CRST syndrome with sicca complex. J Rheumatol 4: 53-58
25. Alspaugh MA, Whaley K (1981) Sjögren's Syndrome. In: Kelly WN, Harris ED, Ruddy S, Sledge CB (eds) Textbook of Rheumatology. WB Saunders, Philadelphia, pp 971-999
26. Alexander EL, Hirsch TJ, Arnett FC, Provost TT, Stevens MB (1982) Ro (SSA) and La (SSB) antibodies in the clinical spectrum of Sjögren's syndrome. J Rheumatol 9: 239-246
27. Fye KH et al. (1976) Association of Sjögren's syndrome with HLA-B8. Arthritis Rheum 19: 883-886
28. Wilson RW, Provost TT, Bias WB, Alexander EL et al. (1984) Sjögren's syndrome. Influence of multiple HLA-D alloantigens on clinical and serologic expression. Arthritis Rheum 27: 1245-1253
29. Fiessinger JN et al. (1978) Salivary immunoglobulins in progressive systemic sclerosis. Biomedicine 28: 298-303
30. Gordon MB, Klein I, Dekker A, Rodnan GP, Medsger TA Jr (1981) Thyroid disease in progressive systemic sclerosis (PSS): increased frequency of glandular fibrosis and hypothyroidism. Ann Intern Med 95: 431-435
31. Rosson RS, Yesner R (1965) Peroral duodenal biopsy in progressive systemic sclerosis. N Engl J Med 272: 391-394
32. Talaat AM et al. (1980) Human respiratory nasal mucosa in progressive systemic sclerosis (scleroderma). An electron microscopic study. J Laryngol Otol 94: 617-627
33. Tsianos EB, Chiras CD, Drosos AA, Moutsopoulos HM (1985) Oesophageal dysfunction in patients with primary Sjögren's syndrome. Ann Rheum Dis 44: 610-613
34. Alexander EL et al. (1983) Sjögren's syndrome. Association of anti-Ro (SS-A) antibody with vasculitis, hematologic abnormalities and serologic hyperreactivity. Ann Intern Med 98: 155-159
35. Oddis CV, Eisenbeis CH, Reidbord HE, Steen VD, Medsger TA Jr (1986) Vasculitis in systemic sclerosis: a subset of patients with the CREST variant, Sjögren's syndrome and neurologic complications. Arthritis Rheum 29: S43 (abstract).

36. Reynolds TB et al. (1971) Primary biliary cirrhosis with scleroderma, Raynaud's phenomenon and telangiectasia. New syndrome. Amer J Med 50: 302-312
37. Clarke AK, Galbraith RM, Hamilton BD, Williams R (1978) Rheumatic disorders in primary biliary cirrhosis. Ann Rheum Dis 37: 42-47
38. Godeau P et al. (1980) Chronic hepatopathy and progressive systemic sclerosis. Frequency of association with Gougerot-Sjögren disease. A report on six new cases. Sem Hop Paris 56: 1895-1900
39. Youinov P et al. (1976) Association of systemic scleroderma, hepatopathy and Gougerot-Sjögren syndrome. 2 cases: coincidence or pathogenic relationship? Nouv Presse Med 5: 1983-1985
40. Albert J et al. (1983) Association of CRST syndrome, Gougerot-Sjögren syndrome, thyroid hyperplasia and chronic persistent hepatitis. Praxis 72: 324-328
41. Miyasaka N et al. (1977) A case of primary biliary cirrhosis associated with Sjögren's syndrome and sclerodactylia. Nippon Shokakibyo Gakkai Zasshi 74: 1392-1397
42. Hauftova D et al. (1982) Primary biliary cirrhosis, CRST syndrome, Sjögren's syndrome and nodular regenerative liver hyperplasia. Cesk Gastroenterol Vyz 36: 429-436
43. Kumagai Y, Shiokawa Y, Medsger TA Jr, Rodnan GP (1984) Clinical spectrum of connective tissue disease after cosmetic surgery. Arthritis Rheum 27: 1-12
44. Saad-Dine Y, Macurak RB, Beasley EW, Ward JA (1981) Hashimoto's thyroiditis, pernicious anemia, Sjögren's syndrome, and CREST syndrome - a case report. J Med Assoc Ga 70: 187-189
45. Segond P et al. (1981) Autoimmune thrombopenia in sclerodermia associated with Gougerot-Sjögren syndrome. Rev Rhum Mal Osteoartic 48: 725-727
46. Sakimura K et al. (1982) A case of Sjögren's syndrome with pulmonary hypertension, hypergammaglobulinemia and thrombocytopenia. Nippon Naika Gakkai Zasshi 10: 71-76
47. Gimeno JV et al. (1985) Pulmonary hypertension in Sjögren's syndrome: an uncommon manifestation. Rev Esp Cardiol 38: 69-71
48. Allard P, Kermarec J, L'Her P, Natali F, Lebarbu M, LeVaqueresse R (1984) Lymphocytic interstitial pneumonia in Gougerot-Sjögren's syndrome with scleroderma. Ann Med Interne (Paris) 135: 431-434
49. Dreiling DA, Soto JM (1976) The pancreatic involvement in disseminated "collagen" disorders. Studies of pancreatic secretion in patients with scleroderma and Sjögren's "disease". Am J Gastroenterol 66: 546-553
50. Farrell DA, Medsger TA Jr (1982) Trigeminal neuropathy in progressive systemic sclerosis. Amer J Med 73: 57-62
51. Lawley TJ, Peck GL, Moutsopoulos HM, Gratwohl AA, Deisseroth AB (1977) Scleroderma, Sjögren-like syndrome, and chronic graft-versus-host disease. Ann Intern Med 87: 707-709
52. Okano Y, Nishikai M, Sato A (1984) Scleroderma, primary biliary cirrhosis, and Sjögren's syndrome after cosmetic breast augmentation with silicone injection: a case report of possible human adjuvant disease. Ann Rheum Dis 43: 520-522
53. Nobunaga M, Oribe K, Ohishi S (1984) A case of scleroderma with Sjögren's syndrome, developed after mammoplasty. Clin Rheumatol 3: 375-379
54. Onbe K, Todoroki S, Anan K, Oribe M, Hashinaga K, Nobunaga T (1978) A case of systemic sclerosis associated with Sjögren's syndrome after breast augmentation (abstract). Nippon Naika Gakkai Zasshi 67: 676-677
55. Sidi Y, Douer D, Pinkhas J (1977) Sicca syndrome in a patient with toxic reaction. JAMA 238: 1951
56. Finch WR, Rodnan GP, Buckingham RB, Prince RK (1980) Bleomycin-induced scleroderma. J Rheumatol 7: 651-659
57. Medsger TA Jr, Masi AT, Rodnan GP, Benedek TG, Robinson H (1971) Survival with systemic sclerosis (scleroderma). A life-table analysis of demographic and clinical factors in 309 patients. Ann Intern Med 75: 369-376

E. Diagnosis and Differential Diagnosis

1. Diagnosis and Differential Diagnosis of Sjögren's Syndrome

T. E. Daniels and N. Talal

Diagnosis

Reports of the clinical components making up what we now call Sjögren's syndrome (SS) have been appearing for more than 100 years (reviewed by Shearn 1971). However, there remains a great need for standardized diagnostic criteria for SS that are acceptable worldwide. A brief review of the definition of SS and the evolution of criteria for its diagnosis illustrates the general problem of syndrome diagnosis and explains some of the variation seen in studies that used different criteria to define SS.

The basis for diagnosing SS during the last 20 years has been the definition presented by Bloch et al. (1965) in their landmark study of 62 patients with generally advanced SS. That definition stated that "Sjögren's syndrome consists of the triad of keratoconjunctivitis sicca ('dry eyes'), xerostomia ('dry mouth'), and rheumatoid arthritis or other connective tissue disease. Salivary or lacrimal gland enlargement may or may not be present". They stated that two of the three major components were sufficient for the diagnosis, and they excluded specific diseases of salivary or lacrimal glands such as lymphoma, sarcoidosis and tuberculosis. This definition, however, leaves criteria for diagnosing keratoconjunctivitis sicca (KCS) and xerostomia unspecified. In patients with advanced SS, the oral and ocular examination findings may be so obvious that further assessment may not have a critical role in diagnosis. However, in patients with mild or even moderately severe disease, symptoms and signs are usually subtle and non-specific, and require objective assessment.

Clinical tests for the ocular and salivary components and criteria for diagnosis of "probable" and "definite" SS were suggested by Feltkamp and van Rossum in 1968 and later modified (Fairfax et al. 1981) in an attempt to better define those components of SS. By these diagnostic criteria, KCS was considered probable if certain eye symptoms were present or the Schirmer tear test positive, and definite if epithelial erosions or filamentary keratitis were present. Xerostomia was considered probable if patients had certain symptoms or their dorsal tongue showed atrophic changes, and definite if either of the above were present along with salivary gland enlargement, punctate sialectasis by sialography, greater than 50% reduction in salivary flow rate measurement, or abnormal findings in salivary gland biopsy. Differences in the specificity and sensitivity of these methods are discussed in Chapter II.A.1. It should be emphasized here that syndromes are arbitrarily defined by the presence or absence of selected criteria. Different criteria will define different patients, and use of alternative diagnostic criteria will increase the size and diversity of the patient pool (Wulff 1981).

Whaley et al. (1973) made minor modifications to the Bloch et al. (1965) definition to establish diagnostic criteria for the 171 patients in their detailed clinical study. They accepted xerostomia (defined as the absence of salivary pooling) or salivary gland enlargement as confirmation of the salivary component of SS. They defined KCS as a reduced rate in an anesthetized Schirmer test plus punctate or filamentary keratitis. Given our present knowledge of the various causes of salivary gland enlargement and dry mouth, continued application of these criteria risks assignment of the diagnosis of SS to patients with KCS whose oral symptoms or salivary enlargement are caused by other disorders.

Noting the unreliability of evaluating patients' symptoms of xerostomia and the diverse causes of dry mouth and reduced salivary flow rate, Daniels et al. (1975) diagnosed the salivary component of SS as the presence of focal sialadenitis in a labial salivary gland biopsy specimen (focus score greater than 1 focus/4 mm^2) after appropriate exclusions (discussed in Chapter II.A.1). A later study (Daniels 1984) showed a significantly stronger correlation between the presence of focal sialadenitis and KCS, or KCS plus a connective tissue disease, than was found for either xerostomia symptoms or reduced parotid flow rate, indicating that histological assessment provided higher disease specificity. In both of these studies, KCS was diagnosed by the presence of characteristic corneal and conjunctival staining with rose bengal, and confirmed by reduced tear meniscus, tear break-up time, and unanesthetized Schirmer test.

Moutsopoulos et al. (1979a) defined the xerostomia of SS with the three criteria of decreased parotid flow rate, abnormal parotid scintigraphy findings and abnormal findings in a labial salivary gland biopsy; and KCS as punctate corneal ulcers and abnormal Schirmer test rate. However, they did not define levels of abnormality for each test, nor state how patients would be classified if less than three of the salivary criteria were abnormal.

Another set of diagnostic criteria for SS was proposed to provide objective criteria for the salivary and ocular components of SS (Manthorpe et al. 1981). The authors defined the "xerostomia" of SS by the presence of at least two of the following three: lymphocytic infiltrates in a labial salivary gland biopsy specimen, unstimulated whole salivary flow rate less than 1.5 ml/15 minutes, and reduced uptake and secretion in salivary scintigraphy. They defined KCS by the presence of at least two of the following three: unanesthetized Schirmer test less than 10 mm/5 minutes, tear break-up time less than 10 seconds and slit lamp-observed corneal epithelial staining by rose bengal with a score greater than 4.

Fox et al. (1986) recently proposed four criteria for diagnosis of SS: 1) KCS by a Schirmer test (<9 mm/5 min) and presence of rose bengal or fluorescein staining; 2) xerostomia by presence of symptoms and decreased basal and stimulated salivary flow rate; 3) lymphocytic infiltrates in labial salivary glands (at least 2 foci/4 mm^2); and 4) presence of rheumatoid factor ($>1:160$), antinuclear antibody ($>1:160$), or positive SS-A or SS-B antibodies. "Possible" SS would be defined by the presence of three of the criteria, and "definite" SS by all four. By excluding the presence of another connective tissue disease as a criterion and by including serological criteria, this proposal offers the first major revision of the Bloch et al. definition of SS. The authors also reaffirm the need to exclude the presence of certain diseases before confirming SS.

Application of these various diagnostic criteria over the last 20 years has led to a heterogeneous group of patients being given the diagnosis of SS. There is a clear need to establish internationally recognized criteria for the diagnosis of SS, both to avoid over-diagnosing this chronic, incurable and potentially progressive disease and to provide a common basis for defining patients in clinical studies.

Primary and secondary Sjögren's syndrome (Table 1)

Regardless of criteria, most clinical studies with large numbers of subjects have observed that patients with SS fall into two main categories: those with another connective tissue disease (usually rheumatoid arthritis) and those without. The latter condition was called "sicca syndrome" by Bloch et al. (1965), but the term is also

Table 1. Distinguishing characteristics of primary and secondary Sjögren's syndrome

Primary Disease
Ocular and oral components but no evidence of other underlying rheumatic disease
HLA-B8, -DR3 positive
Presence of antinuclear antibodies to Ro (SS-A) and La (SS-B)
Secondary Disease
Rheumatoid arthritis or other connective tissue disease with evidence of ocular and/or oral components
Immunogenetic and serologic findings of the accompanying disease (e.g. HLA-DR4 positive if RA)

Table 2. Clinical symptoms and signs associated with Sjögren's syndrome

Salivary component
Symptoms: dry mouth; "cracker sign"; burning oral mucosa. Signs: parotid gland induration or enlargement; cervical or incisal dental caries; oral mucosal erythema; dry, sticky oral mucosal surfaces; reduced stimulated and unstimulated salivary flow rates; focal sialadenitis in minor salivary gland biopsy
Ocular component
foreign body sensation
inability to tear
photophobia
reduced unanesthetized Schirmer test
decreased tear break-up time
filamentary keratitis
decreased tear meniscus
characteristic epithelial staining with rose bengal
Systemic (extraglandular) component
rheumatoid arthritis or other connective tissue disease
pulmonary lymphocytic interstitial infiltrates
interstitial nephritis and/or renal tubular acidosis
purpura - hyperglobulinemic; vasculitic
polymyopathy
neuropathy
chronic liver disease
hypergammaglobulinemia (polyclonal or monoclonal); cryoglobulinemia
presence of autoantibodies (RF, ANA, Ro/SS-A, La/SS-b)

used as a synonym for SS by some investigators (Moutsopoulos et al. 1979b). The names "primary SS" (when another connective tissue disease is absent) and "secondary SS" (when one is present) were introduced by Frost-Larsen et al. in 1978 and further defined by Moutsopoulos et al. (1979a and 1979b). Subsequently, the classification of SS into primary and secondary forms has been widely accepted, making the terms sicca syndrome or "sicca complex" redundant and confusing, and use of these sicca terms should be avoided. The clinical, genetic and serological differences between primary and secondary SS are discussed in other Chapters.

Differential diagnosis of Sjögren's syndrome

Diagnosis of any syndrome usually begins with a clinician identifying a pattern of symptoms and signs suggesting the presence of the syndrome (Table 2). Appropriate clinical and laboratory tests then aid in ruling in or out the diagnosis of other conditions that could produce similar symptoms or signs. The differential diagnosis of SS becomes, then, an analysis of the possible causes of the main components.

Xerostomia

Evaluation of patients complaining of dry mouth symptoms is perhaps the most difficult because it is a common complaint with a variety of causes (Table 3) and several possible means of assessment. Symptoms of dryness may be temporary or permanent, but the most common cause is side effects from one or perhaps a combination of chronically administered drugs (Table 4). Careful review of a patient's current use of prescription and non-prescription drugs should precede the conclusion that symptoms of dry mouth may result from SS.

Salivary gland enlargement

Enlargement or induration of the major salivary glands can also have a variety of causes (Table 5) but occurs much less frequently than oral dryness. Enlargement of

Table 3. Causes of dry mouth (xerostomia)

Temporary
Drug effects
Virus infections
Dehydration (diabetes, trauma)
Psychogenic (fear, depression)
Chronic
Effects of therapeutic irradiation
Sjögren's syndrome
Sarcoidosis
Absent or malformed glands

Table 4. Chronically used drugs causing dry mouth

Psychotherapeutic drugs
Antidepressants (especially tricyclic compounds and MAO inhibitors)
Neuroleptics (especially phenothiazines)
Parasympatholytic drugs
Anti-Parkinsonian (e.g. benztropine, trihexphenidyl)
Antihistamines (e.g. chlorpheniramine, diphenhydramine)
Gastrointestinal ulcer treatment (e.g. propantheline)
Antihypertensive drugs
Many combination preparations or multiple drug prescriptions
Some single drugs (e.g. clonidine)

Table 5. Causes of salivary gland enlargement

Usually unilateral
Primary salivary gland neoplasms
Bacterial infection
Chronic sialadenitis
Usually bilateral
Viral infection (e.g., mumps, influenza, Epstein-Barr, Coxsackie A, Cytomegalovirus)
Sjögren's syndrome (benign lymphoepithelial lesion)
Lymphoma
Sarcoidosis or tuberculosis
Sialadenosis (associated with diabetes mellitus, hyperlipoproteinemia, hepatic cirrhosis, anorexia/bulimia, chronic pancreatitis, acromegaly, or gonadal hypofunction)
Recurrent parotitis of childhood

the parotid or, less frequently, the submandibular gland in SS is usually episodic, waxing and waning over periods of many weeks or months. It may begin, or remain, a unilateral enlargement in a portion of cases, but most are bilateral. In SS (and sarcoidosis), enlarged glands are moderately indurated and usually non-tender to palpation, whereas in sialadenosis the enlarged glands are not indurated and function normally. Accessory salivary gland biopsy usually distinguishes SS from sarcoidosis (Nessan and Jacoway 1979; Daniels 1984). Recurrent parotitis of childhood can be similar to SS except that it is often unilateral, and episodes of swelling last from a few days to several months and may recur several times per year up to puberty.

Ocular symptoms

The initial approach to the dry eye patient begins with the history. Patients may not complain of a dry eye per se, but rather of scratchiness (foreign body sensation), inability to tear, or photophobia. The Schirmer test (or a variant, the Hamano thread test) is used to assess tear production and this is considered abnormal if the wetted area of filter paper is less than 5 mm in 5 minutes. The lids are inspected for normal closure and blink function, and the corneal sensation is tested with a wisp of cotton.

With the slit lamp, the examiner can assess lid position and the tear lake (meniscus) for adequacy. Topical fluorescein is used to look for superficial punctate staining and other corneal surface abnormalities. It is also used to examine the stability of the tear film (tear break-up time); the areas where the tear film breaks down appear dark. Rose bengal stains devitalized epithelium; in KCS there is a characteristic pattern of staining over the lower third of the cornea and adjacent conjunctiva.

Other methods of diagnosis are newer or less generally available. These include assays of tear osmolarity, lysozyme and lactoferrin. Distribution of fluorescein by the tears over time is an investigational method performed with a fluorophotometer.

The various causes of dry eyes are listed in Table 6. Meibomitis, blepharitis and conjunctival inflammation from acquired hypersensitivity to preservatives or other components in artificial tears are relatively common conditions whose symptoms may mimic KCS.

Table 6. Causes of dry eye states

Tear abnormalities
Mucin deficiency (loss of goblet cells)
inflammation: e.g. Stevens-Johnson, pemphigoid
chronic conjunctivitis
toxicity: e.g. burns, drugs
hypovitaminosis A
Aqueous deficiency (loss of lacrimal gland function)
inflammation: e.g. Sjögren's syndrome
congenital absence or malformation
trauma
neurological conditions
Lipid deficiency (loss of Meibomian gland function)
chronic blepharitis
congenital absence or malformation
Eyelid function impairment with poor spread of tear film
Blink abnormality
Lid scarring, including symblepharon
Neurologic abnormality
Surface abnormality of the cornea
Anesthetic cornea
Epithelial irregularity

Table 7. Diagnostic criteria for Sjögren's syndrome

Primary Sjögren's syndrome

1. Keratoconjunctivitis sicca
   a. characteristic corneal and conjunctival epithelial staining with rose bengal observed through a slit lamp, and
   b. reduced tear meniscus and break-up time, or
   c. unanesthetized Schirmer test < 5 mm/5 minutes
2. Focal sialadenitis in an adequate labial salivary gland biopsy specimen with a focus score > 1 focus/4 mm^2 after exclusions

Secondary Sjögren's syndrome

1. Rheumatoid arthritis or other connective tissue disease by established diagnostic criteria, and
2. Either one or both of the criteria for primary Sjögren's syndrome described above

Possible Sjögren's syndrome

1. One of the components of primary Sjögren's syndrome described above, and
2. Presence of any of the following:
   pulmonary lymphocytic interstitial infiltrates
   interstitial nephritis and/or renal tubular acidosis
   purpura-hyperglobulinemic; vasculitic
   polymyopathy
   neuropathy
   chronic liver disease
   hypergammaglobulinemia (polyclonal or monoclonal); cryoglobulinemia; presence of autoantibodies (RF, ANA, Ro-SS-A, La/SS-B)

Criteria for the Diagnosis of Sjögren's Syndrome

The diagnosis of SS can be suspected readily in most patients from the initial history and physical findings. The complaints of inability to swallow a dry bolus of food (the "cracker sign") and an ocular foreign-body sensation ("sandy" or "gritty" eyes) are very useful clues which make for interesting demonstrations to students in the vanishing art of history taking (Table 2). The more objective criteria have already been discussed in other chapters.

We continue to adhere to the basic definition of SS offered by Bloch et al. (1965), while adding specific diagnostic criteria for the diagnosis of KCS and using focal sialadenitis in labial salivary glands (Daniels 1984 and 1986) as the diagnostic criterion for the salivary component of SS (Table 7). In addition, we recognize that diagnosis of any syndrome is not all-or-nothing and that an element of probability exists. Accordingly, we define "possible Sjögren's syndrome" as the presence of either of the components of primary SS, with significant titers of serum autoantibodies or organ system diseases which are seen in frequent association, but not exclusively, with SS (Table 7).

References

Bloch KJ,Buchanan WW, Wohl MJ, Bunim JJ (1965) Sjögren's syndrome: a clinical, pathological, and serological study of sixty-two cases. Medicine 44: 187-231

Daniels TE (1984) Labial salivary gland biopsy in Sjögren's syndrome: assessment as a diagnostic criterion in 362 suspected cases. Arthritis Rheum 27: 147-156

Daniels TE (1986) Salivary histopathology in diagnosis of Sjögren's syndrome. Scand J Rheum (in press)

Daniels TE, Silverman S, Michalski JP, Greenspan JS, Sylvester RA, Talal N (1975) The oral component of Sjögren's syndrome. Oral Surg 39: 875-885

Fairfax AJ, Haslam PL, Pavia D, Sheahan NF, Bateman JRM, Agnew JE, Clarke SW, Turner-Warwick M (1981) Pulmonary disorders associated with Sjögren's syndrome. Q J Med 50: 279-295

Feltkamp TEW, van Rossum AL (1968) Antibodies to salivary duct cells, and other autoantibodies, in patients with Sjögren's syndrome and other idiopathic autoimmune diseases. Clin Exp Immunol 3: 1-16

Fox RI, Robinson C, Curd J, Kozin F, Howell FV (1986) Sjögren's syndrome: Proposed criteria for classification. Arthritis Rheum (in press).

Frost-Larsen K, Isager H, Manthorpe R (1978) Sjögren's syndrome treated with bromhexine: a randomized clinical study. Br Med J 1: 1579-1581

Manthorpe R, Frost-Larsen K, Isager H, Prause JU (1981) Sjögren's syndrome: a review with emphasis on immunological features. Allergy 36: 139-153

Moutsopoulos HM, Mann DL, Johnson AH, Chused TM (1979a) Genetic differences between primary and secondary sicca syndrome. N Engl J Med 301: 761-763

Moutsopoulos HM, Webber BL, Vlagopoulos TP, Chused TM, Decker JL (1979b) Differences in the clinical manifestations of sicca syndrome in the presence and absence of rheumatoid arthritis. Am J Med 66: 733-736

Nessan VJ, Jacoway JR (1979) Biopsy of minor salivary glands in the diagnosis of sarcoidosis. N Engl J Med 301: 922-924

Shearn MA (1971) Sjögren's syndrome. WB Saunders Co, Philadelphia (Major problems in internal medicine, vol 2)

Whaley K, Williamson J, Chisholm DM, Webb J, Mason DK, Buchanan WW (1973) Sjögren's syndrome: I. Sicca components. Q J Med 42: 279-304

Wulf HR (1981) Rational diagnosis and treatment. An introduction to clinical decision making, 2nd edition. Blackwell Scientific Publications, Oxford

III. Laboratory Abnormalities

1. Rheumatoid Factor in Sjögren's Syndrome*

S. Fong, P. Chen, D. A. Carson, and R. I. Fox

Abbreviations
SS Sjögren's syndrome; *WM* Waldenstrom's macroglobulinemia; *RF* rheumatoid factor; *CRI* cross reactive idiotype; *RA* rheumatoid arthritis; *SLE* systemic lupus erythematosus; *CDR* complementarity determining region

Introduction

Rheumatoid factors (RF) are defined by their ability to bind to the Fc portion of IgG molecules. This activity in the sera of rheumatoid arthritis (RA) patients was first noted as an atypical reaction during agglutination tests to detect antibodies to microbial antigens (Rose et al. 1948; Waaler 1940). The antibody nature of RF and its binding to different subclasses of IgG has been the subject of extensive investigations [reviewed in Fong et al. 1984]. As more sensitive tests for RF became available (Carson et al. 1977; Pope & McDuffy 1981; Koopman & Schrohenloher 1980), the presence of this antibody in other autoimmune conditions including Sjögren's syndrome was recognized. Further, certain infectious diseases (Brouet et al. 1974) and B cell malignancies (Kunkel et al. 1961; Kunkel et al. 1973) are associated with RF. Recently, it has been recognized that this "autoantibody" may be synthesized in association with secondary immune responses in normal humans and in animals (Welch et al. 1983; Coulie & Van Snick 1983; Nemazee & Sato 1983). These results have suggested that RF plays a physiologic role in normal immune responses (Grabar 1983; Guilbert et al. 1983) and that persistent stimulation of these cells may lead to their neoplastic transformation (Berard et al. 1981).

In view of RF production in "normal" immune responses, attention has been focused on those factors that induce its synthesis. In mice, at least two distinct methods have been used to induce RF. Injection of pre-formed immune complexes leads to high RF levels (Coulie & Van Snick 1985; Nemazee 1985). This induction requires T cells and mice containing "primed" T cells (i. e., directed against the antigen contained in the pre-formed immune complex) produce higher levels of RF. These results suggest that RF can arise as a result of "hapten-carrier recognition" where the carrier antigen (recognized by specific primed T cells) leads to release of factors that stimulate B cell production of RF. A second method of producing RF is the treatment of B cells with bacterial endotoxin lipopolysaccharide (LPS) (Izui et

* Supported by grants AM 33294 and AM 33983 from the National Institutes of Health and by grants from the Price Family Charitable Foundation and the Kieckhefen Foundation. This is publication number 4383BCR from the Research Foundation of Scripps Clinic.

al. 1979; Dresser 1978). T cells are not required for induction by LPS and RF can be produced in nude mice. The frequency of B cells producing RF in mice responding to immune complexes or LPS has been estimated from 5–15% of the total B cell response (Coulie & Van Snick 1985; Nemazee 1985; Izui et al. 1979; Dresser 1978; Coulie & Van Snick 1983). In contrast, the frequency of cells producing a specific anti-arsonate antibody response has frequency 4×10^{-7} (Manser et al. 1984). The reasons for the high frequency of RF producing cells remains unknown but these findings indicate that the regulation of RF differs from other antigen-specific B cell responses.

Cross Reactive Idiotypes

Idiotypes are serologic markers for the variable region structures of the antibody molecule. Immunoglobulins consist of heavy and light chains; each chain is composed of a "constant" and a "variable" portion. The variable region contains three "framework" regions (that serve to designate subgroups V_κ I, V_κ II, V_κ III, V_κ IV) and three hypervariable regions (also known as complementarity determining regions, CDR). X-ray crystallographic studies indicate that antigens bind to a "pocket" structure formed by the variable region and that amino acid sequences located in the CDR regions are in intimate contact with the antigen [reviewed in (Capra & Fougereau 1983; Rajewsky & Takemori 1983)]. Therefore, the structures that constitute the antibody binding site (i.e., the idiotype) have been the subject of considerable interest.

A powerful tool to study the "idiotype" has been the production of antibodies (termed anti-idiotypes) that react with the antibody combining site. Recently, it has been recognized that anti-idiotype antibodies may react with autoantibodies from different patients with the same disease. Such autoantibodies contain a "cross reactive idiotype" (CRI). Examples of CRI are rheumatoid factor (RF) paraproteins found in Waldenstrom's macroglobulinemia (Kunkel et al. 1973; Kunkel et al. 1974; Ledford et al. 1983) and in SS patients (Fox et al. 1986), anti-DNA antibodies in SLE (Solomon et al. 1983; Atkinson et al. 1985), anti-thyroglobulin antibodies in autoimmune thyroiditis (Matsuyama et al. 1983), and anti-cholinesterase antibodies in myasthenia gravis (Lefvert et al. 1982). CRI also have been observed in non-autoimmune circumstances including anti-tetanus and anti-casein antibodies (Cunningham-Rundles & Cheung 1985). In the case of RF paraproteins in Waldenstrom's macroglobulinema (WM) (Ledford et al. 1983) and anti-DNA antibodies in SLE (Atkinson et al. 1985), the structural basis for CRI results from shared amino acid sequences in the variable region of the light chains. However, very little is known about the site of production of CRI^+ autoantibodies and the factors that regulate the CRI^+ B cells. Recently, we found that RF from 1° SS patients exhibits a CRI and that CRI^+ B cells can be detected in high frequency in minor salivary gland biopsies. As reviewed below, the CRI on RF of SS patients appears closely related to that found on RF paraproteins in WM patients. Therefore, SS patients provide an opportunity to study the regulation of CRI^+ autoantibodies and the factors that may promote the neoplastic transformation of B cells that occurs with high frequency in this disease.

Patient Population

The term "Sjögren's syndrome" (SS) generally refers to the condition of dry eyes/dry mouth resulting from destruction of the lacrimal/salivary gland by lymphoid infiltrates. We have concentrated on a patient population that exhibits features of both autoimmunity (i.e., exhibiting autoantibody production) and lymphoproliferation (i.e., minor salivary gland biopsy with a focus score $> 2\ mm^2$) (Daniels 1984; Fox et al. 1984). It is important that the minor salivary gland biopsy be obtained through histologically normal mucosa since inflammatory oral lesions (i.e., *candidiasis or lichen planus*) can lead to lymphoid infiltrates in the underlying salivary glands (Lundstrom et al. 1982). We have excluded patients with pre-existent lymphoma, graft versus host disease, acquired immune deficiency disease (AIDS) or sarcoidosis.

SS may occur in association with other well recognized autoimmune disorders such as RA, systemic lupus erythematosus (SLE), or progressive systemic sclerosis (PSS); these patients are called secondary SS (2° SS). Also, SS may occur in the absence of these disorders and is termed primary SS (1° SS). In both of these groups, SS patients exhibit a tendency towards lymphoproliferation (as manifest by their destruction of salivary glands and increased risk of lymphoma) (Berard et al. 1981; Kassan et al. 1978) and a systemic autoimmune disorder (i.e., increased frequency of extraglandular involvement including pneumonitis, central nervous system manifestations, nephritis, etc.) (Whaley et al. 1973). In our studies, we have concentrated on 1° SS patients since these individuals generally were not receiving medications such as gold, immunosuppressive agents or glucorticoids that may alter the underlying pathogenetic mechanisms.

Monoclonal Antibody Reactive with a Cross Reactive Idiotype on Rheumatoid Factor from Patients with Sjögren's Syndrome and with Waldenstrom's Macroglobulinemia

Our laboratory and others (Carson & Fong 1983; Greenstein et al. 1984) have developed monoclonal antibodies against a cross reactive idiotype (CRI) present on rheumatoid factor (RF) paraproteins. One monoclonal antibody (MoAb 17-109) was prepared against an IgM-kappa paraprotein with RF activity from a patient ("Sie") with Waldenstrom's macroglobulinemia (WM) and mixed cryoglobulinemia. This MoAb was selected for its ability to bind to the "Sie" but not to IgG myeloma proteins nor to IgM macroglobulinemia molecules lacking RF activity (Carson & Fong 1983). MoAb 17-109 efficiently reacted with intact "Sie" RF and inhibited the binding of this RF to human IgG Fc fragments, suggesting that the idiotype was located in proximity to the antigen binding site. By western immunoblot analysis, the idiotype was localized on kappa light chains of RF paraproteins obtained from WM patients (summarized in Table 1).

Several features are unusual about the RF paraproteins from WM patients. First, the majority of these RF paraproteins contain light chains of the V_κ IIIb subclass with virtually identical amino acid sequence. The high frequency of such similar light chains arising in unrelated patients was surprising (Kunkel et al. 1974; Ledford

Table 1. Reactivity of Antibodies with RF Paraproteins

IgM RFs	Anti-Idiotype Reactivity[a] 17.109	PSL2	PSL3
Sie	+++	++	++
Gar	+++	++	++
Glo	+++	++	++
Got	++	++	++
Neu	–	++	++
Pal	–	++	++
Pom	–	+	–
Wol	–	++	–
Flo	ND	++	++
Lay	–	–	–
Pla	–	ND	ND
Gil	–	ND	ND
Total positive	3	11	8
Total tested	12	12	10
% Positive	25%	92%	80%

[a] For immunoblot analysis, the light and heavy chains of monoclonal IgM RFs were separated by SDS polyacrylamide gel electrophoresis. The separated proteins were electrotransfered to nitrocellulose paper and probed with MoAb 17-109, anti-PSL2 or anti-PSL3 antibodies. The degree of reactivity was assessed by autoradiography with a rabbit anti-mouse Ig followed by ^{125}I-protein A or ^{125}I-protein A alone.

et al. 1983) since this light chain subclass is relatively minor in normal sera (Solomon and McLaughlin 1971). Second, this subclass is not increased in frequency in non-RF paraproteins in WM or multiple myeloma patients (Kunkel et al. 1974); this indicates an association of this subclass with some RF producing cells. Third, MoAb 17-109 reacts with a high proportion of RF paraproteins (Table 1). However, some V_κ IIIb RF paraproteins (i.e., "Wol" and "Neu") failed to react. Thus, the CRI defined by MoAb 17-109 represents a sub-subclass of the V_κ IIIb family. Taken together, these results suggest that CRI$^+$ defined by this MoAb correspond to a highly conserved amino acid sequence and that CRI$^+$ B cells probably have increased tendency towards neoplastic transformation in WM.

RF from patients with primary Sjögren's syndrome (1° SS) also were found to react with MoAb 17-109 (Fox et al. 1986). Examples of western immunoblots are shown in Fig. 1 (lanes D to G). As controls, RF paraproteins (lanes B and C) were reactive while pooled normal human IgG (lane A) was not. In comparison, sera from RA patients lacking SS contained large amounts of RF activity (Fig. 2, lanes A to D) but these RF did not contain detectable reactivity with MoAb 17-109. Studies on sera from patients with RA plus SS (i.e., secondary SS, 2° SS) demonstrated that CRI$^+$ light chains were present but constitute a small proportion of the total RF (i.e., less than 5%) and thus were technically difficult to detect by western immunoblot methods (Fox et al. 1986).

To further quantitate the CRI in sera, we performed direct binding studies of RF to microtiter plates precoated with MoAb 17-109 (Fig. 3). Samples "Sch" and "Sie"

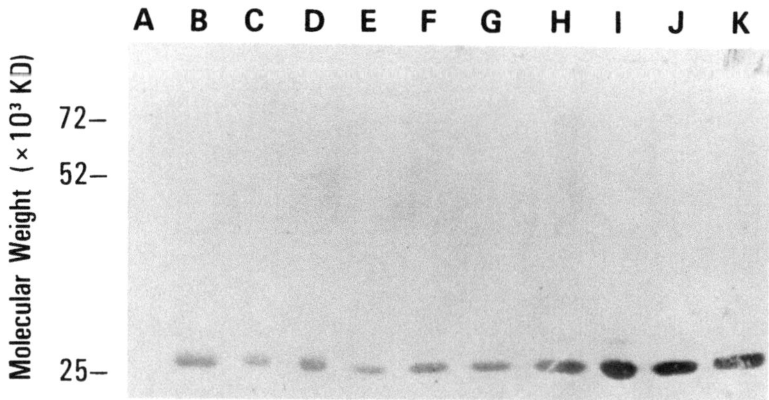

Fig. 1. Monoclonal antibody 17-109 reacts with an epitope associated with light chains. Serum samples from SS patients were enriched for RF activity by passage over and elution from human IgG-Sepharose 4B columns. After elution, SDS gel electrophoresis, and transfer to nitrocellulose, the aliquots were analyzed by the western immunoblotting method with MoAb 17-109 (lanes A to G) or with an anti-human kappa (lanes H to K). *Lane A:* Normal pooled human IgG. *Lanes B to C: IgM-RF "Sie" paraprotein and IgA-RF "Sch" paraproteins, respectively. Lanes D to G:* RF purified from sera of different SS patients. RF samples from the same SS patients were reacted with anti-human kappa (lanes H to K)

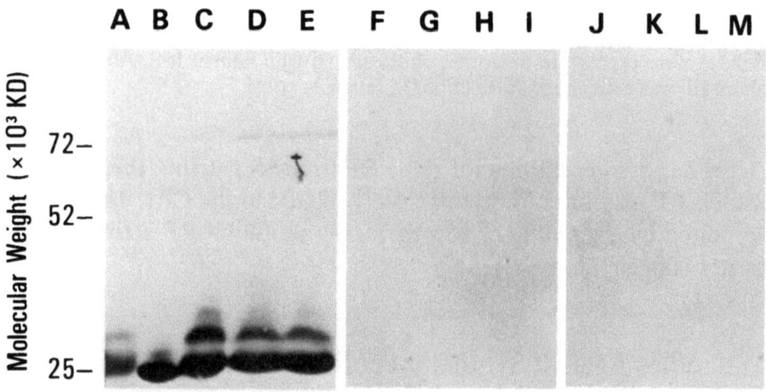

Fig. 2. Reactivity of serum RF samples from RA patients. RF samples from RA patients lacking sicca symptoms were examined using anti-human kappa, MoAb 17-109 or control murine myeloma IgG 2b antibodies using immunoblotting methods to analyze proteins separated on 8% polyacrylamide gels. *Lanes A to D:* RF samples from RA patients plus anti-human kappa. *Lane E:* Pooled normal human IgG (20 μg protein loaded onto gel) plus anti-human kappa. *Lanes F to I:* RF samples from RA patients plus MoAb 17-109. RF samples from RA (lanes L and M) or from SS patients (lanes J to K) were treated with a control murine IgG 2b myeloma protein (MOPC 195)

refer to IgA-RF and IgM-RF paraproteins, respectively, that bear the CRI. Samples A to F are RF from SS patients. The CRI was present in each of the SS samples and was particularly associated with IgA-RF activity. Assuming that the affinity of MoAb 17-109 for the SS RF was comparable to the "Sie" RF (i.e., the immunizing protein), we estimate that 10–20% of the RF in SS patients bears the CRI. If MoAb

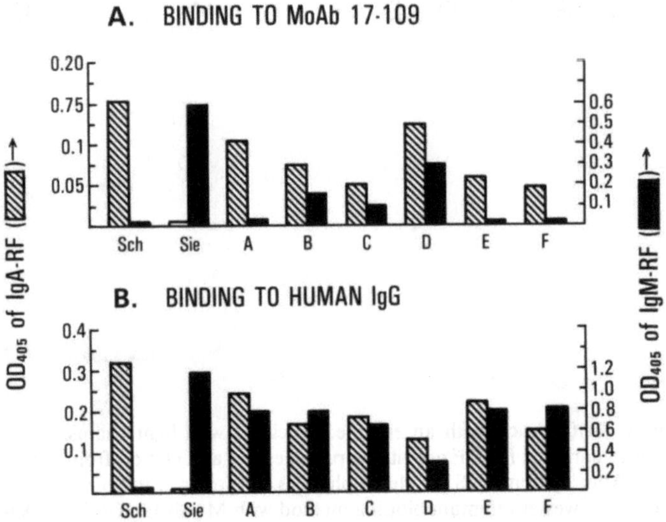

Fig. 3 A, B. Binding of rheumatoid factor to immobilized MoAb 17-109 and to human IgG. **A.** Isotype of RF antibodies binding to MoAb 17-109. IgM-RF paraprotein "Sie" (400 ng/ml), IgA-RF paraprotein "Sch" (400 ng/ml), and RF purified from the serum of SS patients were exposed to microtiter plates precoated with MoAb 17-109. After rinsing, the isotype of bound RF was determined with alkaline phosphatase conjugated anti-human IgM or anti-human IgA antibody. As a control, the binding of RF proteins to control myeloma protein MOPC 195 had O.D.$_{405}$ less than 0.01 units. **B** Isotype of RF molecules binding to human IgG. The same RF preparations as used in frame A were exposed to microtiter plates coated with human IgG. After rinsing, the isotype of bound RF was determined as described in frame A

17-109 has a lower affinity for some RF from SS patients, then a higher proportion of their RF may have idiotypes closely related to the CRI. This latter possibility is supported by the ability of MoAb 17-109 to inhibit RF activity of SS patients by greater than 50%.

Antibodies Against Synthetic Peptides Derived from RF Paraproteins

An additional approach to study CRI is to prepare synthetic peptides from the CDR regions of light chains whose amino acid sequence has previously been determined (Ledford et al. 1983; Kunkel et al. 1974). As described above, RF paraproteins from patients with Waldenstrom's macroglobulinemia are remarkable for their conservation of amino acid sequences in the variable region of their kappa light chains (examples shown in Fig. 4). The light chains derived from nine different RF paraproteins ("Glo" to "Wol") have similar framework regions and only minor amino acid substitutions in the CDR1 or CDR3 regions. The CDR2 region is identical in each of these light chains. In contrast, two other light chains from RF paraproteins ("Pom" and "Lay") had significantly different amino acid sequences.

Synthetic peptides were prepared from the CDR2 and CDR3 region of kappa chains from the RF paraprotein "Sie" (Chen et al. 1984; Chen et al. 1985a; Chen et al. 1985b). These peptides were termed *"PSL2"* and *"PSL3,"* respectively, to denote

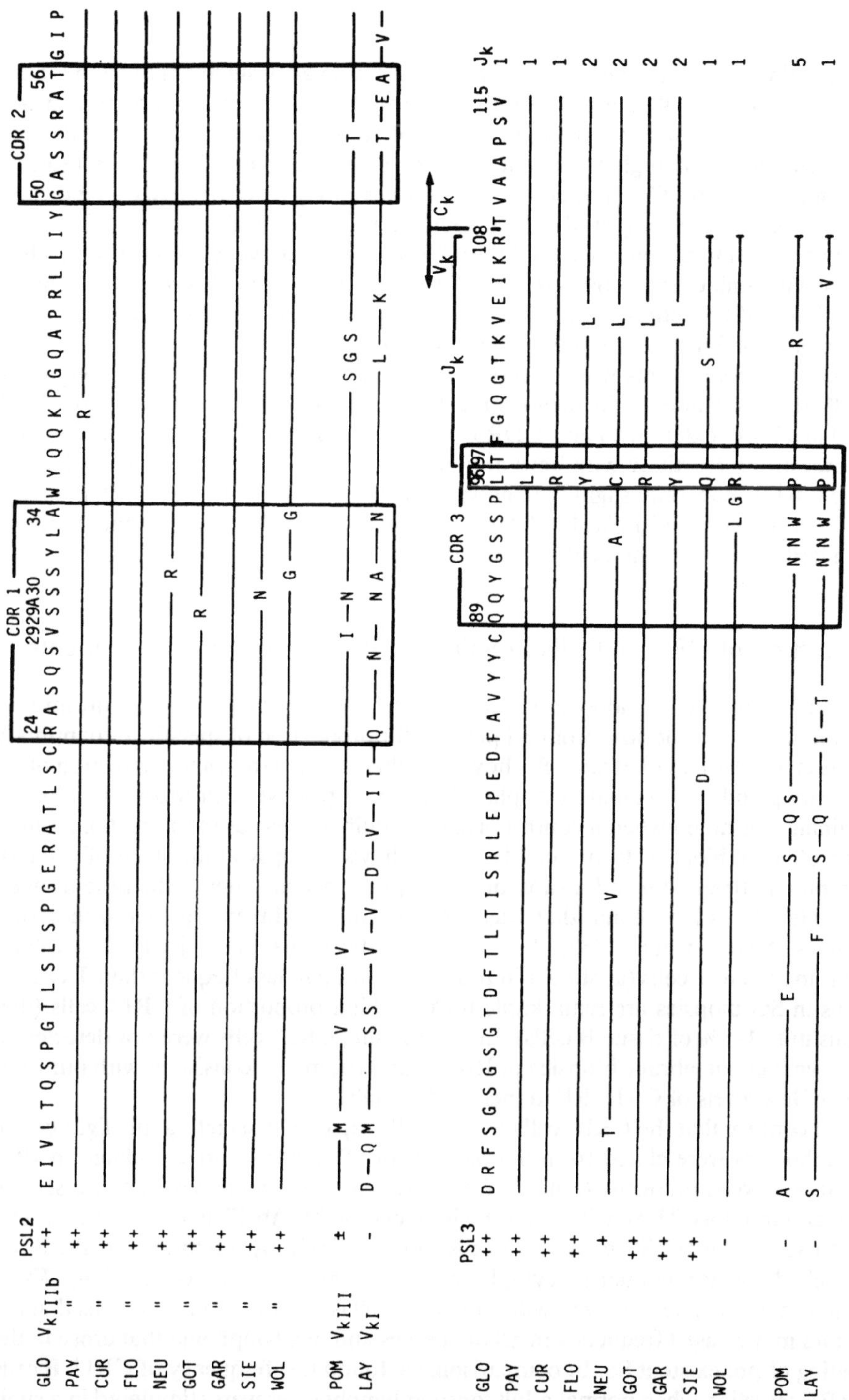

Fig. 4 Amino acid sequence of RF paraproteins from patients with Waldenstrom's macroglobulinemia. The complete V-region and partial C-region are based on previously published results (reviewed in Goñi et al. 1985)

the peptide *S*ie light chain from CDR2 (from amino acids 49 to 61) or from CDR3 (from amino acids 88 to 99). The antipeptide antibodies and immunoblotting methods were used to analyze the light chains of RF paraproteins from patients with Waldenstrom's macroglobulinemia. The results are summarized in Figure 4 (under columns PSL2 and PSL3) where (+ +) indicates strong reactivity and (−) indicates lack of reactivity (Fong et al., 1985; Goñi et al., 1985). Each of the V_{κ} IIIb light chains with similar sequence ("Glo" to "Wol") was reactive with anti-PSL2, while those with amino acid substitutions ("Pom" and "Lay") were less reactive. Reactivity of anti-PSL3 antibody with RF paraproteins was less frequent, consistent with the amino acid differences in the CDR3 region.

RF from SS patients was analyzed with the antipeptide antibodies (Fong et al. 1986) (Fig. 5). These results demonstrate that reactivity was present with anti-CDR2 and to a lesser extent with anti-CDR3 antibody. As a control, the "Sie" paraprotein shows strong reactivity with both antibodies and pooled normal immunoglobulin (IgM, IgG) show only slight reactivity. These findings are consistent with the reactivity of SS RF with MoAb 17-109 and suggest that the CRI in SS patients is due to similarities at the amino acid level in the CDR regions.

Detection of CRI$^+$ B Cells in Salivary Gland Biopsies of SS Patients

The availability of a monoclonal antibody to a CRI provided an opportunity to examine the tissue lesions from SS patients for production of specific autoantibody (Fox et al. 1986). Fig. 6 (frame B) shows lymphocytes in a frozen tissue section of SS salivary gland (SG) contain cytoplasmic material reactive with MoAb 17-109. No staining was noted when a control myeloma antibody was used (frame C). Evaluation of serial biopsies from one SS patient shows a biopsy at the stage of pseudolymphoma (frame D) and a subsequent biopsy two years later at the time of overt non-Hodgkin's lymphoma that was CRI$^+$ (frame E). Taken together with earlier studies (Adamson et al. 1983), these findings indicate that the majority of lymphoid cells in SG are T cells (as shown in frame A); although less frequent than T cells, B cells in SG biopsies are remarkable for their high proportion of CRI$^+$ cells (that constitute 1–5% of tissue B cells). In comparison, CRI$^+$ cells were not detected in the synovial membrane biopsies of RA patients (frame F), consistent with our finding of low levels of CRI$^+$ RF in these individuals.

To confirm that the CRI$^+$ cells were B cells capable of secreting this light chain, lymphocytes were eluted from SG biopsies of SS patients and stimulated in vitro with pokeweed mitogen (Table 2). We found that these lymphocytes could secrete RF and that this RF activity could be inhibited by MoAb 17-109 (Fox et al. 1986). After separating the SG cells into T cells and non-T cells by rosetting, only the B cell enriched fraction contained cytoplasmic CRI$^+$ material (Fox et al. 1986). These results demonstrate reactivity with MoAb 17-109 is due to a CRI on B cells that are found in increased frequency in SS SG tissues and in a lymphoma that arose in the setting of pre-existent SS. In comparison, we found low frequency of CRI$^+$ B cells or RF secretion when normal adult tonsillar lymphocytes were stimulated in a similar manner.

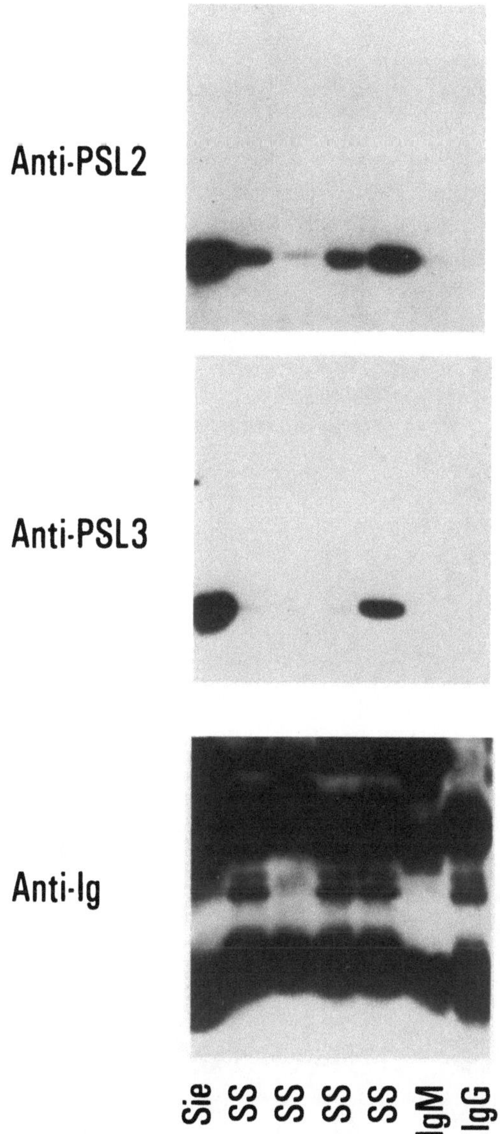

Fig. 5. Immunoblot analysis of Sjögren's syndrome patient serum. Rheumatoid factor was prepared using Sepharose columns containg rabbit IgG. The eluted RF was separated on 8% acrylamide SDS gels and shown to contain both light and heavy chains by western blotting with antihuman Ig antibody (lower panel). The RF was then passed over a MoAb 17-109 Sepharose column. After elution, the CRI^+ RF was separated on SDS/polyacrylamide gels and immunoblots were performed using antibodies against synthetic peptides and ^{125}I-protein A.
Synthetic peptides were derived from the hypervariable regions (complementarity determining region, CDR) of the V_κ IIIb light chain from patient "Sie" (who had RF paraprotein in association with Waldenstrom's macroglobulinemia). The peptide for CDR2 (termed *p*eptide *S*ie *l*ight *c*hain, PSL2) and for CDR3 (i.e., peptide PSL3) were used to prepare specific antibodies used for immunoblotting (top and middle panels, respectively).
Samples analyzed on the gel included the original "Sie" paraprotein and SS samples (derived from four different SS patients). The samples labeled IgG and IgM refer to pooled normal human immunoglobulin preparations. These latter samples were used directly and were not passed over the affinity columns

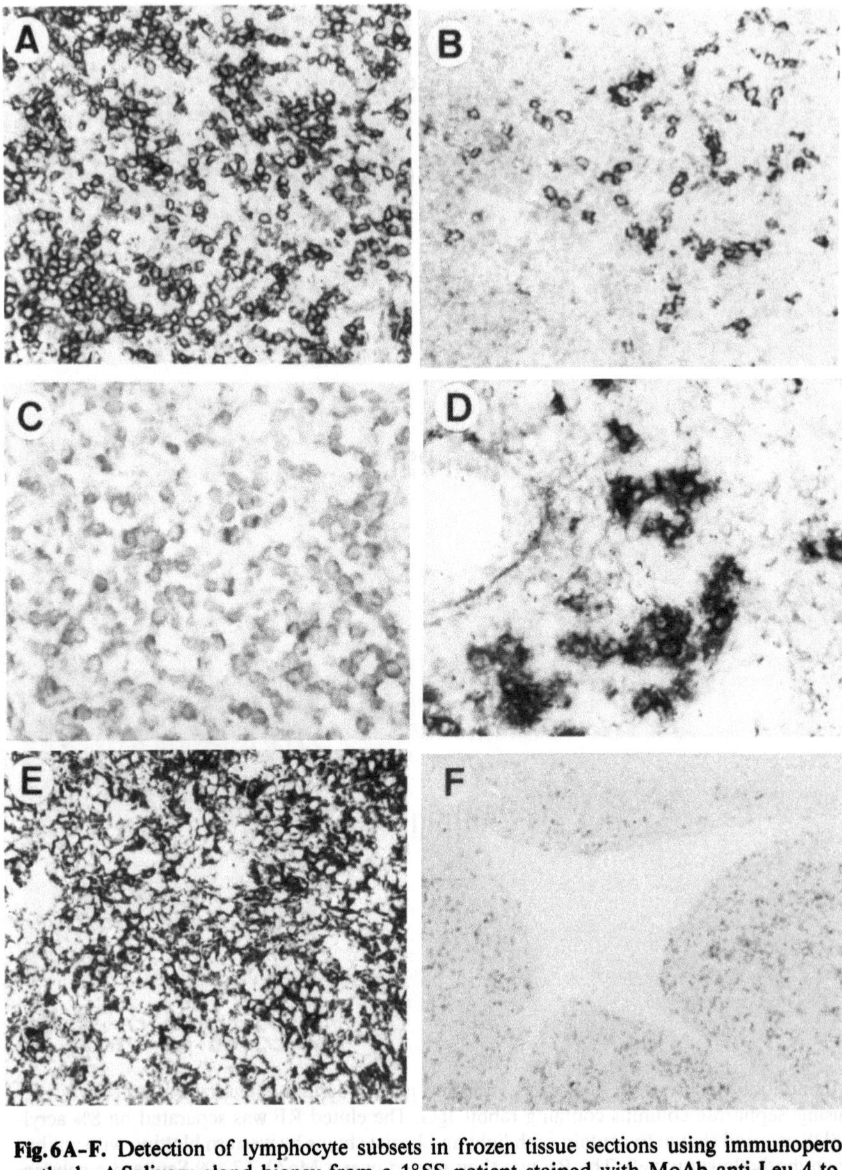

Fig. 6 A–F. Detection of lymphocyte subsets in frozen tissue sections using immunoperoxidase methods. **A** Salivary gland biopsy from a 1° SS patient stained with MoAb anti-Leu 4 to detect mature T cells. **B** and **C** Serial sections of SS salivary gland biopsies stained with MoAb 17-109 (frame B) and control murine myeloma protein (frame C). **D** and **E** Biopsies from the same SS patient (IR) stained with MoAB 17-109 two years prior to the diagnosis of non-Hodgkin's lymphoma (frame D) and at the time of this diagnosis (frame E). **F** RA synovial membrane biopsy reacted with MoAb 17-109 and no significant staining was noted. Original magnification in frames A to E was 500 × and in frame F was 50 ×

Table 2. In Vitro Production of Rheumatoid Factor[a]

Source of Lymphocytes		Secreted RF ($O.D._{405} \times 10^{-3}$)	Percent Inhibition of RF by MoAb 17-109[b]	Percent Cells Stained by MoAb 17-109
A. SS	Patients			
1. DG	SGL	740 ± 20	52	6
	PBL	160 ± 10	65	1
2. MS	SGL	710 ± 30	65	2
	PBL	220 ± 20	-	2
3. ECr	PBL	160 ± 10	70	0.1
4. ECo	PBL	130 ± 10	70	0.3
5. SF	LN	430 ± 40	82	4
Median ± SD		468 ± 240	56 ± 21	2.2 ± 2
B. Controls				
PBL (n = 7)		< 20	-	< 0.01
Tonsils (n = 3)		49 ± 10	-	0.1
Mean ± SD		37 ± 17		

[a] Lymphocytes were cultured for 7 days in the presence of pokeweed mitogen (0.1 μg/ml), and the tissue culture supernatant was analyzed for secreted rheumatoid factor (RF) by ELISA using $O.D._{405}$ absorbance. As reference values, the IgM-RF paraprotein Sie (1000 ng/ml) yielded $O.D._{405} = 0.670$ and control human myeloma proteins lacking RF activity (1000 ng/ml) had $O.D._{405} < 0.020$.

[b] To measure the proportion of RF bearing the 17-109 idiotype, the culture supernatant was pre-mixed with an equal volumn of MoAb 17-109 (100 μg/ml) and then testing for RF activity by ELISA. As a control, a separate aliquot of tissue culture supernatant was pre-mixed with a control murine IgG2 myeloma protein and < 5% inhibition of RF activity was noted.

Speculations on CRI Expression in Sjögren's Patient

The initial reports of CRI^+ light chains with virtually identical amino acid sequences in paraproteins from patients with Waldenstrom's macroglobulinemia were surprising, since kappa chains found in normal sera are extremely heterogeneous. The human genome contains approximately 50 "variable" region genes in germ line configuration as part of the kappa gene complex (Bentley 1983) and additional variable region pseudogenes on other chromosomes (Lotscher et al. 1986). Normal B cell differentiation involves the fusion of a particular "variable" region gene with a "joining" (J) region and a constant region gene. Under the influence of antigen and T cells, the variable region gene undergoes extensive somatic mutation, particularly in the CDR region (Pech et al. 1981). One possible explanation for the existence of CRI in RF of SS or WM patients is that the variable region genes that encode these antibodies have DNA sequence identical (or closely similar) to those in the "germ line". This hypothesis has received support from the recent identification and cloning of a variable region gene from human fetal liver that is predicted to encode a light chain similar to that found in CRI^+ RF (Chen et al. 1986). It is likely that additional factors in SS patients such as specific antigens and T cells play a role in the clonal expansion of CRI^+ B cells.

Conclusion

In summary, RF in 1° SS patients express a CRI that is defined by a MoAb and by synthetic peptides derived from V_{κ} III light chains. This CDR is shared with RF paraproteins found in patients with Waldenstrom's macroglobulinemia and mixed cryoglobulinemia. The CRI can be detected in RA patients lacking sicca but constitutes a much lower proportion of the total RF. B cells containing the CRI can be detected in SG biopsies and CRI^{+} non-Hodgkin's lymphomas arising in the setting of pre-existent SS. The ability to detect and enumerate specific clones of B cells containing the CRI will aid in diagnosis and help in understanding pathogenesis of this autoimmune disorder with a high risk of neoplastic transformation.

Summary

Rheumatoid factor (RF), an autoantibody that has the ability to bind to the Fc portion of IgG, is frequently present in the serum of patients with Sjögren's syndrome (SS). Its role in the disease process is not well understood but its expression at high levels provides a marker of immune dysregulation which is shared with several other autoimmune, infectious and neoplastic diseases. RF from the majority of primary SS patients exhibit a cross reactive idiotype (CRI) defined by a monoclonal antibody (MoAb 17-109). This CRI is located on the kappa light chain by immunoblotting methods and is closely related to the CRI present on RF paraproteins from patients with Waldenstrom's macroglobulinemia (WM). Structural analysis of CRI^{+} light chains using anti-peptide antibodies demonstrated V_{κ} IIIb subclass of kappa chains in the SS RF and WM RF. Although this CRI could be detected in the sera of most RA patients, the proportion of RF bearing the CRI was much lower than in the sera of SS patients. These results suggest the preferential use of particular variable region genes of the kappa light chain in B cells of patients with SS. Thus, CRI expression in SS provides a specific marker to study immune dysregulation of B cells and perhaps identify factors that predispose these patients to increased risk of lymphoid malignancies.

Acknowledgement

We thank Susan Scott and Joe Weber for their excellent technical assistance and our division of rheumatology (Drs. C. Robinson, J. Curd, G. Williams, K. Hench, F. Kozin and E. Tan) and oral medicine (Dr. F. Howell) for allowing us to study their patients.

References

Adamson T, Fox R, Frisman D, Howell F (1983) Immunohistologic analysis of lymphoid infiltrates in primary Sjögren's syndrome using monoclonal antibodies. J Immunol 130: 203–208

Andrews DW, Capra JD (1981) Complete amino acid sequence of variable domains from two monoclonal human anti-gamma globulins of the Wa cross-idiotypic group: suggestion that the J segments are involved in the structural correlate of the idiotype. Proc Natl Acad Sci USA 78: 3799–3803

Atkinson PM, Lampman GW, Furie BC, Naparstek Y, Schwartz RS, Stollar BD, Furie B (1985) Homology of the NH2-terminal amino acid sequences of the heavy and light chains of human monoclonal lupus autoantibodies containing the dominant 16/6 idiotype. J Clin Invest 75: 1138-1143

Bentley DL (1983) Most kappa immunoglobulin mRNA in human lymphocytes is homologous to a small family of germline V genes. Nature 307: 77

Berard C, Greene M, Jaffe E, Magrath I, Ziegler J (1981) A multi-disciplinary approach to non-Hodgkin's lymphoma: NIH conference. Ann Intern Med 94: 218

Brouet J, Clauvel J-P, Danon F (1974) Biological and clinical significance of cryoglobulins: A report of 86 cases. Am J Med 57: 775-782

Capra JD, Fougereau M (1983) Structural correlates of idiotypes. One from column A, one from column B. Immunol Today 4: 177-179

Carson DA, Pasquali J-L, Tsoukas CD, Fong S, Slovin SF, Lawrance SK, Slaughter L, Vaughan JH (1981) Physiology and pathology of rheumatoid factors. Springer Semin. Immunopathol. 4: 161-179

Carson DA, Fong S (1983) A common idiotype on human rheumatoid factors identified by a hybridoma antibody. Mol Immunol 20: 1081-1087

Carson DA, Lawrance S, Vaughan JH, Abraham G (1977) Radioimmunoassay of IgG and IgM rheumatoid factors reacting with human IgG. J Immunol 119: 295

Chen PP, Fong S, Normansell D, Houghten RA, Karras JG, Vaughan JH, Carson DA (1984) Delineation of a cross-reactive idiotype on human autoantibodies with antibody against a synthetic peptide. J Exp Med 159: 1502-1511

Chen PP, Goñi F, Fong S, Jirik F, Vaughan JH, Frangione B, Carson DA (1985 a) The majority of human monoclonal IgM rheumatoid factors express a primary structure-dependent cross-reactive idiotype. J Immunol 134: 3281-3285

Chen PP, Goñi F, Houghten RA, Fong S, Goldfien RD, Vaughan JH, Frangione B, Carson DA (1985 b) Characterization of human rheumatoid factors with seven antiidiotypes induced by synthetic hypervariable-region peptides. J Exp Med 162: 487-500

Chen P, Albrandt K, Orida N, Radoux V, Chen EY, Schrantz R, Liu F, Carson D (1986) Genetic basis for the cross-reactive idiotypes on the light chains of human IgM anti-IgG autoantibodies. Proc Natl Acad Sci USA 83: 8318-8322

Coulie P, Van Snick J (1983) Rheumatoid factors and secondary immune responses in the mouse. II. Incidence, kinetics and induction mechanisms. Eur J Immunol 13: 895-899

Coulie PG, Van Snick J (1985) Rheumatoid factor (RF) production during anamnestic immune responses in the mouse. III. Activation of RF precursor cells is induced by their interaction with immune complexes and carrier-specific helper T cells. J Exp Med 161: 88-97

Cunningham-Rundles C, Cheung M (1985) Cross reacting idiotypes in human sera. Immunol Today 6: 14-16

Daniels TE (1984) Labial salivary gland biopsy in Sjögren's syndrome. Arthritis Rheum 27: 147-156

Dresser DW (1978) Most IgM-producing cells in the mouse secrete autoantibodies (rheumatoid factor). Nature 274: 480-483

Fong S, Carson DA, Vaughan JH (1984) Rheumatoid factor. In: Gupta S, Talal N (eds) Immunology of Rheumatic Diseases. Plenum Publishing Corp., New York pp. 167-196

Fong S, Chen PP, Gilbertson TA, Weber JR, Fox RI, Carson DA (1986) Expression of three cross reactive idiotypes on rheumatoid factor autoantibodies from patients with autoimmune diseases and seropositive adults. J Immunol 137: 122-128

Fong S, Chen PP, Goldfien RD, Jirik F, Silverman G, Carson DA (1985) Recurrent idiotypes of human anti-IgG autoantibodies: their potential use for immunotherapy. In: Singhal SK, Delovitch TL (eds), Mediators of Immune Regulation and Immunotherapy. Elsevier Science Publishing Co., Inc., New York pp. 232-243

Fox RI, Howell FV, Bone RC, Michelson PE (1984) Primary Sjögren's syndrome: Clinical and immunopathologic features. Semin Arthritis Rheum 14: 77-105

Fox RI, Chen PP, Carson DA, Fong S (1986) Expression of a cross reactive idiotype on rheumatoid factor in patients with Sjögren's syndrome. J Immunol 136: 477-483

Goñi F, Chen PP, Pons-Estel B, Carson DA, Frangione B (1985) Sequence similarities and cross-idiotypic specificity of L chains among human monoclonal IgM-K with anti-gammaglobulin activity. J Immunol 135: 4073-4079

Grabar P (1983) Autoantibodies and the physiological roles of immunoglobulins. Immunol Today 4: 337-340

Greenstein J, Solomon A, Abraham G (1984) Monoclonal antibodies reactive with idiotypic and variable-region specific determinants on human immunoglobulins. Immunology 51: 17-23

Guilbert B, Dighiero G, Avrameas S (1983) Naturally occurring antibodies against nine common antigens in human sera. I. Detection, isolation, and characterization. J Immunol 128: 2779-2787

Hieter PA, Maizel JV Jr, Leder P (1982) Evolution of human immunoglobulin K J region genes. J Biol Chem 257: 1516-1522

Izui S, Eisenberg RA, Dixon FJ (1979) IgM rheumatoid factors in mice injected with bacterial lipopolysaccharides. J Immunol 122: 2096-2102

Kassan S, Thomas T, Moutsopolous H, Hoover R, Kimberly R, Budman D, Costa J, Decker J, Chused T (1978) Increased risk of lymphoma in sicca syndrome. Ann Intern Med 89: 888-892

Koopman WJ, Schrohenloher RE (1980) Enhanced in vitro synthesis of IgM rheumatoid factor in rheumatoid arthritis. Arthritis Rheum 23: 985-992

Kunkel HG, Muller-Eberhard HM, Fudenburg HH, Tomasi TB (1961) Gamma globulin complexes in rheumatoid arthritis and certain other conditions. J Clin Invest 40: 117

Kunkel HG, Agnello V, Joslin FG, Winchester RJ, Capra JD (1973) Cross-idiotypic specificity among monoclonal IgM proteins with anti-gammaglobulin activity. J Exp Med 137: 331-342

Kunkel HG, Winchester RJ, Joslin FG, Capra JD (1974) Similarities in the light chains of anti-gamma-globulins sharing cross-idiotypic specificities. J Exp Med 139: 128-136

Ledford DK, Goñi F, Pizzolato M, Franklin EC, Solomon A, Frangione B (1983) Preferential association of kappa-IIIb light chains with monoclonal human IgM-kappa autoantibodies. J Immunol 131: 1322-1325

Lefvert A-K, James RW, Alliod C, Fulpius BW (1982) A monoclonal antiidiotypic antibody against anti-receptor antibodies from myasthenic sera. Eur J Immunol 12: 790-792

Lotscher E, Grzeschik K, Baver H, Pohlenz H, Stranbinger B, Zauchau H (1986) Dispersed human immunoglobulin kappa light chain genes. Nature 320: 456-459

Lundstrom IMC, Anneroth KGB, Bergstedt HF (1982) Salivary gland function and changes in patients with oral lichen planus. Scand J Dent Res 90: 443-458

Manser T, Huang S, Gefter M (1984) Influence of clonal selection on the expression of immunoglobulin variable region genes. Science 226: 1283-1286

Marquart M, Deisenhofer J (1982) The three-dimensional structure of antibodies. Immunol. Today 3: 160-165

Matsuyama T, Fukumori J, Tanaka H (1983) Evidence of unique idiotypic determinants and similar idiotypic determinants on human anti-thyroglobulin antibodies. Clin Exp Immunol 51: 381-386

Nemazee DA (1985) Immune complexes can trigger specific, T cell-dependent, autoanti-IgG antibody production in mice. J Exp Med 161: 242-256

Nemazee DA, Sato VL (1983) Induction of rheumatoid antibodies in the mouse: regulated production of autoantibody in the secondary humoral response. J Exp Med 158: 529-545

Pech M, Hochtl J, Schnell H, Zachau HG (1981) Differences between germ-line and rearranged immunoglobulin Vk coding sequences suggest a localized mutation mechanism. Nature 291: 668-670

Pons-Estel B, Goñi F, Solomon A, Frangione B (1984) Sequence similarities among kappa IIIb chains of monoclonal human IgM kappa autoantibodies. J Exp Med 160: 893-904

Pope RM, McDuffy SJ (1981) IgG rheumatoid factor: Analysis of various species of IgG for detection by radioimmunoassay. J Lab Clin Med 97: 842-853

Rabbitts TH, Bentley DL, Milstein CP (1981) Human antibody genes: V gene variability and CH genes switching strategies. Immunol Rev 59: 69

Rajewsky K, Takemori T (1983) Genetics, expression, and function of idiotypes. Annu Rev Immunol 1: 569-607

Rose H, Ragan C, Pearce E, Lipman M (1948) Differential agglutination of normal and sensitized sheep erythrocytes by sera of patients with rheumatoid arthritis. Proc Soc Exp Biol Med 68: 1-6

Rudikoff S (1983) Immunoglobulin structure-function correlates: antigen binding and idiotypes. Contemp Top Mol Immunol 9: 169-209

Solomon A, McLaughlin CL (1971) Bence Jones proteins and light chains of immunoglobulins. IV. Immunochemical differentiation among proteins within each of the three established k chain classes. J Immunol 106: 120

Solomon G, Schiffenbauer J, Keiser HD, Diamond B (1983) Use of monoclonal antibodies to identify shared idiotypes on human antibodies to native DNA from patients with systemic lupus erythematosus. Proc Natl Acad Sci USA 80: 850–854
Waaler E (1940) On the occurrence of a factor in human serum activating the specific agglutination of sheep blood corpuscles. Acta Pathol Microbiol Scand 17: 172–188
Welch MJ, Fong S, Vaughan JH, Carson DA (1983) Increased frequency of rheumatoid factor precursor B lymphocytes after immunization of normal adults with tetanus toxoid. Clin Exp Immunol 51: 299–305
Whaley K, Webb J, McAvoy B (1973) Sjögren's syndrome 2. Clin Assoc Quart J Med 42: 513–530

2. Autoantibodies in Sjögren's Syndrome

J. B. Harley

Antinuclear antibodies, rheumatoid factor and precipitating autoantibodies were first reported in Sjögren's syndrome almost simultaneously over 25 years ago (Jones 1958; Weissman 1958; Heaton 1959). These findings were quickly exploited by investigators in Glasgow and Bethesda working separately and together. The high prevalence of rheumatoid factor in Sjögren's syndrome was established by Bunim and colleagues (Bloch et al. 1960; Bunim 1961) and is considered elsewhere (see chapter on rheumatoid factor by Robert Fox and Dennis Carson in this volume).

Antibodies binding the cell nucleus are present in over 70% of Sjögren's syndrome patients (Bloch et al. 1960a and 1960b; Bunim 1961; Bloch and Bunim, 1963; Bunim et al. 1964; Bloch et al. 1965; Whaley et al. 1973). Homogeneous, speckled and nucleolar fluorescent patterns are all shown to be common; however, the antigen or antigens which account for the positive nuclear fluorescence have not been directly identified in any case of Sjögren's syndrome. Certainly, Ro/SSA and La/SSB as discussed below must be considered candidates, but antibodies with other specificities have also been found in patients whose clinical illness most closely resembles Sjögren's syndrome. Antibodies to histones (Bernstein et al. 1985) and mitochondria (Whaley et al. 1973) as well as lupus erythematosus (L. E.) cell formation (Bloch et al. 1960b) have been reported. Kurki et al. (1983) has found that 43% of the Sjögren's syndrome patients he tested had IgG antibodies to vimentin which was twice the prevalence he found in rheumatoid arthritis sera and ten times that in normal donors. In addition, anti-erythrocyte, anti-thyroglobulin and anti-prostatic acid phosphatase antibodies have also been appreciated (Bloch et al. 1960; Virji 1985). Anti-salivary gland and anti-salivary gland epithelium antibodies have been reported (Bertram and Halberg 1964; Halberg et al. 1965; MacSween et al. 1967; Feltkamp and van Rossum 1968). How these antibodies are related to pathogenesis or antinuclear antibodies in Sjögren syndrome is presently unknown. If anything, the data suggest that anti-salivary gland autoantibodies protect from salivary gland destruction (Anderson et al. 1973; Whaley et al. 1973).

J. R. Anderson and colleagues (1961) evaluated the precipitins that Jones (1958) had found in exceptional patients (three of 44) against extracts of salivary and submandibular glands. They found precipitins in nine of 29 Sjögren's syndrome sera. Two antigens were identified which were distinguished by reactivity in Oüchterlony double diffusion and by their physical properties. The SjT antigen was found in all tissues tested in addition to salivary gland while the second antigen, SjD, was detected in all extracts but brain, adrenal and liver (probably for technical reasons). SjD which corresponds to Ro(SS-A) was probably not detected in at least heart for technical reasons since this antigen has been found in heart by more recent workers

(Deng et al. 1985; Wolin and Steitz 1984b; Harley et al. 1985a). SjT was more heat sensitive and was destroyed by trypsin while SjD was resistant to trypsin. Both antigenic activities, as found in extracts, were resistant to DNase and RNase (Anderson 1961).

In a subsequent study (Beck et al. 1965) found that the SjD and SjT precipitins were common in primary Sjögren's syndrome (13 and 8 of 16, respectively) while rare in secondary Sjögren's syndrome associated with rheumatoid arthritis (1 and 0 of 18, respectively, for SjD $\chi^2 = 18.0$ with $p < 0.001$ and for SjT $\chi^2 = 9.9$ with $p < 0.01$ using Yates' correction).

These precipitins were later also discovered and characterized by M. Reichlin and colleagues (Clark et al. 1968; Mattioli and Reichlin 1974). Though no direct comparison has been performed, from their physical and serologic properties it may be concluded that SjD corresponds to the Ro antigen and SjT to the La antigen, respectively.

Other laboratories have also independently found precipitating activities. Alspaugh and Tan (1975) found antigenic activities designated SS-A, SS-B and SS-C. By serum exchange SS-A was shown to correspond to Ro and SS-B to La (Alspaugh and Maddison 1979). The respective antigens and antibodies are generally recognized by either of the designations Ro or SS-A and La or SS-B though they are now commonly combined. Alspaugh also found that patients with Sjögren's syndrome in the context of rheumatoid arthritis were less likely to have the anti-SS-A(Ro) or anti-SS-B(La) precipitins.

Efforts to biochemically purify these antigens began with antigen enrichment (Clark et al. 1968; Mattioli and Reichlin 1974; Okarma et al. 1982) and has culminated in the preparation of homogeneous La/SSB (Akizuki et al. 1977a and 1977b; Teppo 1981, Venables et al. 1983; Harley et al. 1984; Stephano 1984; Francoer et al. 1985) and Ro/SSA (Yamagata 1984, Venables et al. 1983b).

La(SS-B) is an RNA-protein complex. By gel filtration, the complex has a molecular weight of near 60 kd. When denatured, the RNA and protein separate. At least some of the antigenicity must be contained in the protein since antigenic peptides have been described at 42 to 46 kd and 29 kd. The smaller peptide has been shown to be a proteolytic product of the larger one (Venables et al. 1983b). Also, a 50 kd La protein has been defined by some workers which was rapidly degraded to a 43 kd peptide in the hands of one group (Reinke and Steitz, 1982; Habets et al. 1983), but this observation was not confirmed by recent *in vitro* translation experiments (Francoeur et al. 1985). Part of the gene coding for the La protein has been cloned and contains at least one of its autoimmune epitopes (Chambers and Keene 1985). The quantitative relationship of this proported autoimmune epitope to the overall anti-La(SS-B) response is not known. Indeed, the fact that reactivity is preserved though the peptide is synthesized in E. coli suggests that the possible posttranscriptional modifications such as phosphorolation of the protein (Pizer et al. 1982) may not contribute to antigenicity of at least this epitope.

The Ro(SS-A) peptide is a 60 kd single chain protein. It shows the unusual property of being only partially denatured by sodium dodecylsulfate leading to an apparent molecular weight of 40 kd (Yamagata et al. 1984). Peptides derived from Ro(SS-A) retain a portion of immune reactivity (R. I. Fox and J. B. Harley, unpublished data).

A major advance in our comprehension of Ro(SS-A) and La(SS-B) structure has come with the application of molecular biological techniques. Protein or ribonucleic acid are radioactively labeled by using the appropriate precursors, then the autoimmune sera are used to immunoprecipitate the binding species. With this strategy, Lerner and Steitz (1979) have been the first to appreciate that the Sm and nRNP antigens bound the U-RNAs. When applied to analyze sera containing anti-Ro/SSA activity five small RNA bands are defined (Lerner et al. 1981 a and 1981 b; Wolin and Steitz 1983 and 1984). These RNA had not been described before they were detected by autoimmune sera. The RNA has been termed hYRNA - h for human and Y for its proported cytoplasmic location. hYRNA is uridine rich and in man four unique RNAs are found between 83 and 112 bases in length, three of which have been sequenced (Hendrick et al. 1981; Kuto et al. 1982; Wolin and Steitz 1983). The 5′ and 3′ base paired ends of the RNA are resistant to digestion with RNase when complexed to the Ro/SSA protein (Wolin and Steitz 1984a). Recently, it has been shown that the hY1 and hY3 genes are in close proximity on the human chromosome (Wolin and Steitz 1983). The hYRNAs are transcripts of RNA polymerase III and are present at about 10^5 copies per cell, less than one percent the total ribosomal RNA. The molecular role of Ro/SSA is not known.

Anti-Ro(SS-A) was first thought to bind the cytoplasm (Clark et al. 1969). Recently, nuclear speckled and particulate patterns (Harman et al. 1983; Wermuth et al. 1985) have been associated withRo(SS-A) precipitins. These results should be applied with caution in clinical practice since the classic "ANA negative" systemic lupus erythematosus patients were Ro(SS-A) precipitin positive (Maddison et al. 1981). Indeed, more than half of sera from patients with the Ro(SS-A) precipitin and without other defined autoantibodies (La(SS-B), nRNP, Sm precipitins, or anti-DNA) do not bind commercially prepared tissue culture cells in the standard antinuclear antibody test (Scopelitis and Biundo 1984; J.B. Harley and M. Reichlin unpublished observations).

A large variety of small RNAs bind the La protein. These include precursor tRNA and 4.5S, 5.0S, 7S and 7-2 RNAs. 5.0S is precursor RNA for ribosomal RNA and 4.5S is partially homologous to the highly repetitive Alu family of DNA sequences (Jelinek et al. 1980). Indeed, electrophoresis of the RNAs immunoprecipitated by anti-La(SS-B) form a few prominent bands on the background of a large number of less abundant RNAs, all of which are between 70 and 130 bases (Lerner et al. 1981; Hendrick et al. 1981; Reinke and Steitz 1982). All La binding RNAs appear to be translation products of RNA polymerase III except for Ul RNA which is an RNA poplymerase II product (Madore et al. 1984). The binding between the La RNAs and the La protein is mediated by three or more terminal uridines at the 3′ end (Francoeur and Mathews 1982; Reddy et al. 1983; Mathews and Francoeur 1984; Stephano 1984).

Certain viral RNAs have also been shown to bind La(SS-B). Two La binding RNAs from each Epstein-Barr virus and adenovirus have been described all which are between 160 and 173 bases (Lerner et al. 1981 a; Lerner et al. 1981 b; Rosa et al. 1981). The leader RNA of vesicular stomititis virus also binds the La protein (Kurilla and Keene 1983). It is suspected that binding of these RNAs to the La protein is part of the reorganization of cellular metabolism that occurs in these viral infections. Indeed, La protein has been thought to be involved in polyadenylation of RNA polymerase II transcripts (Moore and Sharp, 1984). Whether or not binding of the La protein to viral RNAs is important in the autoimmune response of disease states is a subject of much recent interest and special attention has been given to cases of primary Sjögren's syndrome occurring subsequent to viral infections (Whittingham et al. 1985).

The La(SS-B) antigen has recently been localized to the nucleus and nucleolus on different substrates. A murine anti-La(SS-B) monoclonal antibody binds bovine tissue culture cells in a speckled nuclear pattern. This pattern is inhibited by preincubation of the antibody with purified La(SS-B) (Harley et al. 1985). A serum containing a La(SS-B) precipitin has demonstrated an identical staining pattern which was also inhibited by the purified antigen. A similar approach has been used by Graus et al. (1985) to demonstrate that anti-La(SS-B) bound neuronal nucleoli in as much as this binding could be inhibited by La(SS-B). Deng et al. (1981) found that sera precipitating La bound in a speckled pattern in the G_0 phase of the cell cycle but in a nucleolar pattern during G_1 and early S phase. The relation of La(SS-B/SjT) and Ro(SS-A/SjD) to nucleolar staining could well have been suspected from the much older data of K.J. Bloch and colleagues (1965) which is also analyzed below (Table 3).

In addition to precipitation, a number of methods have been developed to measure anti-La(SS-B) and anti-Ro(SS-A) levels in patient sera. Venables and colleagues (1983) developed solid phase and Farr assays to detect anti-La(SS-B). In their hands neither was appreciably more sensitive than precipitation. Solid phase assays for Ro(SS-A) have been hindered by the difficulties in preparation of purified antigen. Nevertheless, highly purified La(SS-B) and Ro(SS-A) have been used in solid phase assays which, in the experience of one group, have been much more sensitive for autoantibodies than precipitation (Harley et al. 1984; Yamagata et al. 1984; Harley et al. 1986a). Indeed, these assays have detected anti-La(SS-B) and anti-Ro(SS-A) in a surprisingly high proportion of normal sera at seven percent and 12.5 to 17.5 percent, respectively (Harley et al. 1984; Gaither et al. 1985). The capacity of normals to synthesize at least anti-La(SS-B) is supported by the observation that lymphocytes from normal donors synthesized IgG anti-La(SS-B) after *in vitro* stimulation with pokeweed mitogen (Mumford et al. 1985).

Of course, any new technology must be approached cautiously. It is clear, however, that solid phase assays can be 100 to 1000 fold more sensitive than precipitation. This methodology is not without disadvantages; in particular, the specificity of the antibody binding is more difficult to establish. Incubation of binding with specifically purified antigen is one strategy that has been used to circumvent this problem (Harley et al. 1986a). Comparison of precipitation with solid phase assays showed a complete concordance for anti-La(SS-B) determination (Harley 1985). Meanwhile, for anti-Ro(SS-A), nearly a quarter of the Sjögren's syndrome patient sera either had low positive solid phase binding and yet formed a precipitin or did not precipitate and had high positive solid phase Ro(SS-A) binding. Comparison of these sera with reference to the other autoantibodies present showed that those sera forming precipitins had higher levels of rheumatoid factor and antinuclear antibody despite having similar anti-Ro(SS-A) and anti-La(SS-B) binding levels (Harley 1985).

Others have used immunoprecipitation with radioactive precursors or immunoblotting to detect autoantibody but direct comparisons with precipitation tests have been rare. M.S. Forman, working in J. Hardin's laboratory (1985), has recently shown that silver staining or ethidium bromide fluorescence can be used instead of radioactivity to detect the RNAs binding Ro(SS-A) or La(SS-B). This method may be safe and simple enough to be clinically useful but it remains more technically involved than the solid phase assays.

The solid phase assays have been hindered by the necessary requirement of purified Ro(SS-A) or La(SS-B). Individual preparations vary in purity and in antibody binding capacity which makes standardization for routine clinical applications difficult. A monoclonal antibody binding La(SS-B) has been used to circumvent this difficulty and has made possible an even more sensitive solid phase assay than those using purified La(SS-B) (Harley et al. 1985b).

Like rheumatoid factor and anti-nuclear antibody, anti-Ro(SS-A) and anti-La(SS-B) cannot be considered specific for Sjögren's syndrome. Over 60 percent of patients with subacute cutaneous lupus have Ro(SS-A) and half of which also have La(SS-B) precipitins (Sontheimer et al. 1982). Approximately 30 and 10 percent of systemic lupus erythematosus patients have Ro(SS-A) and La(SS-B) precipitins respectively (M. Reichlin, 1979). In addition, anti-Ro(SS-A) has been found in rheumatoid arthritis without coexisting Sjögren's syndrome (Boire and Ménard, 1985; Moustopolous et al. 1985). Systemic lupus erythematosus that occurs in C2 deficient individuals is closely associated with Ro(SS-A) precipitins (Provost et al. 1983). Indeed, in a study of 1111 patients with autoimmune disease (Bernstein et al. 1984), though Ro(SS-A) precipitins were commonly present primary Sjögren's syndrome (75 percent) and systemic lupus erythematosus (24 percent), they were also found in myositis (eight percent), idiopathic thrombocytopenic purpura (seven percent), primary biliary cirrhosis (six percent), progressive systemic sclerosis (four percent), chronic active hepatitis in the absence of infection (four percent), and rheumatoid arthritis (3 percent). No other autoantibody has been found in such apparently diverse patients.

Anti-Ro(SS-A) is also common in both expressions of neonatal lupus, the characteristic lupus dermatitis and congenital complete heart block. The natural history of neonatal lupus dermatitis conform with that expected of a disease caused by or associated with an antibody acquired from the mother by placental transfer (Kephart et al. 1981; Miyagaina et al. 1981; Provost 1983; Lumpkin et al. 1985). Also, anti-Ro(SS-A) is found in over 80 percent of causes of complete congenital heart block and recent data suggests that this antibody is blocked or removed from the circulation in affected neonates (Scott et al. 1982; Litsky et al. 1985; Harley et al. 1985a). Mothers of these children may have Sjögren's syndrome, systemic lupus erythematosus, subacute cutaneous lupus erythematosus, or be asymptomatic. Indeed, one of the first known cases of complete congenital heart block was born to a mother reported to have Mikulicz's disease (Aylward 1928; Aiken 1932). Other mothers with Sjögren's syndrome have borne infants with neonatal lupus. These mothers and their infants share identical autoantibodies though Sjögren's syndrome and lupus dermatitis or congenital heart block are quite different clinical manifestations. While it is clear that many mothers with anti-Ro(SS-A) deliver unaffected infants the close association of anti-Ro(SS-A) with the dermatitis and heart disease of neonatal lupus support the notion that these autoantibodies have clinical consequences.

Also supporting the contention that autoantibodies may cause other manifestations of Sjögren's syndrome is a case in which the neonate had primarily distal renal tubular acidosis and urinary concentrating dysfunction as did the mother who had this as a consequence of her primary Sjögren's syndrome (Jordan et al. 1985). The defect persisted in the infant until 10 weeks of age when it spontaneously resolved. Anti-Tamm-Horsfall antibody was detected in both the mother and infant at birth but disappeared from the infant's circulation in parallel with his clinical improvement.

The clinical relationships of autoantibodies to forms of disease expression are the most powerful evidence they are involved in the immunopathogenesis of Sjögren's syndrome. An analysis of Ro(SS-A) in Sjögren's syndrome (Alexander et al. 1983) found close relationships of this precipitin to many clinical and laboratory findings characteristic of the disease (Table 1). Since no effort was made in this study to control for the contribution of other antinuclear antibody specificities or rheumatoid factor, it cannot be concluded that anti-Ro(SS-A) is the major autoantibody accounting for these findings.

The common occurence anti-Ro(SS-A) and anti-La(SS-B) was reinforced by a subsequent study (Harley et al. 1986a) where a sensitive solid phase method was applied and demonstrated that nearly all Sjögren's syndrome patients had at least

Table 1. Clinical and laboratory features in patients with anti-Ro(SS-A) antibodies from E. L. Alexander and colleagues (1983)

Features	Patients with Anti-Ro(SS-A)		
	Positive (n = 33)	Negative (n = 42)	p
Clinical	n	n	
Vaculitis	24	4	0.0005
Salivary gland enlargement	26	15	0.0005
Lymphadenopathy	19	4	0.0005
Purpura	12	1	0.0005
Hematologic[a]			
Anemia	19	6	0.0005
Leukopenia	14	3	0.001
Thrombocytopenia	7	1	0.025
Serologic[b]			
Hyperglobulinemia	21	8	0.0005
Rheumatoid factor	29	17	0.0005
Antinuclear antibody	31	10	0.0005
Cryoglobulinemia	7/13	0/22	0.001
Hypocomplementemia	11	2	0.005

[a] Anemia = hematocrit $<35\%$; leukopenia = <4000 leukocytes/mm^3; thrombocytopenia = $<150{,}000$ platelets/mm^3.
[b] Hyperglobulinemia = serum globulins >4.0 g/dL; rheumatoid factor $\geq 1:80$; antinuclear antibodies $\geq 1:40$; cryocrit $\geq 2\%$; total hemolytic complement <25 units.
Reproduced with permission from the Annals of Internal Medicine (Alexander et al., 1983).

low levels of these autoantibodies (Fig. 1). Purpura, leukopenia, lymphopenia, hypergammaglobulenemia (especially of IgG and IgA), and rheumatoid factor were all associated with anti-Ro(SS-A) and anti-La(SS-B). The relationship with rheumatoid factor was shown to only be present in patients with primary disease ($r=0.63$, $p<0.0001$). Indeed, in this study even though all patients with rheumatoid arthritis and secondary Sjögren's syndrome ($N=16$) had rheumatoid factor, its titer was not related to the level of anti-Ro(SS-A) ($r=0.14$, $p>0.5$) or anti-La(SS-B) ($r=0.15$, $p>0.5$).

How closely hypergammaglobulinemia, rheumatoid factor, antinuclear antibodies, anti-Ro(SS-A) and anti-La(SS-B) are related to one another is a subject of recent study and has prompted a reevaluation of the data from the series of patients at the National Institutes of Health published twenty years ago by K. J. Bloch and his colleagues (1965). These workers performed both bentonite flocculation and γ-globulin sensitized sheep cell agglutination tests for rheumatoid factor. Antinuclear antibodies were determined on mouse and rat liver substrates. The pattern of fluorescence was recorded on the rat liver substrate. Serum was injected subcutaneously in guinea pigs shortly before the intravenous injection of a tissue extract containing antigen to determine passive cutaneous anaphylaxis. SjD (Ro/SS-A) and SjT (La/SS-B) precipitins were determined in these patients and graded by the intensity of the resulting precipitin. The thyroglobulin-coated tanned erythrocyte agglutination test was also performed on these sera.

Sixty-two patients with Sjögren's syndrome were studied. The Spearman correlation coefficients are presented in Table 2. The level of rheumatoid factor as measured by bentonite flocculation was related to the titer of the homogeneous nuclear

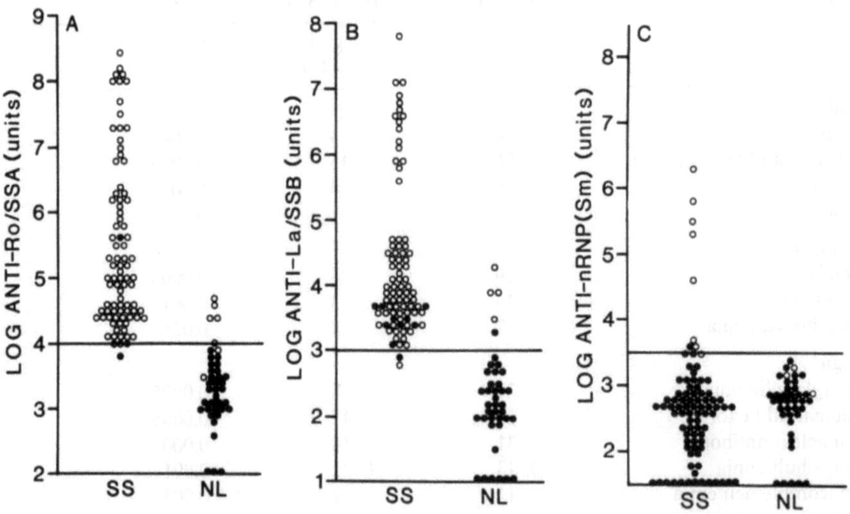

Fig. 1. Relative autoantibody binding concentrations in sera from patients with Sjögren's syndrome (SS) as compared to normal donors (NL). Sera containing specific autoantibody have opened symbols (○) signifying inhibition by preincubation with autoantigen and greater than the indicated threshold of binding units. Sera not sufficiently inhibited by autoantigen are indicated by closed symbols (●). Data are from Harley et al. (1986 a)

Table 2. Relationships between autoantibodies and γ-globulin in Sjögren's syndrome. A reappraisal of data obtained by K. Bloch and colleagues (1965)[a]

		Bentonite Flocculation Test (Titer)	Sensitized Sheep Cell Agglutination (Titer)	Antinuclear Antibody (Titer)	Homogenous Pattern (Titer)	Speckled Pattern (Titer)	Nucleolar Pattern (Titer)	γ-Globulin (mg/ml)	Passive Cutaneous Anaphylaxis
γ-Globulin (mg/ml)	r								0.469
	p								0.0003
	n								56
Bentonite Flocculation (Titer)	r							0.293	0.199
	p							0.021	0.14
	n							62	56
Sensitized Sheep Cell Agglutination (Titer)	r	0.650						0.085	0.123
	p	0.0001						0.53	0.38
	n	57						57	53
Antinuclear Antibody (Titer)	r	0.257	0.354					0.344	0.468
	p	0.078	0.014					0.017	0.0014
	n	48	47					48	44
Homogeneous Pattern (Titer)	r	0.338	0.194	−0.138				0.208	0.185
	p	0.028	0.24	0.43				0.19	0.265
	n	42	39	35				42	39
Speckled Pattern (Titer)	r	−0.045	−0.119	0.383	−0.487			0.390	0.415
	p	0.78	0.47	0.023	0.0011			0.011	0.0087
	n	42	39	35	42			42	39
Nucleolar Pattern (Titer)	r	−0.042	0.160	0.152	−0.158	0.259		0.279	0.405
	p	0.79	0.33	0.38	0.32	0.098		0.074	0.011
	n	42	39	35	42	42		42	39
SjD (Ro/SS-A)	r	0.94	0.029	0.324	0.023	0.164	0.586	0.504	0.527
	p	0.56	0.86	0.057	0.88	0.28	0.0001	0.0007	0.0006
	n	42	39	35	42	42	42	42	39
SjT (La/SS-B)	r	−0.0315	0.0390	0.303	0.105	0.204	0.591	0.439	0.559
	p	0.84	0.82	0.077	0.51	0.20	0.0001	0.0036	0.0002
	n	42	39	35	42	42	42	42	39

[a] Spearman correlation coefficients were derived from the original data (Bloch et al. 1965). In each set of 3 values, the correlation coefficient, r, is presented first followed by the p value and then the number of patients who had both tests performed. The units for each variable are presented in parenthesis except for passive cutaneous anaphyloxis where positive in the original data was given a value of 1 and negative 0 and for SjD and SjT where negative in the original data was converted to 0, weakly positive to 1 and positive to 2.

pattern of antinuclear antibody while the γ-globulin sensitized sheep cell agglutination test was associated with the antinuclear antibody titer on mouse liver. SjD and SjT were strongly associated with one another ($r = 0.783$, $p = 0.0001$, $N = 42$), as has been subsequently shown for Ro(SS-A) and La(SS-B). SjD and SjT were related to the γ-globulin concentration and a relationship with the mouse kidney antinuclear antibody titer is suggested (Table 2). Surprisingly, only the nucleolar antinuclear antibody pattern was related to SjD and SjT precipitins. All six sera with nucleolar bindung had anti-SjD (Ro/SS-A) and were found in primary Sjögren's syndrome patient sera while four of these six also had anti-SjT (La/SS-B). Therefore, in addition to the cytoplasmic and nuclear speckled patterns discussed above, the nucleolar binding must be regarded as potentially related to anti-Ro(SS-A) or anti-La(SS-B). Meanwhile, though 20 of the 62 sera had anti-thyroglobulin, this antibody was not related to any of the other autoantibodies (data are not presented). The capacity of sera to induce passive cutaneous anaphylaxis was related to γ-globulin concentration, antinuclear antibody and the SjD (Ro/SS-A) and SjT (La/SS-B) precipitins. These last results probably reflect that any autoantigen in the extract binding to autoantibody in the serum is capable of causing vascular injury.

In Sjögren's syndrome, especially in its primary form, the association of autoantibodies with each other and hypergammaglobulinemia is especially close (Tables 1, 2 and 3). What connects these responses to one another is not known: they may move in concert, each making a contribution to clinical or laboratory findings, or an individual specificity may be of primary importance in the observed relationships. Evidence supporting both of these possibilities has been found.

Hypergammaglobulinemia is common but not universal in Sjögren's syndrome (Gumpel and Hubbs 1970) and has been related to anti-Ro(SS-A), anti-La(SS-B), rheumatoid factor and antinuclear antibody, especially in primary disease (Alexander et al. 1983; Harley 1986a and 1986b). When a logistic regression analysis was applied to the data published by Harley et al. (1986a), anti-Ro(SS-A), anti-La(SS-B) and rheumatoid factor were related to hypergammaglobulinemia in the single model (Table 3). When overlapping contributions were removed in the multiple model, neither anti-La(SS-B) nor rheumatoid factor made an independent contribution to hypergammaglobulinemia. Anti-Ro/SSA, however, showed a higher logistic regression coefficient and retained a borderline statistical significance ($p = 0.06$).

Table 3. The relationship of Autoantibodies to hyperglobulinemia in primary Sjögren's syndrome by logistic regression

	Single Model[a]		Multiple Model	
	β	p	β	p
Anti-Ro/SSA	0.80	0.0002	1.36	0.06
Anti-La/SSB	0.75	0.0008	0.26	0.69
Rheumatoid Factor	0.001	0.021	−0.0006	0.61

[a] The single model presents the association of each autoantibody level with hyperglobulinemia (>40 gm/dl) without regard to the other two autoantibodies. The multiple model considers the effect of each autoantibody after the effects of the remaining two autoantibodies are removed. β is an estimate of the logistic regression coefficient. Analysis based upon data from Harley et al. (1986a).

Interestingly, the reanalysis of the data from K. Bloch (Table 2) also shows a closer relationship of hypergammaglobulinemia with anti-SjD (Ro/SSA) than with either anti-SjT (La/SSB) or rheumatoid factor as determined by bentonite flocculation or sheep cell agglutination. These observations lead to the conclusion that anti-Ro(SS-A) is the primary autoantibody related to hypergammaglobulinemia in primary Sjögren's syndrome.

Anti-Ro(SS-A) may lead to hypergammaglobulinemia by either being present in high concentrations or by somehow being associated with or otherwise influencing the production of other autoantibodies. At least consistent with the former possibility is the observation that 20 percent of the Sjögren's syndrome patients in a recent series had more than one mg/ml anti-Ro(SS-A) and nine percent had more than 10 mg/ml anti-Ro(SS-A) (Gaither and Harley 1985; Harley et al. 1986a). Analagous data using different methodology has been obtained for the concentration of anti-Sm in systemic lupus erythematosus. Maddison and Reichlin (1979) showed that as much as 20 percent of the total immunoglobulin bound Sm in some sera.

Anti-Ro(SS-A), anti-La(SS-B), rheumatoid factor, and antinuclear antibodies have also been variously related to one another in other recent studies (Alexander 1983; Molina et al. 1985). Attractive explanations for their coincidence include the possibility of multimolecular autoantigenic complexes containing more than one specificity, of cross-reactivity of autoantibodies and of common genetic predisposition for multiple specificities between patients. Eisenberg (1985) has shown that Ro(SS-A) and La(SS-B) may exist as part of the same protein-RNA complex consistent with the hypothesis that their relationship occurs at the level of antigen presentation. Mamula et al. (1985) have presented preliminary data that some anti-IgG antibodies also have anti-Ro(SS-A) activity.

Recently, the genetic composition at the major histocompatibility complex (HLA) has been shown to have an important effect upon the relative quantitative concentrations of these autoantibodies present in sera from patients with primary Sjögren's syndrome (Harley et al. 1986b). Patients who are heterozygous at HLA-DQ for alleles DQ1 and DQ2 have much higher levels of anti-Ro/SSA, anti-La/SSB, rheumatoid factor and antinuclear antibody (Table 4) (Harley et al. 1986b). Gene interaction at HLA-DQ then contributes to higher levels of autoantibodies. There are a number of mechanisms that could explain the observed gene interac-

Table 4. Autoantibodies in primary Sjögrens's syndrome. Comparison of the HLA-DQ1/DQ2 heterozygotes with the remainder of patients

	N	Anti-Ro/SSA (units)	Anti-La/SSB (units)	Antinuclear Antibody (Titer)	Rheumatoid Factor (Titer)
DQ2/DQ2	13	2,120,000	174,000	1:245	1:245
All other allelic combinations at HLA-DQ	35	122,000	9,550	1:83	1:53
p		0.002	0.002	0.06	0.01

Anti-Ro/SSA is expressed as multiples of the limit detection in a solid phase assay, as is anti-La/SSB. The level of significance (p) is determined by least square means. From Harley et al. (1986b)

tion. A locus closely linked to HLA-DQ may be exerting an important influence, but this area of the human chromosome has been extensively studied (Figueroa and Klein 1986) and the important loci are probably known. Moreover, relationships of individual alleles with autoantibody concentrations were much weaker at the closest known locus, HLA-DR (Harley et al. 1986a). Alleles at HLA-DP which is on the other side of HLA-DQ are not in linkage disequilibrium with the HLA-DQ alleles.

If the interaction requires both the expression of a particular gene product from two HLA genes then a mechanism of gene interaction between HLA-DR and HLA-DQ is possible. Nearly all of the HLA-DQ2 positive patients (of the HLA-DQ1/2 heterozygotes) were also HLA-DR3 positive. Therefore, a model of gene interaction between HLA-DR3 and HLA-DQ1 fit the data as well as interaction between HLA-DQ2 and HLA-DQ1.

The most intriguing possibility is that this data does indeed reflect gene complementation by the physical association of multiple polymorphic gene products. Ordinarily, at HLA-DR for example, the α chain is largely invarient so all of the polymorphism is defined by β chain variations. Then only *cis* associations are relevant such as presented in Fig. 2. When, however, variation of both the α and β peptide chains occurs commonly as is the case at HLA-DQ, then two additional molecules may be formed. These result from the combination of the maternal α chain with the paternal β chain and vice versa. These particular *trans* associated molecules are unique to the particular combination of parental gene products, and as in the example presented in Fig. 3, contribute two additional surface molecules with potentially unique properties.

That *trans* associated class II histocompatibility molecules are functionally important in the immune response was first shown in the mouse (Dorf and Benaceraf 1975; Dorf 1978). More recently, the *trans* association of HLA-DQ gene products has been directly demonstrated (Charron et al. 1984 and 1985; Giles et al. 1984; Giles and Capra 1985), though the enhanced autoantibody response found in pri-

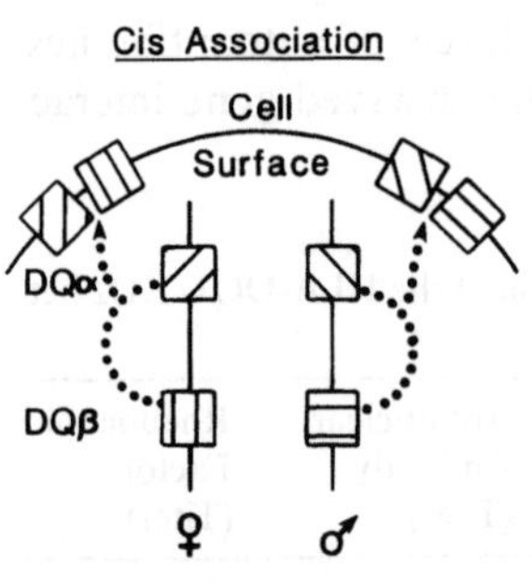

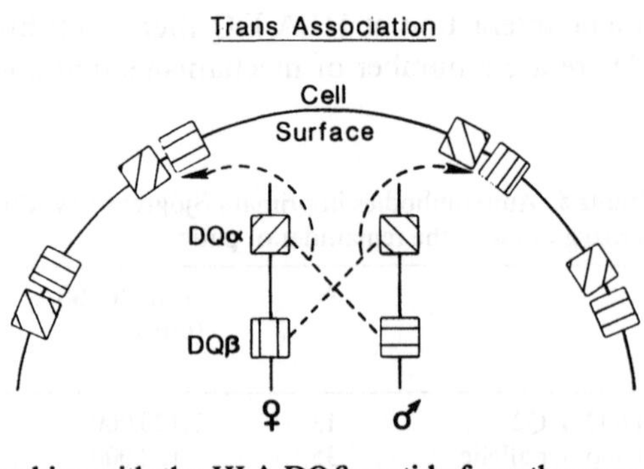

Fig. 2. (left) The HLA-DQα peptide may combine with the HLA-DQβ peptide from the same paternal chromosome by *cis* association to form a functional cell surface HLA-DQ molecule

Fig. 3. (right) The HLA-DQα peptide may combine with the HLA-DQβ peptide coded by the gene from the other paternal chromosome to form a *trans* associated cell surface molecule which are in addition to those surface molecules formed by *cis* association mary Sjögren's syndrome patients heterozygous for HLA-DQ1 and HLA-DQ2 may be the first known example of a consequence of this gene complementation in man.

There is an additional level of complexity at HLA-DQ. Good evidence has been obtained demonstrating the presence of two HLA-DQ α genes and two HLA-DQ β genes (Figuera and Klein 1986). If all four loci are commonly polymorphic then there are up to 16 possible combinations of gene products at HLA-DQ suggesting that the potential complexity of the immune response gene products at this locus is much greater than previously imagined.

Analysis of diseases related to primary Sjögren's syndrome for the importance of gene interaction at HLA-DQ is just beginning. In a preliminary analysis of secondary Sjögren's syndrome, no effect of gene interation at HLA-DQ upon the anti-Ro/SSA or other autoantibody response could be discerned (Harley et al. 1986b). In systemic lupus erythematosus, the anti-Ro/SSA response is also much greater in the HLA-DQ1 and HLA-DQ2 heterozygotes. Anti-La/SSB, on the other hand, is more closely related to the HLA-B8, DR3 haplotype and anti-nRNP(Sm) is greater in HLA-DR4 individuals (Harley et al. 1986c). Whether the differences in genetic composition or mechanisms of disease expression will explain the different HLA associations for the anti-La/SSB response must await further inquiry.

That genetic properties enhance the concentration of a collection of autoantibodies together is consistent with their arising in concert rather than independently of each other. It remains to be seen whether primary relationships can be established for autoantibodies and clinical or laboratory abnormalities. In systemic lupus erythematosus Hochberg and colleagues (1985) have shown that the patients with Ro(SS-A) and La(SS-B) precipitins tend to have HLA-DR3 and to be older while those with Ro(SS-A) alone tend to have HLA-DR2 and to be younger. It is probably important to realize that DR3 is in linkage disequilibrium with DQ2 while DR2 is associated with DQ1.

Special emphasis has been placed upon the relationship of Ro(SS-A) precipitins and vasculitis (Alexander et al. 1982, Molina et al. 1985). In addition to the close clinical association of anti-Ro(SS-A) with vasculitis (Alexander et al. 1982 and 1983), this group has found that the histologic character of the vasculitis varies in association with the Ro(SS-A) precipitin. Two patterns of vasculitis have been recognized - neutrophilic and mononuclear. The mononuclear vasculitis has less than five percent neutrophils and fibrinoid necrosis, lumen occlusion, or extravasation of erythrocytes. The neutrophilic inflammatory vascular disease has more than five percent neutrophils and is indistinguishable from leukocytoclastic vasculitis. These patients also tended to have hyperglobulinemia, antinuclear antibodies, and hypocomplementemia in addition to Ro(SS-A) precipitins (Molina et al. 1985).

Three lines of evidence are consistent with the hypothesis that anti-Ro(SS-A) may be involved in injury to the salivary gland in Sjögren's syndrome but no data support a direct role for anti-Ro(SS-A) or anti-LA(SS-B). Alexander and colleagues (1982) found that a history of parotid swelling was more likely in Ro(SS-A) precipitin positive patients. Penner and Reichlin (1982) were able to recover anti-Ro(SS-A) from the parotid gland of a patient with primary biliary cirrhosis and Sjögren's syndrome. Simultaneous attempts to elute other autoantibodies (anti-mitochondrial and anti-IgG) failed even though they were present in the patient's serum. A similar study was performed in the renal disease of systemic lupus erythematosus and specific enrichment of Ro-anti-Ro immune complexes was found (Maddison and Reichlin 1979). Finally, Miyachi and colleagues (1983) have shown that the presence of Ro(SS-A) precipitins in systemic lupus erythematosus, progressive systemic sclerosis and rheumatoid arthritis is associated with abnormal scialograms.

From his vantage point over a quarter of a century ago, Kurt Bloch and his colleagues (Bloch et al. 1960b) declared, "Sufficient evidence has not yet been collected to support the hypothesis - popular as it may be currently - that this disorder is an expression of autoimmunity." Our understanding has changed and become much more complicated but the mechanisms of pathogenesis and disease perpetuation in Sjögren's syndrome remain unknown. Though autoantibodies are clearly at least associated with extraglandular manifestations such as vasculitis, purpura, and leukopenia, there is less convincing evidence that they are directly involved in the destruction of the salivary and lacrimal glands. The most pressing issues for understanding Sjögren's syndrome which will await the studies of the coming quarter century are questions of etiology and detailed pathogenic processes. The roles that genetic factors and autoantibodies play in these answers will be most interesting.

Acknowledgments

The author appriciates the help and advice of his colleagues, especially of Dr. Morris Reichlin, and the organizations who have chosen to support this work including the Arthritis Foundation, the Veterans Administration, the National Institutes of Health (AM 34159), the Oklahoma Lupus Association, N.A.T.O. and the March of Dimes Birth Defects Foundation (5-507).

References

Alexander EL, Hirsch TJ, Arnett FC, Provost TT, Stevens MB (1982) Ro(SSA) and La(SSB) antibodies in the clinical spectrum of Sjögren's syndrome. J Rheumatol 9: 239-246

Alexander EL, Arnett FC, Provost TT, Stevens MB (1983) Sjögren's syndrome: Association of anti-Ro(SS-A) antibodies with vasculitis, hematologic abnormalities, and serologic hyperreactivity. Ann Intern Med 98: 155-159

Aiken JK (1932) Congenital heart block. Lancet ii: 1375-1379

Akizuki M, Boehm-Truitt MJ, Kassan SS, Steinberg AD, Chused TM (1977a) Purification of an acidic nuclear protein antigen and demonstration of its antibodies in subsets of patients with sicca syndrome. J Immunol 119: 932-938

Akizuki M, Powers R, Holman HR (1977b) A soluble acidic protein of the cell nucleus which reacts with serum from patients with systemic lupus erythematosus and Sjögren's syndrome. J Clin Invest 59: 264-272

Alspaugh M, Maddison PJ (1979) Resulution of the identity of certain antigen-antibody systems in systemic lupus erythematosus and Sjögren's syndrome: an interlaboratory collaboration. Arthritis Rheum 22: 796-798

Alspaugh MA, Tan EM (1975) Antibodies to cellular antigens in Sjögren's syndrome. J Clin Invest 55: 1067-1073

Anderson LG, Tarpley TM, Talal N, Cummings NA, Wolf RO, Schall GL (1973) Cellular-versus-humoral autoimmune responses to salivary gland in Sjögren's syndrome. Clin Exp Immunol 13: 335-342

Anderson JR, Gray KG, Beck JS, Kinnear WF (1961) Precipitating autoantibodies in Sjögren's disease. Lancet ii: 456-460

Aylward RD (1928) Congenital heart block. Br Med J i: 943

Bernstein RM, Bunn CC, Hughes GRV, Francoeur AM, Mathews MB (1984) Cellular protein and RNA antigens in autoimmune disease. Mol. Biol. Med. 2: 105-120
Bernstein RM, Hobbs RN, Lea DJ, Ward DJ, Hughes GRV (1985) Patterns of antihistone antibody specificity in systemic rheumatic disease. I. Systemic lupus erythematosus, mixed connective tissue disease, primary sicca syndrome, and rheumatoid arthritis with vasculitis. Arthritis Rheum 28: 285-293
Bertram U, Halberg P (1964) A specific antibody against the epithelium of the salivary ducts in sera from patients with Sjögren's syndrome. Acta Allerg (Kbh.) 19: 458-466
Biore G, Menard H-A (1985) Clinical significance of anti-SSA(Ro) in rheumatoid arthritis. Arthritis Rheum 28: S47
Bloch KJ, Bunim JJ, Wohl MJ, Zvaifler NJ (1960a) Unusual occurrence of multiple tissue component antibodies in Sjögren's syndrome. Trans Ass Amer Phys 73: 166-175
Bloch KJ, Wohl MJ, Ship II, Oglesby RB, Bunim JJ (1960b) Sjögren's syndrome. I. Serologic reactions in patients with Sjögren's syndrome with and without rheumatoid arthritis. Arthritis Rheum 3: 287-297
Bloch KJ, Buchanan WW, Wohl MJ, Bunim JJ (1965) Sjögren's syndrome. A clinical pathological, and serological study of sixty-two cases. Medicine (Baltimore) 44: 187-231
Bunim JJ (1961) Heberden oration. A broader spectrum of Sjögren's syndrome and its pathogenic implications. Ann Rheum Dis 20: 1-10
Bunim JJ, Buchanan WW, Wertlake PT, Sokolof L, Bloch KJ, Beck JS, Alepa FP (1964) Clinical staff conference. Clinical, pathologic and serologic studies in Sjögren's syndrome. Ann Intern Med 61: 509-530
Chambers JC, Keene JD (1985) Isolation and analysis of cDNA clones expressing human lupus La antigen. Proc Natl Acad Sci USA 82: 2115-2119
Clark GM, Reichlin M, Tomasi TB (1968) Characterization of soluble cytoplasmic antigen reactive with sera from patients with systemic lupus erythematosus. J Immunol 102: 117-122
Charron DJ, Lotteau V, Turmel P (1984) Hybrid HLA-DC antigens provide molecular evidence for gene complementation. Nature 305: 813-815
Charron DJ, Lotteau V, Turmel P (1985) Hybrid HLA-DC/DS antigens: Molecular evidence for gene trans-complementation. *In* "histocompatibility Testing 1984" (ED Albert, MP Baur, M Mayr, eds). Heidelberg: Springer Verlag. Deng JS, Takasaki Y, Tan EM (1981) Nonhistone nuclear antigens reactive with autoantibodies. Immunofluorescent studies of distribution in synchronized cells. J Cell Biol 91: 654-660
Deng JS, Santheimer RD, Gilliam JN (1985) Expression of Ro/SS-A antigen in human skin and heart. J Invest Derm 85: 412-416
Dorf ME (1978) Complementation of H-2-linked genes controlling immune responsiveness. Springer Semin. Immunopathol 1: 171-206
Dorf ME, Benacerraf B (1975) Complementation of the H-2 linked Ir genes in the mouse. Proc Natl Acad Sci USA 72: 3671-3075
Eisenberg RA (1985) Association of the Ro and La antigenic determinant. Immunodiffusion analysis of human spleen extract. J Immunol 135: 1707-1713
Feltkamp TEW, van Rossum AL (1983) Antibodies to salivary duct cells, and other autoantibodies, in patients with Sjögren's syndrome and other idiopathic autoimmune diseases. Clin Exp Immunol 3: 1-16
Figueroa F, Klein J (1986) The evaluation of MHC class II genes. Immunol Today 7; 78-81. Forman MS, Nakamura M, Mimori T, Gelpi C, Hardin JA (1985) Detection of antibodies to small nuclear ribonucleoproteins and small cytoplasmic ribonucleoproteins using unlabeled cell extracts. Arthritis Rheum 28: 1356-1361
Francoeur AM, Chan EKL, Garrels JI, Mathews MB (1985) Characterization and purification of lupus antigen La, an RNA binding protein. Molec Cellular Biol 5: 586-590
Gaither KK, Harley JB (1985) Affinity purification and immunoassay of anti-Ro/SSA. Protides Biol Fluids 33: 343-346
Giles RC, Capra JD (1985) Biochemistry of MHC class II molecules. Tissues Antigens 26: 57-68
Giles RC, DeMars RC, Chang C, Capra JD (1985) Allelic polymorphism and transassociation of molecules encoded by the HLA-DQ subregion. Proc Natl Acad Sci (USA) 82: 1776-1780
Graus F, Cordon-Cardo C, Bonfa E, Elkon KB (1985) Immunohistochemical localization of La nuclear antigen in brain. Selective concentration of the La protein in neuronal nucleoli. J Neuroimmunology 9: 307-319

Gumpel JM, Hobbs JR (1970) Serum immune globulins in Sjögren's syndrome. Ann Rheum Dis 29: 681-683

Halberg P, Bertram U, Soberg M, Nerup J (1965) Organ antibodies in disseminated lupus erythematosus. Acta Med Scand 178: 291-299

Habets WJ, den Brok JH, Boerbooms AMT, Van de Putte LBA, van Venrooij WJ (1983) Characterization of the SS-B(La) antigen in adenovirus-infected and uninfected HeLa cells. Europ J Mol Biol 2: 1625-1631

Harley JB (1985) Autoantibodies in Sjögren's syndrome: comparison of autoantibody determination methods show that antinuclear antibody and rheumatoid factor are associated with Ro/SSA precipitin formation. Protides Biol Fluids 33: 343-346

Harley JB, Yamagata H, Reichlin M (1984) Anti-La/SSB antibody is present in some normal sera and is coincident with anti-Ro/SSA precipitins in systemic lupus erythematosus. J Rheumatol 11: 309-314

Harley JB, Kaine JL, Fox OF, Reichlin M, Graber B (1985 a) Ro/SSA antibody and antigen in congenital complete heart block. Arthritis Rheum 28: 1321-1325

Harley JB, Rosario MO, Tamagata H, Fox OF, Koren E (1985 b) Immunologic and structural studies of the lupus/Sjögren's syndrome autoantigen, La/SSB, with a monoclonal antibody. J Clin Invest 76: 801-806

Harley JB, Alexander EL, Bias WB, Fox OF, Provost TT, Reichlin M, Yamagata M, Arnet FC (1986 a) Anti-Ro(SS-A) and anti-La(SS-B) in patients with Sjögren's syndrome. Arthritis Rheum 29: 196-206

Harley JB, Reichlin M, Arnett FC, Alexander EL, Bias WB, Provost TT (1986 b) Gene interaction at HLA-DQ enhances autoantibody production in primary Sjögren's syndrome. Science 232: 1145-1147

Harmon CE, Deng JS, Peebles CL, Tan EM (1984) The importance of tissue substrate in the SS-A/Ro antigen-antibody system. Arthritis Rheum 27: 166-172

Heaton JM (1959) Sjögren's syndrome and systemic lupus erythematosus. Brit Med J i: 466-469

Hendrick JP, Wolin S, Rinke J, Lerner MR, Steitz JA (1981) Ro small cytoplasmic ribonucleoproteins are a subclass of La ribonucleoproteins: further characterization of the Ro and La small ribonucleoproteins from uninfected mammalian cells. Mol Cell Biol 1: 1138-1149

Hochberg MC, Boyd RE, Ahearn JM, Arnett FC, Bias WB, Provost TT, Stevens MB (1985) Systemic lupus erythematosus: a review of clinico-laboratory features and immunogenetic markers in 150 patients with emphasis on dermatographic subsets. Medicine (Baltimore) 64: 285-295

Jelinek WR, Toomey TP, Leinwand L, Duncan CH, Biro PA, Chondary PV, Weissman SM, Rubin CM, Houck CM, Deininger PL, Schmidt CW (1980) Ubiquitous, interspersed repeated sequences in mammalian genomes. Proc Natl Acad Sci USA 77: 1398-1402

Jones BR (1958) Lacrimal and salivary precipitating antibodies. Lancet ii: 773-735

Jordan SC, Sakai R, Tabak MA, Ettenger RB, Cohen AH, Fine RN (1985) Induction of neonatal renal tubular dysfunction by transplacentally acquired IgG from a mother with Sjögren's syndrome. J Pediat 107: 566-569

Kato N, Hoshino H, Harada F (1982) Nucleotide sequence of 4.5s RNA (C8 or hY5) from HeLa cells. Biochem Biophys Res Commun 108: 363-370

Kephart D, Hood A, Provost TT. Neonatal lupus: serologic findings. J Invest Derm 77: 331-333

Kurilla MG, Keene JD (1983) The leader RNA of vesicular stomatitis virus is bound by a cellular protein reactive with anti-La lupus antibodies. Cell 34: 837-845

Kurki P, Helve T, Virtanen I (1983) Antibodies to cytoplasmic intermediate filaments in rheumatic diseases. J Rheumatol 10: 558-562

Lerner MR, Andrews NC, Miller G, Steitz JA (1981 a) Two small RNAs encoded by Epstein-Barr virus and complexed with protein are precipitated by antibodies from patients with systemic lupus erythematosus. Proc Natl Acad Sci USA 78: 805-809

Lerner MR, Boyle JA, Hardin JA, Steitz JA (1981 b) Two novel classes of small ribonucleoproteins detected by antibodies associated with lupus erythematosus. Science 211: 400-402

Litsky SE, Noonan JA, O'Connor WN, Cottrill CM, Mitchell B (1985) Maternal connective tissue disease and congenital heart block. Demonstration of immunoglobulin in cardiac tissue. N Engl J Med 312: 98-100

Lumpkin LR, Hall J, Hogan JD, Tucker SB, Jordan RE (1985) Neonatal lupus erythematosus: a report of three cases associated with anti-Ro/SSA antibodies. Arch Dermatol 121: 377-381

MacSween RNM, Goudie RB, Anderson JR, Armstrong E, Murray MA, Mason DK, Jasani MK, Boyle JA, Buchanan WW, Williamson J (1967) Occurence of antibody to salivary duct epithelium in Sjögren's disease, rheumatoid arthritis and other arthritides: a clinical and laboratory study. Ann Rheum Dis 26: 402-411

Maddison PJ, Reichlin M (1977) Quantitation of precipitating antibodies to certain soluble nuclear antigens in SLE: their contribution to hypergammaglobulinemia. Arthritis Rheum 20: 819-824

Maddison PJ, Provost TT, Reichlin M (1981) Serological findings in patients with "ANA-negative" systemic lupus erythematosus. Medicine (Baltimore) 60: 87-94

Maddison PJ, Reichlin M (1979) Deposition of antibodies to a soluble cytoplasmic antigen in the kidneys of patients with systemic lupus erythematosus. Arthritis Rheum 22: 858-863

Maddison PJ, Skinner RP, Vlachoyiannopoulos P, Brennand DM, Hough D (1985) Antibodies to nRNP, Sm, Ro(SSA), and La(SSB) detected by ELISA: their specificity in connective tissue disease sera. Clin Exp Immunol 62: 337-345

Madore SJ, Wieben ED, Pederson T (1984) Eukaryotic small ribonucleoproteins: anti-La human autoantibodies react with U1 RNA-protein complexes. J Biol Chem 259: 1929-1933

Mamula M, Fox OF, Harley JB (1985) Cross-reactivity of Ro/SSA and immunoglobulin G. Arthritis Rheum 28: S37

Mathews MB, Francoeur AM (1982) Interaction between VA RNA and the lupus antigen La: formation of a ribonucleoprotein *in vitro*. Proc Natl Acad Sci USA 79: 6772-6776

Mattioli M, Reichlin M (1974) Heterogenity of RNA protein antigens reactive with sera of patients with systemic lupus erythematosus. Arthritis Rheum 17: 421-429

Miyachi K, Naito M, Maeno Y, Suzuki S, Hamamoto T, Sugiura M, Kasahava M, Torikai K, Umeda H (1983) Sialographic study in patients with and without antibodies to Sjögren's syndrome A (Ro). J Rheumatol 10: 387-394

Miyagawa S, Kitamura W, Yoshioka J, Sakamoto K (1981) Placental transfer of anticytoplasmic antibodies in annular crythema of newborns. Arch Dermatol 117: 569-572

Molina R, Provost TT, Alexander EL (1985) Two types of inflammatory vascular disease in Sjögren's syndrome. Differential association with seroreactivity to rheumatoid factor and antibodies to Ro(SS-A) and with hypocomplemantemia. Arthritis Rheum 28: 1251-1258

Moore CL, Sharp PA (1984) Site-specific polyadenylation in a cell-free reaction. Cell 36: 581-591

Moutsopoulos HM, Skopouli FN, Sarras AK, Tsampoulos C, Mauridis AK, Constantopoulos SH, Maddison PJ (1985) Anti-Ro(SS-A) positive rheumatoid arthritis (RA): a clinico serological group of patients with high incidence of D-penicillamine side effects. Ann Rheum Dis 44: 215-219

Mumford P, Room GRW, Venables PJW, Maini RN (1985) IgG antibodies to SS-B(La), RNP/Sm and DNA are produced by PWM-stimulated normal human lymphocytes in culture. Rheumatol Int 5: 109-112

Ouarma TB, Krueger JA, Holman HR (1982) Analysis of speckled fluorescent antinuclear antibody test antisera using electrofocused nuclear antigens. J Clin Invest 70: 296-303

Penner E, Reichlin M (1982) Primary biliary cirrhosis associated with Sjögren's syndrome: evidence for circulating and tissue deposited Ro/anti-Ro immune complexes. Arthritis Rheum 25: 1250-1253

Pizer L, Deng JS, Sternberg R, Tan EM (1983) Characterization of a phosphoprotein associated with the SS-B/La nuclear antigen in adenovirus-infected and uninfected KB cells. Mol Cell Biol 7: 1235-1245

Provost TT (1983) Neonatal lupus. Arch Dermatol 119: 619-622

Provost TT, Arnett FC, Reichlin M (1983) Homozygous C2 Deficiency, lupus erythematosus, and anti-Ro(SS-A) antibodies. Arthritis Rheum 26: 1279-1282

Reichlin M (1979) Newly defined serologic systems in systemic lupus erythematosus and dermatomyositis. Inter J Derm 18: 602-607

Reinke J, Steitz JA (1982) Precursor molecules of both human 5S ribosomal RNA and transfer RNAs are bound by a cellular protein reactive with anti-La lupus antibodies. Cell 29: 149-159

Reddy R, Henning P, Tan EM, Busch H (1983) Identification of a La protein binding site in a RNA polymerase III transcript (4.51 RNA). J Biol Chem 258: 8352-8356

Rosa MD, Gottlieb E, Lerner MR, Steitz JA (1981) Striking similarities are exhibited by two small Epstein-Barr virus-encloded ribonucleic acids and the adenovirus-associated ribonucleic acids VAI and VAII. Molec Cell Biol 1: 785-796

Santheimer RD, Maddison PJ, Reichlin M, Jordon RE, Stasny P, Gillam JM (1982) Serologic and

HLA associations in subacute cutaneous lupus erythematosus, a clinical subset of lupus erythematosus. Ann Intern Med 97: 664-671

Scopelitis E, Biundo JJ (1984) Inconsistent staining of HEp-2 cells with anti-SS-A antibody. Arthritis Rheum 27: 1318-1320

Scott JS, Maddison PJ, Taylor PV, Esscher E, Scott O, Skinner RP (1982) Connective-tissue disease, antibodies to ribonucleoprotein and congenital heart block. N Engl J Med 309: 209-212

Stefano JE (1984) Purified lupus antigen La recognizes an oligouridylate stretch common to the 3′ termini of RNA polymerase III transcripts. Cell 36: 145-154

Teppo A-M (1981) Enzyme immunoassay of antibodies to Sjögren's syndrome B antigen. Clin Chem 27: 1341-1345

Venables PJW, Charles PJ, Buchanan RRC, Fi T, Munford PA, Schrieber L, Room GRW, Maini RN (1983 a) Quantitation and detection of isotypes of anti-SS-B antibodies by ELISA and Farr assays sing affinity purified antigens: an approach to the investigation of Sjögren's syndrome and sytemic lupus erythematosus. Arthritis Rheum 26: 146-155

Venables PJW, Smith PR, Maini RN (1983 b) Purification and characterization of the Sjögren's syndrome A and B antigens. Clin Exp Immunol 54: 731-738

Virji MA (1985) Circulating prostatic acid phosphatase-immunoglobulin complexes in Sjögren's syndrome. Clin Chem Acta 151: 223-230

Weissmann G (1958) Sjögren's syndrome. Review of the literature and report of a case with achalasia of the esophagus. Am J Med 24: 475-481

Wermuth DJ, Goeghegan WD, Jordan RE (1985) Anti-Ro/SSA antibodies. Association with a particulate (large speckled like thread) immunofluorescent nuclear staining pattern. Arch Dermatol 121: 335-338

Whaley K, Chisholm DM, Goudie RB, Downie WW, Dizk WC, Boyle JA, Williamson J (1969) Salivary duct autoantibody in Sjögren's syndrome: correlation with focal sialadenitis in the labial mucosa. Clin Exp Immunol 4: 273-282

Whaley K, Webb J, McAvoy BA, Hughes GRV, Lee P, MacSween RNM, Buchanan WW (1973) Sjögren's syndrome. 2. Clinical associations and immunological phonomena. Quart J Med (New series) 17: 513-548

Whittingham S, McNeilage J, MacKay IR (1985) Primary Sjögren's syndrome after infectious mononucleosis. Ann Intern Med 102: 490-493

Wolin SL, Steitz JA (1983) Genes for two small cytoplasmic Ro RNAs are adjacent and appear to be single copy in the human genome. Cell 32: 735-744

Wolin SL, Steitz JA (1984 a) The Ro small cytoplasmic ribonucleoproteins: identification of the antigenic protein and its binding on the Ro RNAs. Proc Natl Acad Sic USA 81: 1996-2000

Wolin SL, Steitz JA (1984 b) The Ro small cytoplasmic ribonucleoprotein particle: structures and clues to the pathogenesis of congenital heart block. Clin Res 32: 470 A

Yamagata H, Harley JB, Reichlin M (1984) Molecular properties of the Ro/SSA antigen and ELISA for quantification of antibody. J Clin Invest 74: 625-633

3. Immunogenetics of Sjögren's Syndrome

D. L. Mann

Introduction

Probably every disease known to be present in man has been examined in the context of expression of alleles of the human major histocompatability complex (MHC). This gene complex, located on chromosome 6, controls the expression of cell surface glycoproteins which have antigenic determinants that can be identified by serologic (HLA typing) and cellular tests (mixed lymphocyte reactions) in the laboratory. Recognizing the high degree of polymorphism of the histocompatability antigens, investigators reasoned that the polymorphism may be disease related. The diseases which have shown the highest frequency of association with MHC antigens are the autoimmune diseases.

In retrospect, this may seem logical in that it is now known that certain gene products of the MHC play a significant (if not absolute) role in the control of the immune response (Schwartz and Shreffler 1980). In addition to providing evidence for an association of MHC alleles with a particular disease, the use of HLA typing allows identification in some instances of genetic markers for susceptibility to particular diseases [such as congenital adrenal hyperplasia (Chrousos et al. 1982)] by virtue of linkage with other genes on chromosome 6.

Sjögren's syndrome was one of the first autoimmune diseases where it was demonstrated that certain of the HLA antigens were present in higher frequency in the diseased population compared to the frequency of the antigen in nondiseased individuals (Chused et al. 1977; Fye et al. 1978). This association was identified prior to a complete understanding of the gene complex that controls the expression of the HLA antigens, particularly the portion that controls expression of what is now known as the DR region.

In order to better understand and interpret the results of analysis of HLA frequencies and the genetic and immunologic implications of this association, a brief explanation and description of the MHC and its products is in order.

The Human Major Histocompatability Gene Complex

Over twenty years ago, a number of investigators recognized the presence of lymphocyte cell surface antigenic determinants that had the genetic characteristics of allelic expression. It was soon recognized that these antigenic determinants were similar in many respects to the histocompatibility antigens which had been described in mice. The human histocompatibility antigens were then found to be controlled by several loci which were located on the short arm of the sixth chromosome. Antigens first identified were part of what is now known as the HLA-A, B and C antigens and designated as a group as Class I antigens. A series of international workshops resulted in the development of antisera, which identifies the alleles of the Class I products. These products have a molecular weight of 44,000 kilodaltons and are associated in the cell membrane with B-2 microglobulin.

The definition of multiple alleles at each locus raised the question as to the biologic function of these molecules. Extensive studies in mice and studies in man demonstrated that these determinants were histocompatability antigens. However, transplantation is a surgical exercise and not a normal biologic event. It was predicted that these determinants might play some role in protection or susceptibility to diseases. As investigators were developing reagents to serologically detect the alleles of the Class I antigens, it was found that individuals could be phenotyped by observing the blastogenic response of their lymphocytes to lymphocytes from another individual in a one-way mixed lymphocyte reaction (Bradley and Festenstein 1978). These reactions were found to be independent of, but linked to, the HLA Class I determinants. These observations led to the identification of what is now known as the HLA-D determinants that are defined by mixed lymphocyte reactions. In the process of investigating the reaction to human sera to T and B lymphocytes, we found that certain antibodies reacted selectively against B cell and not against T cell from the same individual (Mann, Abelson, Harris and Amos 1979). These antisera were subsequently found to recognize determinants which were carried on B cells, monocytes, and activated T cells. These antisera defined a product of the major histocompatibility complex which became known as the HLA-DR antigens (Mann, Abelson, Henkart, Harris and Amos 1975). These antigens were originally thought to be controlled by a single locus. However, using immunoprecipitation techniques we (Mann et al. 1979), as well as others, found that the HLA-DR antigens are carried on molecules of 34,000-29,000 dalton molecular weight and are controlled by more than one locus in the major histocompatibility complex (Shackelford et al. 1981; Karr et al. 1982). The second locus controlling the expression of serologically detectable determinants is now known as DQ. Subsequent to this, a new locus or region was identified using mixed lymphocyte response (Shaw et al. 1980) and found to map distinct from the DR and DQ. This locus has been given the designation of DP. Thus, the three distinct gene regions of the HLA-D region are known as DQ, DR and DP. Each region has 1-2 alpha genes encoding for the 34,000 molecular weight glycoprotein and at least 4 beta genes encoding for a 29,000 molecular weight glycoprotein. The entire composition of the DR region is now being elucidated with DNA sequence analysis.

HLA Association with Sjögren's Syndrome

The early reports of HLA association with Sjögren's syndrome demonstrated an increased frequency of the serologically defined HLA-B8 antigen and the DW3 determinant (defined by mixed lymphocyte reaction) (Fye et al. 1978; Manthorpe et al. 1981) in individuals with this desease. These same antigens were also found in increased frequency in several other diseases which were thought to have an autoimmune pathogenesis (Chused et al. 1978). With the capability of seriologically detecting the different alleles of the HLA-DR region, studies were performed to compare the frequency of expression of certain HLA-DR antigens in primary and secondary Sjögren's syndrome (Moutsopoulos et al. 1979; Moutsopoulos et al. 1980). As discussed in other sections of this book, secondary Sjögren's syndrome is distinguished from primary Sjögren's syndrome in that the former is associated with other autoimmune diseases. In our initial studies, we found and reported that HLA-DRW3, the serologically defined antigen (which is now known as HLA-DR3), was significantly increased in frequency in the patient population with primary Sjögren's syndrome, compared to the frequency of this antigen in the normal population (Moutsopoulos et al. 1978). It is well recognized that the B8, DR3 antigens are in linkage disequalibrium which most probably accounts for the original HLA-B8 association with the disease. The increased frequency of the DW3 allele, determined by mixed lymphocyte reactions, in patients with Sjögren's syndrome is a reflection of an association between the DW3 and the serologically defined DR3 antigen. In addition to the observation that the DR3 allele was increased in frequency in this disease, we also observed that there were other antisera (which reacted with specific B lymphocyte antigens) reacting with increased frequency compared to of reaction frequencies in the normal population. These sera appeared to be detecting either a supertypic determinant on the molecule bearing HLA-DR3 or a determinant controlled by other genes. These sera did not react with patterns that were consistent with the definition of the DR antigen (Mann et al. 1979). This was particularly true in Sjögren's syndrome. These alloantisera were subsequently found to define a determinant on molecules distinct from DR bearing molecules (Karr et al. 1982) which was called MT2 which has been renamed and is now called DRW52.

The results of studies demonstrating an increased frequency of the HLA-B8, DR3, DW52 antigens in patients with primary Sjögren's syndrome compared to the frequency of these antigens in the normal population is shown in Table 1. This table also shows the frequency of DR4 and DQW1 in the patient population with primary Sjögren's syndrome. The frequency of the DR4 antigen was decreased compared to the frequency of this antigen in the normal population. Other HLA-DR antigens appeared with essentially the same frequencies in patient and normal populations. Another antigen which appears to play some role in Sjögren's syndrome is

Table 1. HLA alloantigens that differ in frequency in primary Sjögren's syndrome compared to the normal population

HLA alloantigens	% in Normal N=293	% in primary Sjögren's Syndrome N=27	P-value
B8	19	59	0.01
DR3	23	66	0.01
DR4	27	11	NS
DRW52	53	81	0.05
DQW1	55	68	NS

DQW1, originally defined by an alloantisera (Ia-715) which reacts with molecules which are products of genes distinct from HLA-DR (Shackelford et al. 1981). The relevance of this particular determinant to primary Sjögren's syndrome will be discussed when considering the results of the family studies.

We also found that there were differences in antigen frequencies comparing patients with primary Sjögren's syndrome and patients with secondary Sjögren's syndrome, the latter individuals with clinical manifestations of other autoimmune diseases. These differences were an increased frequency of HLA-DR4 in patients with secondary Sjögren's syndrome. The HLA-DRW52 antigen was also found to be increased in frequency in patients with secondary Sjögren's syndrome. A summary and comparison of altered HLA-DR antigen frequencies in primary and secondary Sjögren's syndrome is presented in Table 2. The comparisons that are considered are antigen frequencies found in patients with Sjögren's syndrome with Raynaud's phenomenon (SSRP) and patients with Sjögren's syndrome with rheumatoid arthritis (SSRA). HLA-DR3 is increased in frequency in both primary Sjögren's syndrome (SS), and SSRP, and decreased in frequency in patients with SSRA. In contrast, DR4 was increased in frequency in patients with SSRP and SSRA compared to the frequency of this antigen in patients with SS. The DRW52 determinant or MT2 determinant, was increased in frequency in all patients with Sjögren's syndrome, primary or secondary. DQW1 was increased in frequency in patients with SS compared to the patients with SSRA. There was an intermediate frequency in patients who had SSRP. These results indicated quite clearly that Sjögren's syndrome presenting with other diseases, have frequencies of both HLA-DR3 and HLA-DR4 which appear to associate with a particular disease. The common determinant, which is increased frequencies in all of the patients, is DRW52. The DQ1 specificity is elevated in frequency only in the patients with primary Sjögren's syndrome compared to the patients with rheumatoid arthritis and probably represents a negative association with this secondary disease.

In another study, Wilson et al. (1984) examined HLA antigen frequencies in patients with primary Sjögren's syndrome, Sjögren's syndrome with rheumatoid arthritis, Sjögren's syndrome with systemic lupus erythematosus, and a group of individuals with nonspecified connective tissue diseases which are associated with

Table 2. Comparison of HLA-DR alloantigens that differ in frequencies in primary Sjögren's syndrome (SS) and secondary Sjögren's syndrome in patients with Raynaud's phenomenon (SSRP) and rheumatoid arthritis (SSRA)

HLA-DR alloantigen	% SS (N=27)[a]	% SSRP (N=15)[a]	% SSRA (N=12)[a]
DR3	66	80[b]	8
DR4	11	73[c]	66[c]
DRW52	81	93	92
DQW1	68[d]	46	8

[a] Number in each group.
[b] Significant increase compared to SSRA ($p < 0.001$)
[c] Significant increase compared to SS ($p < 0.008$)
[d] Significant increase compared to SSRA ($p < 0.003$)

Sjögren's syndrome. These results essentially confirmed the results which we had previously reported on patients with primary Sjögren's syndrome and secondary Sjögren's syndrome. Fifty percent of the patients with primary Sjögren's syndrome had DR3 and this antigen was found in 13% of the patients with Sjögren's syndrome and rheumatoid arthritis. The frequency of HLA-DR3 in patients with systemic lupus erythematosus and Sjögren's syndrome was approximately that found in the normal population (25%). Eighty percent of the patients with connective tissue disease and Sjögren's syndrome had the DR3 determinant. A striking increase in frequency in the MT2 or DRW52 determinant was found in all of the patients with Sjögren's syndrome with either the primary or secondary disease. These investigators further compared the association of HLA antigens with two antibodies found in sera in patients with Sjögren's syndrome that are directed against two antigenic determinants on ribonucleic acids called SS-A and SS-B. The individuals who had developed antibodies against SS-A and SS-B appeared to have a higher frequency of HLA-DR3 than those individuals who did not have antibodies to this ribonucleic acid antigen. However, there was also an increased frequency of HLA-DR2 in those individuals who were DR3 negative who developed antibodies to SS-B but not SS-A. These results indicated that the development of antibodies to ribonucleic acids were associated with the DR allotypic determinants in diseased individuals.

We have had the opportunity to study three families with Sjögren's syndrome occuring in more than 1 member of the family (Mann and Moutsopoulus 1983). The results of HLA typing individuals in these families revealed the same associations that were found when examining HLA alloantigen frequencies in the populations of individuals with primary Sjögren's syndrome. These results are summarized in Fig. 1. In Family 1, the affected individuals were a mother and a daughter. In this family, the C haplotype from the mother was inherited by the affected daughter. The A haplotype was inherited from the father. These two haplotypes carry the DR2, DQW1, and DRW6, DRW52 and DQW1, respectively. The D haplotype in the mother was also DQW1. One disease free sibling shared these same antigens on a different haplotype (B) with the affected individual. A similar combination of HLA-DR antigens was found in Family 2. In this family, three out of six members had primary Sjögren's syndrome and one individual had Sjögren's syndrome with rheumatoid arthritis. All individuals affected with the primary disease inherited the A and D haplotypes from the parents. The individual with the secondary disease inherited the AC haplotypes. The A haplotype carried the DR3, DRW52 antigens, and the D haplotype, DR1, DQW1. The individual with secondary Sjögren's syndrome inherited the C haplotype which expressed the HLA-DR4 antigen. In Family 3, a mother and daughter were affected. In this family, the C haplotype was inherited by the affected offspring from the mother. This C haplotype carried the DRW6, DRW52, DQW1 antigens. In these families, it appears that combinations of antigens defining distinct haplotypes were unique in the individuals who had the disease. All the individuals who had primary Sjögren's syndrome carried a combination of the DQ1 and DRW52 antigens. With one exception, disease-free family members typed for one another of these antigens, however, the combination was absent. In the one individual who had Sjögren's syndrome with rheumatoid arthritis, the DR4 antigen appeared, again similar to that observed in population studies.

Sjogren's Syndrome Family 1

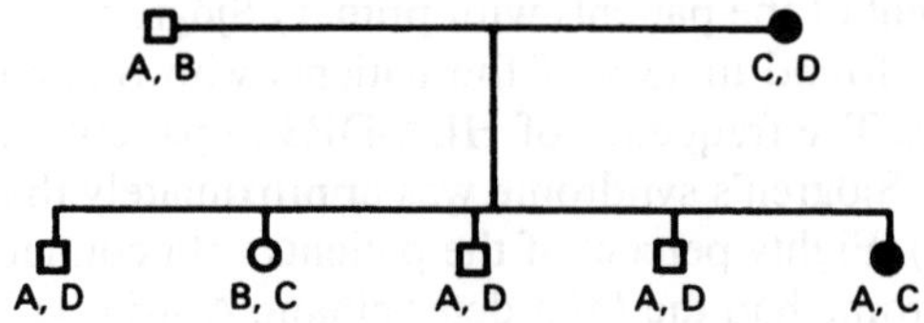

A. HLA A2	B44	Cw4	DR2	DQW1	
B. HLA A2	B40	Cw1	DR2	DQW1	● Primary S.S.
C. HLA A3	B7	Cw-	DRw6	DRW52 DQW1	
D. HLA A1	B17	Cw-	DR7	DQW1	

Sjogren's Syndrome Family 2

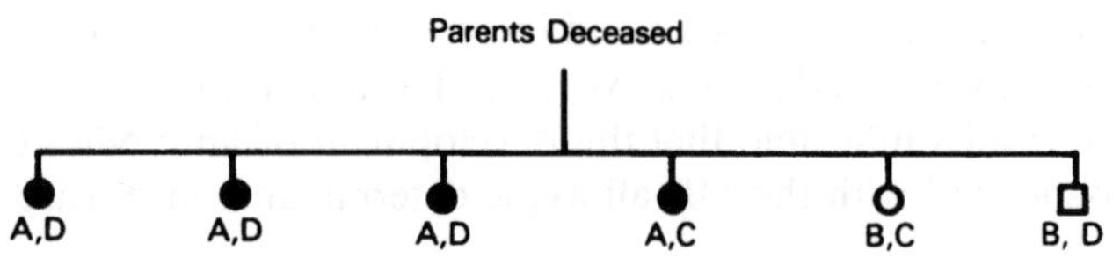

A. HLA A1	B8	Cw3	DR3	DRW52	● Primary S.S.
B. HLA A3	B18	-	DR2	DQW1	
C. HLA 2	B40	Cw6	DR4	-	● Secondary S.S.
D. HLA A11	B19	-	DR1	DQW1	

Sjogren's Syndrome Family 3

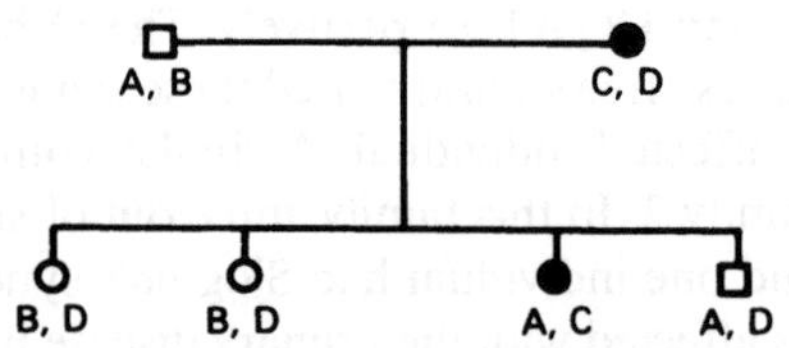

A. HLA A1	B8	Cw3	DR3	DRW52	● Primary S.S.
B. HLA A22	B8	Cw1	DR3	DRW52	
C. HLA A23	Bw38	-	DRw6	DRW52 DQW1	
D. HLA Aw34	B27	-	DR1	DRW52	

Fig. 1. Results of HLA typing of 3 families with more than one member with primary or secondary Sjögren's syndrome

Conclusion and Projections

To summarize the results of the studies, it appears that certain major histocompatability complex genes play a contributing role in the susceptibility of an individual to develop Sjögren's syndrome, be it the primary disease or Sjögren's syndrome associated with other autoimmune disorders.

It is quite clear that the HLA-DR52 antigen has a high frequency in all patients with Sjögren's syndrome whether or not they present with the primary disease or other associated diseases which are thought to be immunologic in origin. Our results demonstrated this to be true in individuals with primary Sjögren's syndrome, Sjögren's syndrome with Raynaud's phenomenon, as well as individuals with Sjögren's syndrome and rheumatoid arthritis. The studies of Wilson et al. (1984) have also demonstrated that HLA-DRW52 is elevated in frequency in individuals with the above mentioned diseases as well as in individuals with Sjögren's syndrome and other connective tissue disorders. In the discussion of the genetic implications or reasons for elevations of this antigen, Wilson et al. (1984) suggested that the gene(s) for this determinant were in the region that is now known as DQ. Recent evidence clearly indicates that this antigen is expressed or found on products that are encoded for by DR $\alpha 1$, $\beta 2$ genes. HLA-DR 3, which is found to have a high association with the primary Sjögren's syndrome and to a lesser extent, association with other diseases of which Sjögren's syndrome is a component, is also a product of the DR region being encoded for by the $\alpha 2$, $\beta 2$ genes. In contrast, HLA-DQW1 is encoded for by the DQ locus and specifically by the $\alpha 2$, $\beta 2$ genes. The results of our studies as cited as well as those of Wilson's, strongly indicate that the combination of expression of genes in the DR locus appear to be contributing to the development of this disease. In addition, our results suggest that the HLA-DQ locus may also confer a susceptibility factor in the development of Sjögren's syndrome.

Thus, the results of the HLA-typing studies in populations of individuals with primary as well as secondary Sjögren's syndrome, as well as the family studies indicate that the major histocompatability complex is a genetic marker for these diseases. Furthermore, it is also quite clear that these genes are not markers exclusively for primary and secondary Sjögren's syndrome as the frequency of HLA-DRW52 is approximately 55% in the North American Caucasian population. Certainly, the frequency of the diseases, which we are discussing are orders of magnitude less. It would seem likely that these genes and/or their products play a contributory role rather than a primary role in the development of this disease.

The role of HLA antigens in the immune response has been elicidated in part. It is quite clear, from a variety of studies, that these determinants act as restriction elements in communication between antigen-presenting cells, B and T lymphocytes. In mice, IA molecules (homologs of HLA-DR), clearly control the animal's ability to respond to defined antigens. In man, direct demonstration of response and nonresponse to individual antigenic determinants has not been directly demonstrated which may be due in part to the complexity of the HLA-DR region. This is pointed out in studies on the human response to pork and beef insulin where the former differs from human insulin by a single amino acid (Kahn et al. 1983). The results of these studies demonstrated an association of the immune response to insulin antigens and HLA-DR antigen which was relative and not absolute (Mann et al. 1983). It seems likely that in diseases such as Sjögren's syndrome or in other autoimmune diseases, combinations of HLA-DR antigens provide the immunological environment for the response which results in the disease process. One possibility is that this response is an autoimmune reaction to certain target organs where alteration of the cell surface structures occur as a result of viral infections. In Sjögren's syndrome, glandular tissue may become the target for this autoimmune response. At the level of antigen recognition, one role the HLA-DR molecules might play is that certain combinations of individual genes when expressed, make recognition of a particular antigenic determinant much more likely which in turn results in an autoimmune reaction. Another possibility is that HLA-DR genetic polymorphisms occur at a level not recognized by serologic analysis. This polymorphism, functioning at a molecular level, results in a substantial alteration in the immune response such that autoimmune reactions occur. This latter hypothesis is testable using available HLA-D region molecular probes.

Many of the individuals with a variety of autoimmune diseases have antibodies to nucleic acids. The association of the HLA-DR phenotype with the ability to develop antibodies detecting certain specific antigenic determinants on nucleic acids was demonstrated by Wilson et al. (1984). It is likely that such antibodies develop as the result of the breakdown of cells targeted for destruction rather than being pathogenic in and of themselves. This conclusion is, however, not based on experimental evidence.

There is some evidence that the HLA-DQ region effects development of suppressor cell function. In certain instances, lack of suppression may effect B-cell proliferation. Polyclonal B-cell activation is frequent in patients with Sjögren's syndrome. It is possible that specific genes of the MHC DR region control or regulate this activiation and that these gene products identified as HLA-DQW1 play a role in this regulatory process. Activated B cells are often found in the salivary glands of patients with active disease and may be participating in the autoimmune destruction of these tissue. This polyclonal B-cell activation is most probably the precursor of the malignant transformation of B cells which progress to the lymphomas that are seen frequently in patients with Sjögren's syndrome. We have recently found that a variety of oncogenes that are found in B-cell tumors are activated in B cells from patients with autoimmune diseases (Boumpas, Mark, Mann, unpublished observations). One of these oncogenes has related DNA sequences that map to the X chromosome (G. Mark, personal communication). Since Sjögren's syndrome is primarily a disease of females, we might speculate that a gene(s) on the X chromosome has some regulatory role in development of this autoimmune disease.

In order to solve the puzzles of this disease we will need to identify an etiologic agent which effects cells of the target glands and causes an autoimmune reaction to these cells. This autoimmune reaction may be found only in individuals with specific MHC class II molecules which occur together with abnormalities of regulatory genes found on another chromosome.

References

Bradley BA, Festenstein H (1978) Cellular typing. Br Med Bull 34: 223–233

Chrousos GP, Loriaux LD, Mann D, Cutler GB (1982) Late onset of 21-hydroxylase deficiency in an allelic variant of congenital adrenal hyperplasia characterized by attenuated clinical expression and different HLA haplotype association. Horm Res 16: 193–200

Chused TM, Kassan SS, Opelz G, Moustsopoulos HM, Terasaki PI (1977) Sjögren's syndrome associated with HLA-DW3. N Engl J Med 296: 895–897

Fye KH, Terasaki PI, Michalski JP, Daniels TE, Opelz G, Talal N (1978) Relationship of HLA-DW3 and HLA-B8 to Sjögren's syndrome. Arthritis Rheum 21: 337–342

Kahn CR, Mann D, Rosenthal AS, Galloway JA, Johnson AH, Mendell N (1983) The immune response to insulin in man: interaction of HLA alloantigens and the development of the immune response. Diabetes 31: 716-723

Karr RW, Kannapell CC, Stein JA, Gebel HM, Mann DL, Duquesnoy RJ, Fuller TC, Rodey GE, Schwartz BD (1982) Molecular relationships of the human B cell alloantigens MT2, MB3, MT4 and DR5. J Immunol 128: 1809-1818

Mann DL, Abelson L, Harris S, Amos DB (1975) Detection of antigens specific for "B" lymphoid cultured cell lines with human alloantisera. J Exp Med 142: 84-89

Mann DL, Abelson L, Henkart P, Harris SD, Amos DB (1975) Specific human B lymphocyte alloantigens (L-B) linked to HL-A. Proc Natl Acad Sci USA 72: 5103-5106

Mann DL, Kaufman J, Orr H, Robb R, Strominger J (1979) Serologic and structural studies of DR related antigens. Transplant Proc Vol XI: 668-673

Mann DL, Mendell N, Kahn CR, Johnson AH, Rosenthal A (1983) In vitro lymphocyte proliferation response to therapeutic insulin components: evidence for genetic control by the human major histocompatability complex. J Clin Invest 72: 1130-1138

Mann DL, Moutsopoulos HM (1983) HLA-DR alloantigens in different subsets of patients with Sjögren's syndrome and in family members. Ann Rheum Dis 42: 533-536

Manthrope R, Morling N, Platz P, Ryder LP, Svejgaard A, Thomsen M (1981) HLA-D antigen frequencies in Sjögren's syndrome: differences between primary and secondary forms. Scand J Rheumatol 10: 124-128

Moutsopoulos HM, Chused TM, Johnson AH, Knudsen B, Mann DL (1978) B lymphocyte alloantigens in sicca syndrome. Science 199: 1441-1442

Moutsopoulos HM, Mann DL, Johnson AH, Chused TM (1979) Genetic differences between primary and secondary sicca syndrome. N Engl J Med 301: 761-763

Moutsopoulos HM, Chused TM, Mann DL, Klippel JH, Fauci AS, Frank MM, Lawley TJ, Hamberger MI (1980) Sjögren's syndrome (Sicca syndrome): Current issues. Ann Intern Med 92: 212-226

Schwartz BD, Shreffler DC (1980) Genetic influence on the immune response. In: Parker CW (ed) Clinical Immunology. WB Saunders Co, Philadelphia, pp 49-85

Shackelford DA, Mann DL, van Rood JJ, Ferrara GB, Strominger JL (1981) Human B cell alloantigens DC1, MT1 and LB12 are identical to each other but distinct from the HLA-DR antigen. Proc Natl Acad Sci USA 78: 4566-4570

Shaw S, Pollack MS, Payne SM, Johnson AH (1980) HLA-linked B-cell alloantigens of a new segregant series: population and family studies of the SM antigens, Hum Immunol 1: 177-183

Wilson RW, Provost TT, Bias WB, Alexander L, Edrow DW, Hochberg MC, Stevens MB, Arnett FC (1984) Sjögren's syndrome: influence of multiple HLA-D region alloantigens on clinical and serological expression. Arthritis Rheum 27: 1245-1253

4. The Relationship Between Anti-RO (SS-A) Precipitin Antibody Positive Sjögren's Syndrome and Anti-RO (SS-A) Precipitin Antibody Positive Lupus Erythematosus*

T. T. PROVOST, E. L. ALEXANDER, and M. REICHLIN

Introduction

The relationship between Sjögren's syndrome and various connective tissue diseases has intrigued clinicians for several decades. During the past decade, our extensive clinical laboratory studies of the anti-Ro (SS-A) and anti-La (SS-B) precipitin antibodies have suggested a close relationship between anti-Ro (SS-A) precipitin positive lupus erythematosus and anti-Ro (SS-A) precipitin positive Sjögren's syndrome. These studies indicate that these two anti-Ro (SS-A) precipitin positive disorders are much more closely related immunopathologically than our current nosology would indicate. We postulate that high titered Ro (SS-A) antibody patients (as measured by gel double diffusion) and designated in this chapter as anti-Ro (SS-A) precipitin antibody positive Sjögren's syndrome and anti-Ro (SS-A) precipitin antibody positive SLE patients may share similar, if not identical immunogenetic backgrounds, most likely in the D region of the major histocompatibility complex and that this similar immunogenetic background is probably responsible, at least in part, for the close relationship of these two entities.

Clinical Associations

During our initial studies on the clinical specificities of the anti-Ro (SS-A) and anti-La (SS-B) precipitin antibodies, we first became aware of an association between anti-Ro (SS-A) precipitin antibody positive lupus erythematosus and Sjögren's syndrome (Maddison et al. 1978). Our initial studies comparing the clinical features of anti-Ro (SS-A) precipitin antibody positive lupus patients with anti nRNP positive and precipitin antibody [Sm, nRNP, Ro (SS-A) and La (SS-B)] negative systemic lupus erythematosus patients indicated that Sjögren's syndrome, photosensitivity and lupus skin disease may be more common in anti-Ro (SS-A) precipitin antibody positive lupus patients (Table 1). A similar association was also found when we examined a group of 41 ANA negative, anti-Ro (SS-A) precipitin antibody positive lupus patients (Maddison et al. 1981). In this study, we detected that 4 (10%) of these ANA negative (mouse liver substrate), anti-Ro (SS-A) precipitin antibody positive lupus patients also had historical and clinical features of Sjögren's syn-

* This work was supported by U.S. Public Health Service grants HL34723, RO1 AM25650, AO970101, and AO991905 from the National Institutes of Health and a grant from the Kroc Foundation.

Table 1. Clinical features in systemic lupus patients with anti-Ro (SS-A), anti-nRNP and no precipitating antibodies (Maddison et al. 1978)

Clinical feature	Ro n=38	NRNP n=30	No precipitating AB n=26
Lupus dermatitis	32 (84%)	16 (53%)	18 (69%)
Photosensitivity	16 (42%)	5 (17%)	4 (15%)
Sjögren's	6 (16%)	0 (0%)	0 (0%)

n = number

drome. [It must be emphasized that at that time in our studies, detailed questioning and lip biopsies were not performed to examine for occult Sjögren's syndrome.]

The clinical association of anti-Ro (SS-A) precipitin antibody positive systemic lupus erythematosus with Sjögren's syndrome has also recently been strengthened by our and other investigators, studies comparing the serologic and clinical features of patients with young versus late onset lupus erythematosus (Cattaggio et al. 1984; Hochberg et al. 1985). These studies have clearly demonstrated that lupus erythematosus occurring in young adults (i.e. ≤22 years of age) is frequently characterized by the presence of native DNA antibodies, renal disease and the HLA-DR2 phenotype. In marked contrast, late onset lupus erythematosus (i.e. lupus beginning after the onset of 50) is characterized by the presence of anti-La (SS-B) and or anti-Ro (SS-A) precipitin antibodies, the HLA-DR3 phenotype and the frequent clinical appearance of lung and neuropsychiatric manifestations. There is a parallel increase in the frequency of anti-Ro (SS-A) precipitin antibody positivity, Sjögren's syndrome and the HLA-DR3 phenotype (a HLA phenotype commonly seen in Sjögren's syndrome) with increasing age of onset of lupus erythematosus (Table 2).

Further observations that suggest a close relationship between lupus erythematosus and Sjögren's syndrome have been provided by studies of family pedigrees of Sjögren's syndrome patients which demonstrate an increased frequency of lupus erythematosus among relatives. For example, in a study of the autoimmune diseases among 51 primary Sjögren's syndrome patients, we found that 18 (35%) of the probands had a positive family history of autoimmunity. In two proband's families (5%), lupus erythematosus was the autoimmune disease (Reveille et al. 1984). Con-

Table 2. Parallel increase in frequency of Sjögren's syndrome, anti-Ro (SS-A) precipitin positivity and HLA-DR3 phenotype with increasing age of lupus erythematosus onset (Hochberg et al. 1985)

Manifestation	AGE (years)		P-value
	≤22	≥50	≤22 vs. ≥50
Sjögren's syndrome in SLE	11%	37%	0.01
Anti-Ro (SS-A) positivity in SLE	18%	47%	0.08
HLA-DR3	24%	52%	0.1
HLA-DR2	48%	16%	0.05%

versely, the most common associated autoimmune disease among SLE patients, in families with multiple members with SLE, is Sjögren's syndrome (Reveille et al. 1983). In family members of 20 patients with both SLE and Sjögren's syndrome, 6 (30%) probands had a positive family history for autoimmunity. In one family (5%) the autoimmune disease was primary Sjögren's syndrome and in 2 (10%) systemic lupus erythematosus (Reveille et al. 1984).

Recent studies have indicated that 75% of homozygous C2 deficient patients with a lupus-like syndrome are anti-Ro (SS-A) precipitin antibody positive (Provost et al. 1983). Rynes et al. have recently reported anti-Ro (SS-A) and anti-La (SS-B) precipitin antibody positive identical twin girls with a homozygous C2 deficiency (Rynes et al. 1986). One of the sisters had SLE; the other SLE and Sjögren's syndrome. Thus, despite a presumably similar HLA haplotype (A25, B18, DR2) and the presence of the anit-Ro (SS-A) and anti-La (SS-B) precipitin antibodies, these two identical twins had clinically different expressions of their diseases.

Serologic Studies

Specificity and Frequency of Anti-Ro (SS-A) Precipitin Antibody in Lupus and Sjögren's Syndrome

In addition to these clinical data demonstrating the association of Sjögren's syndrome with anti-Ro (SS-A) precipitin antibody positive systemic lupus erythematosus, studies have demonstrated that patients with anti-Ro (SS-A) precipitin antibody positive lupus and anti-Ro (SS-A) precipitin antibody positive Sjögren's syndrome have a great deal of serologic similarities. Extensive studies by several groups including ours have documented that the anti-Ro (SS-A) and anti-La (SS-B) precipitin autoantibodies are highly, but imperfectly specific for connective tissue diseases (Clark et al. 1969; Maddison et al. 1978; Bernstein et al. 1985). The overwhelming majority of patients demonstrating either of these two precipitin autoantibodies have either lupus erythematosus and/or Sjögren's syndrome. For example, in one large study, we detected a frequency of only 0.1% (6/5000) of anti-Ro (SS-A) precipitin antibody positivity among non-connective tissue disease hospitalized patients (Maddison et al. 1978). (Five of these 6 anti-Ro (SS-A) precipitin antibody positive patients, with no evidence of connective tissue disease, were 60 years old or greater and no specific testing was done to rule out an occult Sjögren's syndrome). More recent studies by the Colorado group examining approximately 750 pregnant women have detected a 0.5% frequency of anti-Ro (SS-A) precipitin antibody positivity amongst these asymptomatic individuals (Harmon et al. 1984). Thus, these studies employing gel double diffusion to detect the presence of the anti-Ro (SS-A) precipitin antibody have indicated that this antibody system has a high degree of specificity for both Sjögren's and lupus erythematosus and is rarely present in normal individuals.

Similar extensive published studies examining the specificity of the anti-La (SS-B) precipitin antibody system in normal populations have not been published. Our extensive studies, however, indicate that this antibody system only infrequently occurs in the absence of the anti-Ro (SS-A) precipitin antibody. Thus, we believe with a great deal of confidence, that this antibody system also demonstrates a high degree of specificity for Sjögren's syndrome and systemic lupus erythematosus.

Studies in our and other laboratories have indicated that the anti-Ro (SS-A) precipitin antibody is found in approximately 25-30% of systemic lupus erythematosus patients (Maddison et al. 1978; Synkowski et al. 1982; Scopelitus and Biundi 1980). The anti-Ro (SS-A) precipitin antibody system is also found in approximately 40-45% of Sjögren's syndrome patients (Alexander et al. 1982; Alexander and Provost 1981). The anti-La (SS-B) precipitin antibody is found in approximately 10% of SLE and a variable percentage of Sjögren's syndrome patients (Alexander et al. 1982; Alexander and Provost 1981). Most recent studies using ELISA technology have detected abnormal quantities of anti-Ro (SS-A) and anti-La (SS-B) antibodies in almost all patients with Sjögren's syndrome (Harley et al. 1986). Most important is the fact that only a very few normal individuals, by this very sensitive technique, possess abnormal quantities of either of these two autoantibodies. (For a complete discussion, see chapter on Autoantibodies in Sjögren's Syndrome by J. B. Harley in this volume.)

Association with Rheumatoid Factor

In addition to the strong association of the anti-La (SS-B) with the anti-Ro (SS-A) antibodies, we have also detected that there is a strong association between the presence of the anti-Ro (SS-A) precipitin antibody and rheumatoid factor activity (Table 3). For example, in several studies of anti-Ro (SS-A) precipitin antibody positive lupus erythematosus patients, we have detected that approximately 70% of patients demonstrated rheumatoid factor activity (Maddison et al. 1978; Maddison et al. 1981). In many instances this was high titer (>640). By contrast, we found that only 26% of our anti-nRNP antibody positive and 12% of precipitin antibody negative lupus patients possessed rheumatoid factor activity (Maddison et al. 1978).

Studies of both primary and secondary Sjögren's syndrome have also revealed a similar increased frequency of rheumatoid factor activity. For example, in one study of 75 primary and secondary Sjögren's syndrome patients, 61% of the anti-Ro (SS-A) precipitin antibody positive patients possessed rheumatoid factor activity (Alexander et al. 1982). Other studies examining only primary Sjögren's syndrome patients have confirmed this relationship of anti-Ro (SS-A) precipitin antibody positivity with rheumatoid factor activity (Alexander and Provost 1983; Molina et al. 1985).

Table 3. Laboratory features associated with anti-Ro (SS-A) precipitin positivity in systemic lupus erythematosus and Sjögren's syndrome (Maddison et al. 1978; Alexander and Provost 1983)

Laboratory features	SLE	Sjögren's syndrome
Rheumatoid factor	70%	63%
Hypergammaglobulinemia	61%	64%
Cytopenia	37%	21%

Rheumatoid factor activity, frequently high titered, is also detected in anti-Ro (SS-A) precipitin antibody positive mothers of neonatal lupus infants. In a series of 10 mothers of neonatal lupus infants, we detected that 7 (70%) were rheumatoid factor positive (Watson et al. 1984).

The exact relationship of the rheumatoid factor activity to anti-Ro (SS-A) precipitin antibody positivity is unknown at the present time. However, recent intriguing data by Harley's group have suggested that anti-Ro (SS-A) antibodies may also react with epitopes on IgG and thus, anti-Ro (SS-A) antibodies may also possess rheumatoid factor activity (Mamula et al. 1985).

Other Laboratory Similarities

Also as demonstrated in Table 3, anti-Ro (SS-A) precipitin antibody positive lupus and anti-Ro (SS-A) precipitin antibody positive Sjögren's syndrome patients also frequently demonstrate hypergammaglobulinemia (Maddison et al. 1978; Alexander et al. 1983). (See chapter on Autoantibodies in Sjögren's syndrome in this volume for a further discussion). Cytopenia (neutropenia, lymphopenia and thrombocytopenia) also appear to frequently occur in anti-Ro (SS-A) precipitin antibody positive lupus and Sjögren's syndrome patients (Maddison et al. 1978; Alexander et al. 1982).

Neonatal Lupus

The studies of neonatal lupus provided us with strong additional evidence of the close relationship between Sjögren's syndrome and anti-Ro (SS-A) precipitin antibody positive lupus erythematosus. Neonatal lupus infants and their mothers almost always possess anti-La (SS-B) and or anti-Ro (SS-A) percipitin antibodies (Franco et al. 1981; Watson et al. 1984). The antibodies are produced in the mother and transferred to the infant in utero. The manifestations of neonatal lupus are the development of transient polycyclic annular lupus lesions (highly reminiscent of subacute cutaneous lupus erythematosus lesions (Sontheimer and Gilliam, 1979) and isolated congenital heart block. The cutaneous lupus skin lesions and the anti-La (SS-B) and anti-Ro (SS-A) precipitin antibody positivity in the infant's sera disappear within the first six months of life. The isolated congenital heart block which appears to be the result of an inflammatory process, however, persists.

The clinical manifestations of the neonatal lupus infant's mothers are varied. As depicted in Table 4, most of the mothers at the time of the birth of their affected offspring are asymptomatic (Lee et al. 1983; Watson et al. 1984). Approximately 20%, however, demonstrate features of lupus erythematosus and another 20% have Sjögren's syndrome. Thus, we have very strong evidence that an anti-Ro (SS-A) precipitin antibody positive mother with sicca signs and symptoms can transfer to her unborn infant specific antibodies [Ro (SS-A) and La (SS-B)] which are then associated with the development in the infant of classic polycyclic annular cutaneous lupus features. This experiment of nature also provides a great deal of evidence to suggest a cause and effect relationship between the development of cutaneous lupus lesions and the anti-Ro (SS-A) and anti-La (SS-B) antibodies.

Table 4. Summary of clinical features of anti-Ro (SS-A) and anti-La (SS-B) precipitin antibody positive mothers of infants with neonatal lupus erythematosus (Lee et al. 1984; Watson et al. 1984)

Clinical features	Number
Asymptomatic	12
Lupus erythematosus	3
Sicca signs and symptoms	5

Central Nervous System Disease in Sjögren's Syndrome

We have detected the presence of central nervous system disease in association with Sjögren's syndrome (Alexander et al. 1982b; Alexander et al. 1982c). Our studies have indicated a very high association of central nervous system disease in Sjögren's syndrome patients demonstrating cuteneous vasculitis (Molina et al. 1985b). Although brain biopsy material is limited, very preliminary studies indicate that the central nervous disease is induced by a vasculopathy (de la Monte et al. 1983; Alexander and Provost, unpublished observations). This vasculopathy is characterized by endothothelial swelling, focal necrosis of small blood vessel walls, extravastion of red blood cells, a microglial proliferation in the areas around the diseased blood vessel, hemosiderin laden macrophages and hemosiderin deposits. These lesions are found throughout the brain. The presence of extravasated red blood cells, hemosiderin laden macrophages and free hemosiderin in the tissues indicate that many of these lesions are acute as well as chronic.

Despite the fact that many of these lesions are occurring in patients who demonstrate cutaneous vasculitis, the vasculopathy in the brain of Sjögren's patients is characterized by a paucity of inflammatory cells in and about the diseased blood vessels. This vasculopathy resembles the type of vasculopathy described by Johnson and Richardson in central nervous system lupus erythematosus (Johnson and Richardson 1968). (For a more complete description, see the chapter on Central and Peripheral Nervous System Involvement in Sjögren's syndrome by E. A. Alexander in this volume).

Immunogenetic Studies

Our studies have demonstrated that at least 90% of primary and secondary Sjögren's syndrome patients possess the HLA DRw52 phenotype (Wilson et al. 1984) (Table 5). This is a supertypic specificity found on the beta chain of HLA DR3, DR4, Dw6, and Dw8 alloantigens. This HLA DRw52 phenotype is also found with increased frequency in systemic lupus erythematosus patients. For example, 64% of 87 Caucasian SLE patients were HLA-DRw52 positive compared to 46% of 600 Caucasian controls, $P < 0.01$ (Arnett et al. 1984). At the present time our preliminary data suggest that it is anti-Ro (SS-A) precipitin antibody positive late onset SLE patients with Sjögren's syndrome who frequently have the HLA

Table 5. Immunogenetic relationship between anti-Ro (SS-A) precipitin positive SLE and anti-Ro precipitin positive Sjögren's syndrome patients (Watson et al. 1984; Alvarellos et al. 1984; Wilson et al. 1984)

	HLA phenotypes		
	DR_2	DR_3	HLA-Dw52
Neonatal lupus (n=18)	27%	73%[a]	91%[a]
Anti-Ro (SS-A) positive SLE (n=29)	62%[a]	45%[a]	73%
Anti-Ro (SS-A) positive 1° SS (n=23)	39%	74%[a]	96%[a]
Controls (n=600)	24%	25%	46%

[a] statistically significant
n = number of patients

DRw52 phenotype (Hochberg et al. 1985; Wilson et al. 1984). For example, 14 of 16 SLE-SS patients (88%) compared to 39 of 74 SLE patients without an accompanying Sjögren's syndrome (53%) were HLA-DRw52 positive. $P < 0.02$ (Wilson et al. 1984). It is also important to note that mothers of neonatal lupus infants also have a statistically significant increased frequency of the HLA DRw52 phenotype (Watson et al. 1984; Lee et al. 1984).

In addition, our studies indicate that the Ro (SS-A) precipitin antibody is associated with the HLA DR2 and DR3 phenotypes. At least, 95% of anti-Ro (SS-A) precipitin antibody positive SLE and 85–90% of anti-Ro (SS-A) precipitin antibody positive Sjögren's syndrome patients possess either or both of these HLA - DR phenotypes (Alvarellos et al. 1983; Wilson et al. 1984). Our studies indicate that the highest titers of the anti-Ro (SS-A) antibody are found in those individuals who possess the HLA DR3 phenotype (Harley et al. 1986). On the other hand, the La (SS-B) antibody is generaly found in association with the HLA-DR3 and not the HLA-DR2 phenotype (Alvarellos et al. 1983; Wilson et al. 1984). For example, in a study of 102 1° and 2° SS patients, 18 patients were anti-La (SS-B) precipitin antibody positive and of these 13 were HLA-DR3 positive P value <0.006 (Wilson et al. 1984).

The immunogenetic, clinical and serological features of anti-Ro (SS-A) precipitin antibody positive patients with both systemic lupus erythematosus and Sjögren's syndrome (SLE/SS) are presented in Table 6. Note that all the SLE/SS patients possessed either the HLA-DR2 or DR3 phenotype and six of seven tested SLE/SS patients were HLA-DRw52 positive. For a comparison of HLA frequencies in anti-Ro (SS-A) precipitin antibody positive lupus and anti-Ro (SS-A) precipitin antibody positive Sjögren's syndrome patients see Table 5. Also, compare the serologic features of these SLE/SS patients with anti-Ro (SS-A) precipitin antibody positive lupus and anti-Ro (SS-A) precipitin antibody positive Sjögren's syndrome patients in Table 3.

In summary, our HLA studies suggest an association of similar HLA-DR region alleles with the expression of high titered Ro (SS-A) antibody (i.e. anti-Ro (SS-A) precipitin antibody positive Sjögren's syndrome and anti-Ro (SS-A) precipitin antibody positive lupus erythematosus). Thus, we reason it is highly conceivable that

Table 6. Immunogenetic and serologic features of eight anti-Ro (SS-A) precipitin positive SLE/ Sjögren's syndrome patients (Ahearn et al. 1982; Provost et al. 1986)

Patients	Increased Globulin	Rheumatoid Factor	HLA-DR	HLA-DRw52
1	+	+	3.6	+
2	+	+	3.6	+
3	+	+	3	+
4	+	+	2.3	+
5	+	–	2.4	–
6	+	+	3	+
7	+	+	2.7	nT
8	–	+	2.3	+

nT = not tested

many of the similarities between anti-Ro (SS-A) precipitin antibody positive lupus erythematosus and anti-Ro (SS-A) precipitin antibody positive Sjögren's syndrome may have an immunogenetic basis.

Longitudinal Clinical Studies of Anti-Ro (SS-A) Precipitin Positive Lupus and Anti (SS-A) Precipitin Positive Sjögren's Syndrome Patients

The longitudinal studies of anti-Ro (SS-A) precipitin antibody positive SLE and anti Ro (SS-A) precipitin antibody positive Sjögren's syndrome patients have provided us additional evidence to support our hypothesis that there is a close pathologic relationship between anti-Ro (SS-A) precipitin antibody positive SLE and anti-Ro (SS-A) precipitin antibody positive Sjögren's syndrome. During the past decade, we have detected a small group of patients who after several years of Sjögren's syndrome, have suddenly developed cutaneous manifestations of lupus erythematosus. The cutaneous lupus lesions generally resemble the cutaneous lesions seen in subacute cutaneous lupus erythematosus (SCLE) (Sontheimer et al. 1979). Seventy percent of SCLE patients are anti-Ro (SS-A) precipitin antibody positive. We have also seen a small number of patients who originally demonstrated classic anti-Ro (SS-A) precipitin antibody positive cutaneous lupus lesions (SCLE) and then subsequently lost all of the cutaneous features of lupus erythematosus and now have Sjögren's syndrome. The following are several examples of these two types of observations:

E. P. - This is a 65 year old Caucasian female who had noted dry eyes and a dry mouth for a number of years. At least five years after the onset of sicca symptoms, this patient developed classic, subacute cutaneous lupus erythematosus lesions involving the face, V of the neck and back. These lesions were characterized as widespread, annular, and polycyclic. There was slight scale formation, absence of telangectasia, and follicular plugging (Fig. 1).

Laboratory studies demonstrated that the patient possessed the anti-Ro (SS-A)

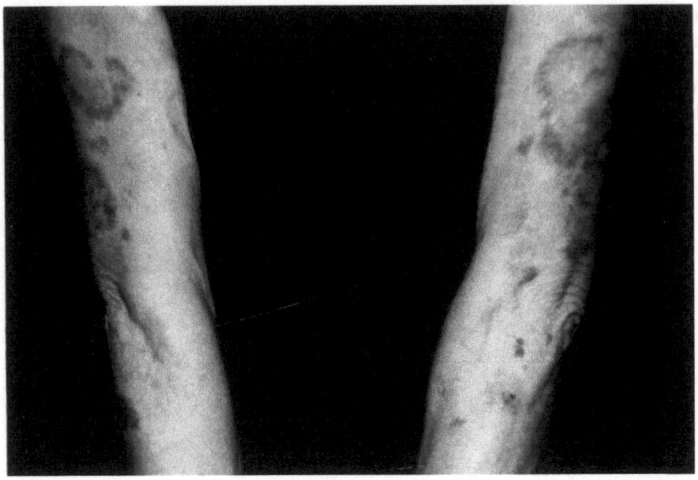

Fig. 1. Classic annular lupus lesions developing on the extensor surfaces of arms in an anti-Ro (SS-A) precipitin antibody positive patient, E. P., approximately five years after the onset of symptoms of Sjögren's syndrome. These cutaneous lupus lesions are identical to those lupus lesions described as subacute cutaneous lupus erythematosus (SCLE). At least 70% of SCLE patients are antiRo (SS-A) precipitin antibody positive (Sontheimer et al. 1982)

precipitin antibody and a lip biopsy displayed the characteristic features of Sjögren's syndrome.

This case illustrates the fact that the signs and symptoms of Sjögren's syndrome in a Ro (SS-A) precipitin antibody positive patient may antedate the development of classic anti-Ro (SS-A) precipitin antibody positive subacute cutaneous lupus lesions by years.

L. L. - This is a 28 year old Caucasian female with a five year history of a leukocytoclastic angiitis of the lower extremities and a lip biopsy documented Sjögren's syndrome. Serologic testing revealed the presence of both the anti-Ro (SS-A) and anti-La (SS-B) precipitin antibodies. She also had a rheumatoid factor titer of greater than 256.

Her first pregnancy was normal. Soon after her first pregnancy, the patient complained of joint pains and was eventually treated with 10 mg of Prednisone.

During her second pregnancy, the patient noted the development of erythematous lesions on her right forearm which gradually subsided. Physical examination of the mother, however, revealed a patchy, slightly erythematosus lupus dermatitis over her right forearm. There was no involvement of her face or other areas of the body.

The patient's second pregnancy resulted in the birth of a child with the classic cutaneous features of neonatal lupus. Serologic examination of the baby revealed both the anti-Ro (SS-A) and anti-La (SS-B) precipitin antibodies.

This is a very fascinating case because it demonstrates two features associated with anti-Ro (SS-A) precipitin antibody positivity. These are: 1) that an anti-Ro (SS-A) positive Sjögren's patient may subsequently develop cutaneous lupus lesions and 2) that an anti-Ro (SS-A) positive mother with Sjögren's syndrome may give birth to a child with a neonatal lupus syndrome.

R. M. - This is a 73 year old Caucasian female who was first seen and evaluated in 1984. She had sicca symptoms of many years duration and dryness of all the mucous membranes was observed. During the previous nine months, the patient had been seen and evaluated at two other hospitals. These previous hospitalizations had demonstrated a compression fracture of the L-1 vertebrae, proteinuria, renal tubular acidosis, primary hypothyroidism, splenic and renal calcifications, anemia of chronic disease, arthritis, alopecia and erythematous skin lesions. The patient had also during this time frame developed ataxia and course tremors of her hands. Computer axial tomography (CAT) scans had revealed pontine and cerebellar atrophy. In addition to these findings, hyperpigmented macular lesions were noted over the lower extremities. On questioning, the patient revealed that these had been present for the past 25-30 years. A biopsy of these, according to the patient, in the late 1950's had revealed a vasculitis. The patient was diagnosed as having aortic insufficiency and, subsequently, developed congestive failure which initially, promptly responded to digitalization and diuretics.

Laboratory studies revealed anti-Ro (SS-A) and anti-La (SS-B) precipitating antibodies were detected. Rheumatoid factor was present in a titer of 1:80.

In the spring of 1985, the patient developed typical annular lesions of subacute cutaneous lupus erythematosus. At the present time, the patient's clinical course is dominated by her cardiac problems. She has developed gross congestive failure, poorly responsive to Digoxin and diuretics.

This complex case is significant because this patient has had long standing Sjögren's syndrome, perhaps for as long as two to three decades. In addition, there is evidence that her disease was complicated by vasculitis of the lower extremities. Subsequently, the patient developed renal tubular acidosis and possibly elements of Fanconi's syndrome; primary hypothyroidism and neurologic involvement. Most recently, this anti-Ro (SS-A) and anti-La (SS-B) precipitin antibody positive Sjögren's syndrome patient has developed the characteristic cutaneous lesions of subacute cutaneous lupus erythematosus.

S. D. - This is a 49 year old Caucasian female who gave a history of two years of a photosensitive dermatitis involving the arms, chest, and face. The dermatitis was described as being confluent, erythematous, polycyclic, scaly, with plaques demonstrating central clearing and hyperpigmentation. The lesions involved the dorsal portions of the forearms, hands, upper arms, chest, and back. The impression at that time was discoid lupus erythematosus. The dermatitis responded to a short course of oral prednisone and a steroid cream. Serologic studies revealed a negative ANA and the presence of the anti-Ro (SS-A) precipitin antibody.

One year later, she was referred to our institution for evaluation. At that time, she gave a history of arthralgias of the elbows and feet the previous 7-8 months. She also complained of weakness and fatigue. In addition, she gave a history of recent memory loss characterized by forgetting tasks in the middle of their performance. She also gave a history of drinking constantly (four pots of coffee per day and took water to bed with her).

Physical examination at that time revealed dry mucous membranes. A lip biopsy revealed the characteristic features of Sjögren's syndrome.

Cognitive functions demonstrated a mild memory attention defect. Cerebral spinal fluid examination revealed a normal IgG index with the presence of two IgG oligoclonal bands. Subsequently, this patient developed several focal central nervous system lesions including dysarthria and mild left hemiparesis. Nuclear magnetic resonance scanning demonstrated several occipital and frontal attenuated areas as well as a previous left periventricular area of infarction.

This case demonstrates the onset of an anti-Ro (SS-A) precipitin antibody positive, intensely photosensensitive lupus dermatitis two years prior to the onset of definite signs and symptoms in Sjögren's syndrome. In addition, the Sjögren's syndrome was accompanied by central nervous system involvement.

J. D. - This is a 51 year old Caucasian female who gave a history of approximately one and a half years of myalgias and arthralgias. After an evaluation by a rheumatologist who discovered a weakly positive anti-nRNP precipitin antibody and an antinuclear antibody titer of ≥ 160, a diagnosis of undifferentiated connective tissue disease was made. She was, subsequently, treated with low doses of Prednisone.

In the late spring of 1984, she consulted a dermatologist for urticaria-like lesions. Physical examination at that time revealed a classic livido reticularis pattern over both lower extremities. A biopsy of one of the urticarial lesions demonstrated a leukocytoclastic angiitis.

Subsequently, she was referred to our institution for evaluation. Physical examination at that time revealed in addition to the chronic, persistent, urticaria-like lesions, a lupus-like dermatitis characterized by erythema, scaling, slight hypopigmentation and telangectasia over the dorsal aspects of her forearms. The remainder of the physical examination was within normal limits. Serologic examination at that time revealed a positive antinuclear antibody titer of ≥ 160 and the presence of anti-nRNP and anti-Ro (SS-A) precipitin antibodies.

In the first week of November 1984 the patient, while attending a farm exhibit, was exposed to bright sunlight. Soon after, she developed an explosive onset of a classic, subacute cutaneous lupus dermatitis over her shoulders, neck, and anterior chest. During this period of time, the patient also complained of dryness of her mouth and eyes and, subsequently, developed a partial right hemiparesis. A lip biopsy demonstrated the characteristic finding of Sjögren's syndrome.

This patient's disease began as an undifferentiated connective tissue disease and then she developed the characteristic features of an anti-Ro (SS-A) precipitin antibody positive subacute cutaneous lupus erythematosus. Now the predominant clinical picture in this patient is Sjögren's syndrome.

J. C. - This is a 40 year old Caucasian female with a history of fatigue, malaise, arthralgias and cutaneous lesions, dating since childhood. At the age of 11, she awoke one morning with difficulty in flexing her knees and was noted to have knee and ankle effusions. A diagnosis of rheumatic disease was made. During her teens, she became aware of sun sensitivity, skin eruptions, and generalized myalgias after sunlight exposure. An intermittent malar rash was also present. In her late teens, a blood test for rheumatoid factor was positive. This teenage illness was characterized predominantly as an arthritic condition characterized by arthralgias in the MCP joints, wrists, tempro mandibular joints, neck, knees, and ankles.

During her late twenties, she developed more signs and symptoms of joint disease consisting of erythema and effusions. She was evaluated at another institution on several occasions. On one occasion, the complaint was unexplained fever. The joint pains and malaise were treated with low doses of corticosteroids and the symptoms regressed quickly. Because of episodic fevers, skin eruptions, arthritis, and arthralgias, together with malaise and fatigue, a diagnosis of systemic lupus erythematosus was made. Subsequently, she developed many sore throats and noted the onset of dryness of her eyes. She also stated that she was forced to use commercial eyedrops because of the dryness of her eyes and gave a history of drinking large quantities of fluid because of the dryness in her mouth. She also noted a marked increase in the number of dental caries. In addition to these progressive symptoms, the patient noted increasing problems with her memory. She noted that as a legal secretary she had to take many notes in order not to confuse orders from a variety of lawyers working in the law office. This memory problem had begun approximately two years before and was now becoming very critical.

Her pregnancy history is interesting in that her second child, a son, was born with a heart block (3:1).

On physical examination, she demonstrated the classic lesions of subacute cutaneous lupus erythematosus involving predominantly her neck, anterior chest, back, and arms. Serological evaluation revealed an ANA positive at a 1:160 titer anti-Ro (SS-A) and anti-La (SS-B) precipitin antibodies were present.

This patient demonstrates the development of a connective tissue disease process over two and a half decades. Initially, the connective tissue disease was predominantly an arthritic condition and, subsequently, a clear cut diagnosis of subacute cutaneous lupus erythematosus and Sjögren's syndrome has emerged simultaneously during the third decade of this patient's life. This anti-Ro (SS-A) positive woman also during her second pregnancy, gave birth to a child with neonatal lupus manifesting itself as a congenital heart block.

Summary

It is our hypothesis that high titered anti-Ro (SS-A) antibody patients as represented by anti-Ro (SS-A) precipitin antibody positive lupus and anti-Ro (SS-A) precipitin antibody positive Sjögren's syndrome have a much closer pathologic relationship than our current nosology indicates. The weight of the evidence, although incomplete as detailed above, strongly suggests that in addition to sharing similar serology, Ro (SS-A) precipitin positive lupus and Sjögren's syndrome patients probably share the same immunogenetic background; that anti-Ro (SS-A) precipitin antibody positive Sjögren's syndrome patients may give birth to neonatal lupus infants; that there is a striking parallel increase in the frequency of Sjögren's syndrome, and anti-Ro (SS-A) precipitin antibody positivity, with increasing age of onset of lupus erythematosus; that the central nervous system vasculopathy in Sjögren's syndrome appears to be indistinguishable from the vasculopathy of central nervous system lupus erythematosus and that patients with long-standing anti-Ro (SS-A) precipitin antibody positive Sjögren's syndrome may suddenly develop cutaneous lupus erythematosus lesions and vice versa.

It is anticipated, if our hypothesis is correct, that in the future, cDNA probes will detect DNA nucleotide homologies in the HLA-DR region of these anti-Ro (SS-A) precipitin antibody positive lupus and anti-Ro (SS-A) precipitin antibody positive Sjögren's syndrome patients. The mechanism(s), however, responsible for determining the clinical expression of the disease in these anti-Ro (SS-A) precipitin antibody positive patients is totally unknown at this time.

References

Alexander EL, Provost TT (1981) Ro (SS-A) and La (SS-B) antibodies. Springer Seminars in Immunopathology 4: 253-273

Alexander EL, Craft C, Moser R, Dorsch C, Provost TT, Alexander GE (1982a) Necrotizing spinal arteritis in Sjögren's syndrome: Association with nervous system complications. Arth Rheum 28: 1341-1347

Alexander EL, Hirsch TJ, Arnett FC, Provost TT, Stevens MB (1982b) Ro (SS-A) and La (SS-B) antibodies in the clinical spectrum of Sjögren's syndrome. J Rheumatology 9: 239-246

Alexander EL, Provost TT, Stevens MB, Alexander GE (1982c) Neurologic complications of primary Sjögren's syndrome. Medicine 61: 247-257

Alexander EL, Arnett FC, Provost TT, Stevens MB (1983) Sjögren's syndrome: Association of anti-Ro (SS-A) antibodies with vasculitis, immunologic abnormalities and serologic hyperreactivity. Ann Int Med 98: 155-159

Alexander EL, Provost TT (1983) Cutaneous manifestations of primary Sjögren's syndrome: A reflection of vasculitis and association with anti-Ro (SS-A) antibodies. J Invest Dermatol 80: 386-391

Alvarellos A, Ahearn JM, Provost TT, et al (1983) Relationship of HLA-DR and MT antigens to autoantibody expression in systemic lupus erythematosus. Arth Rheum 26: 1533-1535

Arnett FC, Reveille JD, Wilson RW, Provost TT, Bias WB (1984) Systemic lupus erythamtosus: Current state of the genetic hypothesis. Seminars in Arth Rheum 14: 24-35

Bernstein RM, Bunn CC, Hughes GRV, Francoeur AM, Mathews MB (1984) Cellular Protein and RNA Antigens in Autoimmune Disease. Mol Biol Med 2: 105-120

Cattaggio LJ, Skinner RP, Smith G, Maddison PJ (1984) Systemic lupus erythematosus in the elderly: The clinical and serological characteristics. J Rheumatology 11: 175-181

Clark G, Reichlin M, Tomasi TB (1969) Characterization of a soluble cytoplasmic antigen reactive with sera from patients with systemic lupus erythematosus. J Immunol 102: 117-121

de la Monte SM, Hutchins GM, Gupta PK (1983) Polymorphous meningitis with atypical mononuclear cells in Sjögren's syndrome. Ann Neurology 14: 455

Franco HL, Weston WL, Peebles C, Forstot SL, Phanaphak P (1981) Autoantibodies directed against sicca syndrome antigens in the neonatal lupus syndrome. J Amer Acad Dermatol 4: 67-72

Harley JB, Alexander EL, Bias WB, Fox OF, Provost TT, Reichlin M, Yamagata H, Arnett FC : Anti-Ro (SS-A) and anti-La (SS-B) in Sjögren's syndrome. Arth Rheum (in press)

Harmon CE, Lee LA, Huff JC, Norris DA, Weston WL (1984) The frequency of antibodies to the SS-A/Ro antigen in Pregnancy Sera. Arth Rheum 27: 520

Hochberg MC, Boyd RE, Ahearn JM, Arnett FC, Bias WB, Provost TT, Stevens MB (1985) Systemic lupus erythematosus: A review of clinicolaboratory features and the immunogenetic markers in 150 patients with emphasis on demographic subsets. Medicine 64: 285-295

Johnson RT, Richardson EP (1968) Neurologic manifestations of systemic lupus erythematosus: A clinical pathologic study of 24 cases and review of the literature. Medicine 47: 337-369

Lee LA, Bias WB, Arnett FC, Provost TT, Weston WL (1983) Immunogenetics of the neonatal lupus syndrome. Ann Int Med 99: 592-596

Maddison PJ, Mogavero HS, Provost TT, Reichlin M (1978) Clinical significance of autoantibodies to a soluble cytoplasmic antigen in systemic lupus erythematosus and other connective tissue diseases. J Rheumatology 6: 189-195

Maddison PJ, Provost TT, Reichlin M (1981) Serological findings in patients with "ANA negative" systemic lupus erythematosus. Medicine 60: 87-94

Mamula M, Fox OF, Harley JB (1985) Cross-reactivity of Ro (SS-A) and Immunoglobulin G. Arth Rheum 28: 537

Molina R, Provost TT, Alexander EL (1985a) Two types of inflammatory vascular disease in Sjögren's syndrome: Differential association with seroreactivity to rheumatoid factor and antibodies to Ro (SS-A) and with hypocomplementemia. Arth Rheum 28: 1251-1258

Molina R, Provost TT, Alexander EL (1985b) Peripheral inflammatory vascular disease in Sjögren's syndrome: Association with nervous system complications. Arth Rheum 28: 1341-1347

Provost TT, Arnett FC, Reichlin M (1983) Homozygous C2 deficiency, lupus erythematosus and anti-Ro (SS-A) antibodies. Arth Rheum 26: 1279-1283

Reveille JD, Bias WB, Winkelstein JA, Provost TT, Dorsch C, Arnett FC (1983) Familial systemic lupus erythematosus: Immunogenetic studies in eight families. Medicine 62: 21-35

Reveille JD, Wilson RW, Provost TT, Bias WB, Arnett FC (1984) Primary Sjögren's syndrome and other autoimmune diseases in families: Prevalence and immunogenetic studies in six kindred. Ann Int Med 101: 748-756

Rynes R, Reichlin M, Harley J (1986) SLE, complement component C2 deficiency, anti-Ro (SS-A) and anti-La (SS-B) antibodies. Arth Rheum (in press)

Scopelitis E, Biundo JJ, Alspaugh MA (1980) Anti SS-A antibodies and other antinuclear antibodies in systemic lupus erythematosus. Arth Rheum 23: 287-292

Sontheimer RD, Thomas JR, Gillian JN (1979) Subacute cutaneous lupus erythematosus. A cutaneous marker for a distinct lupus erythematosus subset. Arch Dermatol 115: 1409-1415

Sontheimer RD, Maddison PJ, Reichlin M, et al (1982) Serologic and HLA associations in subacute cutaneous lupus erythematosus. Ann Int Med 97: 664-671

Synkowski DR, Reichlin M, Provost TT (1982) Serum autoantibodies in systemic lupus erythematosus and correlation with cutaneous features. J Rheumatology 9: 380-385

Watson RM, Lane AT, Barnett NK, Bias WB, Arentt FC, Provost TT (1984) Neonatal lupus erythematosus: A clinical, serological and immunogenetic study with review of the literature. Medicine 63: 362-378

Wilson R, Provost TT, Bias WB, Alexander EL, Edlow DW, Hochberg MC, Stevens MB, Arnett FC (1984) Sjögren's syndrome: Influence of multiple HLA-D region alloantigens on clinical and serological expression. Arth Rheum 27: 1245-1253

5. Immunologic Abnormalities in Sjögren's Syndrome

H. M. Moutsopoulos and N. Talal

The field of autoimmunity, like immunology itself, is undergoing rapid change due to progress in cellular immunology and molecular biology. The old concept that individuals are tolerant to self because of the elimination of "forbidden" clones during fetal development was abandoned almost a decade ago. Normal healthy individuals have B lymphocytes capable of reacting with self antigens through Ig receptors. Such cells can be triggered to proliferate and secrete autoantibodies of a wide range of specificities. This potential for autoimmunity exists in everyone and has important implication for immunopathology.

Autoimmune disease are multifactorial in origin and generally attributable to a breakdown in normal immunoregulatory control mechanisms. The precise contributions of genetic, viral, endocrine, psychoneurologic and other factors to autoimmune disorders is still largely unknown and beyond the scope of this chapter (Talal 1985).

Two major phenomena characterize Sjögren's syndrome (SS) as an autoimmune disease: 1) the chronic lymphocytic infiltrate of the exocrine glands leading to the appelation "autoimmune exocrinopathy" (Strand and Talal 1980) and 2) the B-lymphocyte hyperreactivity manifest as multiple circulating autoantibodies and immune complexes (Alspaugh et al. 1976, Lawley et al. 1979).

Immunoregulation

T cell activation requires appropriate presentation of antigen on the surface of an antigen presenting cell (APC), usually a macrophage strongly expressive of class II histocompatability cell surface antigens (Fig. 1). These cell surface molecules, collectively called Ia (or DR in man), are now known to be the products of several IR gene loci in the Major Histocompatibility Complex (MHC) (I-A and I-E in the mouse; DP, DQ and DR in man). Each molecule is composed of an α and β chain. There are several α and seven β chain gene loci. The Ia molecules are capable of functionally, perhaps physically, interacting with foreign antigens to activate T cells in conjunction with the secretion of the macrophage product interleukin-1 (IL-1).

The helper/inducer T-cell (OK T4) responds to IL-1 and to antigen on APCs (Fig. 1) to produce interleukin-2 (IL-2), a critical immune hormone that interacts with specific receptors on T-cells and natural killer (NK) cells to mediate lymphocyte proliferation, γ interferon production and the production of other lymphokines that regulate B-cells (e.g., B cell growth and differentiation factors). IL-2 produc-

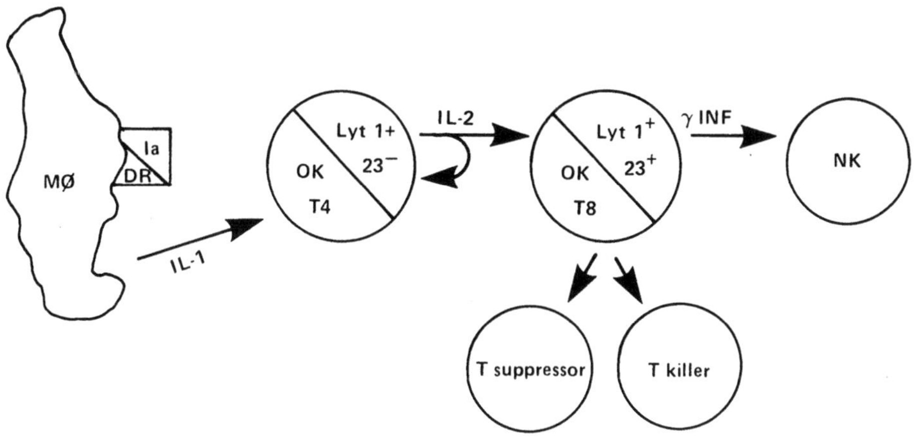

Fig. 1. T-lymphocyte depended immune response

tion and response is deficient in many autoimmune conditions including SS (Miyasaka et al. 1986, in press).

Interferon induces the expression of class II molecules on APCs and has been postulated as the cause of aberrant Ia expression on thyroid cells in thyroiditis (Bottazzo et al. 1983). Such expression could convert parenchymel cells into APCs which might then lead to aberrant immune reactions locally and target-organ specific autoimmunity. A local virus infection has been proposed as the stimulus for this interferon production.

Localization of activated B-cells

The number of B-lymphocytes spontaneously secreting immunoglobulins in SS and SLE peripheral blood and bone marrow was determined by a plaque forming cell assay (Fauci and Moutsopoulos 1981). Peripheral blood B-lymphocytes from SS patients and normal controls, unlike lymphocytes from SLE patients, did not spontaneously secrete increased amounts of immunoglobulins. The same was observed with bone marrow B-lymphocytes. Thus, the activated B-cells in SLE patients are widely distributed while in SS patients they home to organs such as the exocrine glands or the spleen. In this regard, it was previously demonstrated by Talal et al (1970) that the B-lymphocytes infiltrating the labial minor salivary glands of SS patients synthesize great amounts of immunoglobulins and also rheumatoid factor, vastly different from that seen with control salivary glands. Furthermore, minor salivary glands of patients with primary SS and controls were examined for intracytoplasmic immunoglobulin (Lane et al. 1983) using the peroxidase-antiperoxidase bridge technique. Plasma cells were the principal cell type demonstrating positive staining. The majority of plasma cells infiltrating the minor salivary glands containing IgG in contrast to controls which contained IgA. A recent study (Segerberg-Konttinen 1986) demonstrates by activation marker phenotype, ultramorphology and DNA synthesis that the activated cells in the salivary gland lesions, although few in total number, are B-cell in origin. Thus, the infiltrated exocrine gland tissues in SS may be a major site of B-cell activation.

Immunoregulatory cell studies

The polyclonal B-cell activation that occurs in autoimmunity probably arises from multiple mechanisms, some dependent and some independent of T cells. To examine the possible contribution of T cells, several studies have examined immunoregulatory cell phenotypes and function in the peripheral blood and infiltrating lymphocytes of SS patients.

Peripheral blood lymphocyte studies

Patients with primary SS and either glandular or extraglandular involvement were studied with regard to absolute number of total lymphocytes, T-cells and immunoregulatory T-cell subpopulations, B-cell numbers and function and suppressor cell capabilities. This group of patients with primary SS had absolute total lymphocytes, T-cell and B-cells not different from normal controls (Moutsopoulos et al. 1980). These results, however, are in contrast to some previous studies which have demonstrated a T-lymphocytopenia in SS patients (Talal et al. 1974; Moutsopoulos et al. 1976). They agree, however, with Van Boxel et al. (1973) who described a normal percentage of circulating T-cells in SS patients.

Only three of ten patients with glandular SS but nine of eleven with extraglandular SS had proportions of T-cells bearing receptors for the Fc portion of IgG lower than the normal range (Moutsopoulos et al. 1980). This initial finding was similar to findings in patients with SLE (Morimoto 1978). Overnight trypsinisation of the peripheral blood mononuclear cells from SS but not SLE patients resulted in normalization of the percentage of these cells showing that this phenomenon was due to an immunoglobulin occupying the Fc-γ receptor.

There have been several studies (Morimoto et al. 1982; Fox et al. 1987; Miyasaka et al. 1983) using monoclonal antibodies to defined lymphocyte subsets in the peripheral blood. In general, a decrease in suppressor T-cells occurs only when there is an accompanying systemic rheumatic disease or when severe extraglandular disease is present.

Phenotypes of the lymphocytes in the infiltrates of the labial minor salivary glands

Initially T- and B-lymphocytes were enumerated in the salivary glands using specific antiserum to immunoglobulin and rosetting assays with complement-coated erythrocytes (Talal et al. 1974; Tannenbaum et al. 1975). Talal et al. (1974) using heteroserum to thymocytes found a predominance of T-cells only in very large foci of lymphocytes. Chused et al. (1974) reported a predominance of B-cells in the lymphoid infiltrates of the minor salivary glands from SS patients based on the pyrinophilic staining of the cells. Today, however, it is known that activated T-cells can demonstrate pyrinophilic staining due to their increased RNA synthesis (Potvin 1979; Palutke et al. 1980).

The development of monoclonal antibodies permitted more sophisticated studies of the lymphoid cells infiltrating the minor salivary glands (Morimoto et al. 1982; Fox et al. 1982; Lindhal et al. 1985; Moutsopoulos et al. 1986). All investigators agree that the predominant cell in the infiltrates of the minor salivary gland is one bearing the T-helper/inducer phenotype. There are fewer suppressor than helper T cells. B-cells make up approximately 20% of the total infiltrative population (Table 1).

Parotid gland and submandibular gland biopsy specimens were also examined. The majority of lymphocytes were again helper T-cells while suppressor T-cells and B-cells were in the same ratios as in the minor salivary glands (Fox et al. 1982, 1983). Thus, the lymphoid infiltrates in the minor salivary glands appear representative of the ones affecting the major salivary glands.

Using the Leu-7 and Leu-11 monoclonal antibodies, we and others were unable to demonstrate NK cells in the infiltrates, while Leu-7 and Leu-11 positive cells were identified in the peripheral blood of SS patients (Fox et al. 1985a; Moutsopoulos et al. 1986). The absence of this cell cannot be explained by the preferential loss of the Leu-7 epitope from the lymphocytes infiltrating the minor salivary glands because these cells also did not react with the monoclonal antibody-F_{45} (Fox et al. 1985a). This antibody recognizes a distinct epitope on the same molecule. Also the case of "masked" epitopes by immunoglobulins or other proteins was ruled out by incubation of cell suspensions from the labial biopsies at 37 °C for two hours (Fox et al. 1985).

Using the monoclonal OKM_1 antibody (Lindhal et al. 1985; Moutsopoulos et al. 1986) it was observed that less than 5% of the cells in the round cell infiltrates were stained. The absence of polymorphonuclear leukocytes in the lesion suggested that these are monocytes/macrophages. This poor representation of monocyte/macrophage in the histopathologic lesion of SS was further substantiated by enzyme-histochemical studies (Dalakas, personal communication).

Previous studies have suggested a defective monocyte/macrophage function in SS patients. Sixty percent of patients have an abnormal clearance of ^{51}Cr-labelled

Table 1. Reactivity of the lymphocytes in the infiltrates of the labial minor salivary glands with monoclonal antibodies (Moutsopoulos et al. 1986)

Monoclonal Antibodies		% Stained Cells
Leu-4	(T-lymphocytes)	55-75
Leu 3a	(T-helper/inducer cells)	45-55
Leu 2a	(T-suppressor cells)	10-20
Leu 14	(B-lymphocytes)	20-35
Leu-7	(NK Cells)	<5
OKM_1	(monocyte/macrophage)	<5
OKIa	(anti-HLA-DR)	70-100

IgG-sensitized autologous erythrocytes (Hamberger et al. 1979), a measure of reticuloendothelial system function. Moreover, patients with glandular disease tended to have normal clearances while clearance was abnormal in patients with systemic (extraglandular) disease. There was no correlation between clearance and serum immune complex levels, complement levels, or rheumatoid factor titers. These findings suggest an abnormality of the normal functional activity of Fc-receptors in patients with extraglandular SS. This could predispose to the continued circulation of immune complexes allowing for increased tissue deposition.

Miyasaka et al. (1981) reported a deficient response in the autologous mixed lymphocyte reaction in the majority of SS patients due in some to a defect in stimulatory macrophages (Miyasaka 1983). In other patients, the defect could be attributed to an inadequate response of T-cells, probably related to an impaired production of IL-2 (Fox et al. 1985b).

Finally, using the monoclonal antibody OK-Ia as well as anti HLA-DR it was shown that more than 90% of the cells in the infiltrates were stained positive (Fox et al. 1982; Lindhal et al. 1985; Moutsopoulos et al. 1986). HLA-DR positive cells may be B-lymphocytes, monocytes or in vitro activated T-cells (Lampson et al. 1980; Yu et al. 1980). Since B-cells and monocytes/macrophages are the minority population in the SS infiltrates whereas T-cells predominate, this finding suggests that the T-cells are activated in the SS lesions. Supporting evidence comes from IL2 production and T-cell activation markers in the pseudolymphomatous lesions in SS (Fox et al. 1983).

In addition, OK-Ia and anti HLA-DR antibodies intensively stained the epithelial cells (ducts and acini) in SS lesions, particularly in areas close to the round cell infiltrates. This phenomenon was not observed in normal salivary gland tissues (Lindhal et al. 1985; Moutsopoulos et al. 1986).

Conclusions

The immunopathologic findings in SS salivary glands and peripheral blood are summarized in Tables 2 and 3. The lesions contain a predominance of activated T-helper/inducer cells, a dramatic B-lymphocyte hyperreactivity, an inappropriate HLA-DR expression of the glandular (ducts and acini) tissues and a reduced number of macrophages and NK cells. On the basis of these findings, the following hypothesis can be proposed (Fig. 2). An unknown causative agent infects the salivary glands in an individual genetically susceptible to Sjögren's syndrome. The infection can be transient or persistent, perhaps the latter if macrophage function is

Table 2. Immunologic findings in the salivary glands

Many DR+ glandular epithelial cells
Many T helper cells expressing activation markers
Activated B cells
Production of monoclonal immunoglobulins
Absence of NK cells

Table 3. Immunologic findings in the peripheral blood

Polyclonal hypergammaglobulinemia
Autoantibodies (ANA+ and RF+)
Anti-Ro (SS-A) and anti-La (SS-B)
Monoclonal immunoglobulins
Deficient IL-2 production
Decreased NK cell function

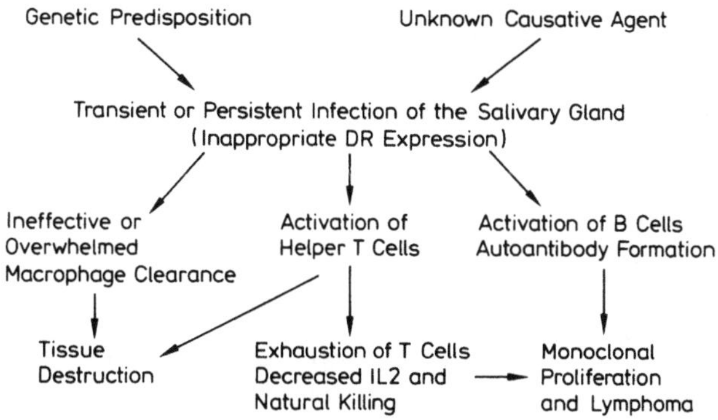

Fig. 2. Pathogenesis of Sjögren's syndrome

overwhelmed or otherwise ineffective. It sets in motion a chain of immunologic events which includes the inappropriate expression of DR which may render salivary gland epithelium capable of functioning as antigen presenting cells. This inappropriate HLA-DR expression leads to T-cell activation. The activated T-cells, perhaps through interferon-γ, further induce HLA-DR expression in the glandular cells. B cells also become activated perhaps both through the actions of helper T-cells but perhaps also through intrinsic mechanisms such as occurs with EB virus infection. The unleashing of this uncontrolled immune response results in autoantibody formation and tissue destruction through a variety of mechanisms. An eventual exhaustion of immune capability through defective IL2 and NK cell function then predisposes to monoclonal B-cell proliferation and malignant lymphoma.

References

Adamson III TC, Fox RI, Frisman DM, Howell FV (1983) Immunohistologic analysis of lymphoid infiltrates in primary Sjögren's syndrome using monoclonal antibodies. J Immunol 130 (1): 203

Alspaugh MA, Talal N, Tan EM (1976) Differentiation and characterization of autoantibodies and their antigens in Sjögren's syndrome. Arth Rheum 19: 216–222

Anderson LG, Cummings NA, Asofsky R, Hylton MB, Tarpley TM Jr, Tomasi TB Jr, Wolf RO, Schall GL, Talal N (1972) Salivary gland immunoglobulin and rheumatoid factor synthesis in Sjögren's syndrome. Natural history and response to treatment. Am J Med 53: 456–463

Bottazzo GF, Pujol-Borrell R, Hanafusa T, Feldman M (1983) Role of aberrant HLA-DR expression and antigen presentation in induction of endocrine autoimmunity. Lancet 2: 1115–1119

Chisholm DM, Mason DK (1968) Labial salivary gland biopsy in Sjögren's disease. J Clin Pathol 21: 656–660

Chused TM, Hardin JA, Frank MW et al (1974) Identification of cells infiltrating the minor salivary glands in patients with Sjögren's syndrome. J Immunol 112: 641-646
Fauci A, Moutsopoulos H (1981) Polyclonally triggered B-cells in the peripheral blood of normal individuals and in patients with SLE and primary Sjögren's syndrome. Arth Rheum 24: 557-584
Fox R, Carstens S, Fong S et al. (1982) Use of monoclonal antibodies to analyze peripheral blood and salivary gland lymphocyte subsets in Sjögren's syndrome. Arth Rheum 25: 419-422
Fox R, Adamson TC III, Fong S, Robinson CA, Morgan ED, Robb JA, Howell FV (1983) Lymphocyte phenotype and function in pseudolymphoma associated with Sjögren's syndrome. J Clin Invest 72: 52-62
Fox R, Hugli T, Lanier L et al (1985a) Salivary gland lymphocytes in primary Sjögren's syndrome lack lymphocyte subsets defined by Leu-7 and Leu-11 antigens. J Immun 135: 207-214
Fox R, Theofilopoulos AN, Altman A (1985b) Production of Interleukin 2 (IL-2)by salivary gland lymphocytes in Sjögren's syndrome. Detection of reactive cells by using antibody directed to synthetic peptides of IL-2. J of Immunol 135 (5): 3109-3115
Hanafusa T, Pujoi-Borrell R, Chiovato L et al (1985) Aberrant expression of HLA-DR antigen on thyrocytes in Graves' disease: relevance for autoimmunity. Lancet 2: 1111-1115
Hamburger MI, Moutsopoulos HM, Lawley TJ et al (1979) Sjögren's syndrome: a defect in reticuloendothelial system Fc-receptor-specific clearance. Ann Intern Med 91: 534-538
Lane HC, Callihan TR, Jaffe RS et al (1983) Presence of intracytoplasmic IgG in the lymphocyte infiltrates of the minor salivary glands of patients with primary Sjögren's syndrome. Clin Exp Rheum 1: 237-239
Lampson L, Levy R (1980) Two populations of Ia-like molecules on human B-cell line. J Immunol 125: 293-299
Lawley T, Moutsopoulos HM, Katz SI, Theopilopoulos AN, Chused TM, Frank MM (1979) Demonstration of circulating immune complexes in Sjögren's syndrome. J Immunol 123: 1382-1387
Lindhal G, Hedfors E, Klareskog L, Forsum U (1985) Epithelial HLA-DR expression and T-lymphocyte subsets in salivary glands in Sjögren's syndrome. Clin Exp Immun 61: 475-482
Miyasaka N, Sauvezie B, Pierce D et al (1981) Decreased autologous mixed lymphocyte reaction in Sjögren's syndrome. J Clin Invest 66: 928-933
Miyasaka N, Sauvezie B, Raff H et al (1983) T-cell macrophage subset interactions and decreased autologous mixed lymphocyte reaction in Sjögren's syndrome. Rheum Int 3: 13-17
Miyasaka N, Murota N, Yamaoka K, Sato K, Yamada T, Nishido T, Okuda M (1986) Interleukin-2 defect in the peripheral blood and the lung in patients with Sjögren's syndrome. Clin Exp Immunol 65: 497-505
Morimoto CT (1978) Loss of suppressor T-lymphocyte function in patients with systemic lupus erythematosus (SLE). Clin Exp Immunol 32: 125-133
Morimoto C, Reinherz E, Nadler L et al (1982) Comparison of T- and B-cell markers in patients with Sjögren's syndrome and SLE. Clin Immunol Immunopathol 22: 270-277
Moutsopoulos HM, Fye KH, Sawada S et al (1976) In vitro effect of thymosin on T-lymphocyte rosette formation in rheumatic diseases. Clin Exp Immunol 26: 563-573
Moutsopoulos HM, Mann DL, Johnson AH, Chused TM (1979) Genetic differences between primary and secondary sicca syndrome. N Eng J Med 301: 761-763
Moutsopoulos H, Fauci A (1980) Immunoregulation in Sjögren's syndrome. Influence of serum factors on T-cell subpopulations. J Clin Invest 65: 519-528
Moutsopoulos HM, Hooks JJ, Chan CC et al (1986) HLA-DR expression by labial salivary gland tissues in Sjögren's syndrome. Ann Rheum Dis 45: 677-683
Palutke M, Tabaczka P, Weise RW et al (1980) T-cell lymphomas of large cell type. A variety of malignant lymphomas: "Histiocytic" and mixed lymphocyte "histiocytic". Cancer 46: 87-93
Potvin C (1979) A simple, modified methyl green pyronin Y stain for DNA and RNA in formalin-fixed tissues. Lab Med 10: 772-782
Sakane T, Steinberg AD, Green I (1978) Studies of immune functions of patients with systemic lupus erythematosus: I. Dysfunction of suppressor T-cell activity related to impaired generation of rather than response to suppressor cells. Arth Rheum 21: 657-664
Segerberg-Konttinen M, Bergroth V, Jungell P, Malmstrom M, Nordstrom D, Sane J, Immonen I, Konttinen YT (manuscript submitted) Lymphocytes activation in Sjögren's syndrome
Shoenfeld Y, Schwarz RS (1984) Immunologic and genetic factors in autoimmune diseases. N Engl J Med 311: 119-129

Strand V, Talal N (1980) Advances in the diagnosis and concept of Sjögren's syndrome (autoimmune exocrinopathy). Bull Rheum Dis 30: 1046-1052

Talal N (1985) Endocrine, viral and genetic factors in autoimmune diseases. Immunopath and Immunother Letters 1 (4): 3-5

Talal N, Asofsky R, Lightbody P (1970) Immunoglobulin synthesis by salivary gland lymphoid cells in Sjögren's syndrome. J Clin Invest 49: 49

Talal N, Sylvester R, Greenspan J et al (1974) T- and B-lymphocytes in peripheral blood and tissue lesions in Sjögren's syndrome. J Clin Invest 53: 180-190

Talal N (1976) Disordered immunologic regularion and autoimmunity. Transplant Rev 31: 240-263

Tannbenbraum H, Pinkus G, Anderson L et al (1975)Immunologic characterization of the mononuclear cell infiltrates in RA synovia and in lip biopsies from patients with Sjögren's syndrome. Arth Rheum 18: 305-314

Van Boxel J, Hardin JA, Green I, Paul WE (1973) Multiple heavy chain determinants on B-lymphocytes in Sjögren's syndrome. N Eng J Med 289: 823-826

Yu D, McCune J, Fu K et al (1980) Two types of Ia-positive T-cells, J Exp Med 152: 895-903

6. Animal Models of Sjögren's Syndrome*

R. W. HOFFMAN and S. E. WALKER

Abbreviations

CFA Complete Freund's Adjuvant; *NZB* New Zealand Black; *NZW* New Zealand White.

Sjögren's syndrome was first recognized by Henrich Sjögren (1933) as the triad of keratoconjunctivitis sicca, xerostomia and rheumatoid arthritis. Based upon unique clinical, immunologic and genetic features, two distinct forms of Sjögren's syndrome, primary and secondary, have since been recognized (Bloch et al. 1965; Fox et al. 1984; Moutsopoulos et al. 1980). The primary form is keratoconjunctivitis sicca associated with xerostomia, whereas secondary Sjögren's syndrome is the triad of keratoconjunctivitis sicca, xerostomia and a connective tissue disease (Fox et al. 1984; Kaplinsky et al. 1980; McAdam et al. 1976; Whaley and Alspaugh 1985). Sjögren's syndrome is of interest because it is a common autoimmune disease with significant morbidity (Moutsopoulos et al. 1980). Although extensive studies have provided a large body of information concerning autoantibody production, immune complexes, immunoregulation and immunogenetics, the etiology of Sjögren's syndrome is not known. Appropriate animal models could greatly advance our understanding of the pathogenesis and treatment of this disorder.

Characteristics of Ideal Animal Models of Sjögren's Syndrome

In the past three decades, a number of investigators have examined models of Sjögren's syndrome which might exhibit clinical, pathologic and immunologic features similar to human disease. The ideal animal model should have the clinical hallmarks of dry eyes and dry mouth, and the lacrimal and salivary glands should have mononuclear inflammatory cell infiltration with destruction of normal ductal epithelium and epimyoepithelial island formation. Typical serologic abnormalities such as hyperglobulinemia, antinuclear antibodies, antibodies to extractable nuclear antigens SS-A (Ro) and SS-B (La), and rheumatoid factor should be present.

* Supported by the Medical Research Service of the Veterans Administration and grant 2R01 AM25868 from the National Institutes of Health, U.S. Public Health Service.

Induction of Experimental Sialoadenitis

Investigators have taken several approaches to develop experimental Sjögren's syndrome. A variety of animals have been injected with salivary gland extracts in complete Freund's adjuvant in an attempt to induce experimental sialoadenitis, rats sensitized with foreign protein have been challenged with antigens instilled into the parotid duct, and rats and mice have been injected with antisera raised in rabbits immunized with salivary glands or saliva. Most of these studies, performed prior to recent advances in cellular immunology, did not explore basic mechanisms of autoimmune sialoadenitis. Recent reports of mice with chronic graft-versus-host disease, however, suggested that salivary gland inflammation could be induced as part of a generalized autoimmune diathesis.

Adjuvant Models

Adjuvant models of Sjögren's syndrome are described in Table 1.

Beutner and colleagues (1961) attempted to produce sialoadenitis by injecting New Zealand White rabbits with saline extracts of rabbit submaxillary salivary

Table 1. Adjuvant models of experimental sialoadenitis

Animal	Substances injected	Results	Reference
Rabbits	Submax + CFA	Produced antibodies, no sialoadenitis	Beutner et al. 1961
Cat	Parotid + CFA	Dose-related sialoadenitis	McCabe 1961
Guinea pig	Submax + CFA	Sialoadenitis in treated and control animals; inflammation probably nonspecific	Chan 1964; Kurata et al. 1969
Guinea Pig	Adjuvants (carbonyl iron, Bortadella pertussus vaccine)	Focal areas of inflammation	Whaley and MacSween 1974
Rats	Submax + CFA + Bortadella pertussus vaccine	Sialoadenitis severe if mature female donated submax; T cell depletion decreased sialoadenitis	Sharawy and White 1978; White and Casarett 1974; White 1976
Rats	Submax + CFA	Sialoadenitis; immunoflourescence of duct cell cytoplasm	Dean and Hiramoto 1984
Mice (thymectomized)	Submax + CFA	Thy 1.2$^+$, Lyt 2$^+$ cells infiltrated submax and parotid	Hayashi 1985
Mice	Salivary gland + CFA	Autoimmune SL/Ni strain developed severe sialodenitis	Takeda and Ishikawa 1983

gland in complete Freund's adjuvant. This early attempt to induce sialoadenitis did not succeed; inflammatory changes were not found in submaxillary glands of the recipients. However, circulating antibodies were induced. Sera from 3 of 7 injected animals fixed complement in the presence of rabbit submaxillary gland extract, and sera from 6 animals agglutinated tanned red blood cells coated with rabbit "submaxillary globulin".

In a series of similar experiments, McCabe (1961) demonstrated that repeated injections of cat parotid gland in complete Freund's adjuvant produced pathological changes characteristic of Sjögren's syndrome in cats. In one animal which received a single injection of extract, parotid tissue contained a small focus of lymphocytes and an epimyoepithelial island. Cats receiving at least 4 injections had progressively more severe parotid inflammation. All 10 immunized animals were hyperglobulinemic, possibly due to the nonspecific effect of repeated immunization, but circulating antibodies to parotid tissue were not demonstrated in a hemagglutination assay. Adjuvant-injected control animals had no sialoadenitis or hyperglobulinemia.

A number of early experiments revealed the limitations of adjuvant-induced sialoadenitis in guinea pigs. Treated animals usually developed minor inflammatory changes which were not specific for lacrimal and salivary glands, and epimyoepithelial islands were not present. Inflammation bore no relationship to the immunization schedule; in some instances, infiltrates were found in animals injected with adjuvant alone.

Chan (1964) attempted to produce experimental autoimmune sialoadenitis by injecting guinea pigs with homogenized guinea pig submaxillary glands in phenol-saline mixed with complete Freund's adjuvant. Fourteen of 30 immunized animals developed sialoadenitis in at least one salivary gland. The pathologic lesions, which resembled Sjögren's syndrome, consisted of inflammatory mononuclear cell infiltration of ducts and acini. However, epimyoepithelial island formation was absent. In this model, severity of the lesions was not related to number of immunizations or the time interval following immunization. Sialoadenitis was found in submaxillary glands from two control animals injected only with complete Freund's adjuvant; therefore, injecting salivary gland plus adjuvant may have produced a nonspecific inflammatory response.

In a separate series of experiments, syngeneic and allogeneic salivary gland lipoprotein extracts plus complete Freund's adjuvant were injected into guinea pigs and controls received extracts of xenogeneic organs other than salivary glands (rabbit or human liver, pancreas, kidney, spleen, adrenal or thyroid). Sixteen of 25 recipients developed focal periductal lymphocytic infiltrates in the parotid and lacrimal glands, but submaxillary glands were spared. Scattered lymphocytic infiltrates were also found in the kidney, testis, adrenal, thyroid and liver of the experimental group. No lesions were found in control animals (Kurata et al. 1969).

In a subsequent study, Whaley and MacSween (1974) produced sialoadenitis in guinea pigs injected with a variety of adjuvants (complete Freund's adjuvant, carbonyl iron, Bortadella pertussis vaccine) alone or in combination. The affected glands were characterized pathologically by focal periductal mononuclear cell infiltration of glandular tissue without epimyoepithelial island formation. Injections of salivary gland extract in complete Freund's adjuvant, however, did not produce inflammatory changes.

T lymphocytes participate in induction of inflammation in the rat adjuvant model (Sharawy and White 1978; White and Casarett 1974). Lewis rats immunized with a saline extract of allogenic submaxillary tissue in complete Freund's adjuvant and injected with Bordetella pertussis vaccine at the time of immunization developed sialoadenitis. Severity of lesions was influenced by age and sex of donor rats. Extracts from mature female rats produced multiple inflammatory lesions characterized by foci of mononuclear inflammatory cells adjacent to ducts without destruction of epithelium. Extracts from males and immature animals produced a milder form of sialoadenitis. Abnormalities were not present in other salivary glands or lacrimal glands. Rats which were made T cell deficient by thymectomy, whole body irradiation and reconstitution with syngeneic bone marrow cells had decreased occurrence of experimental sialoadenitis (12% in T cell deficient mice versus 80% in sham-thymectomized controls). However, passive transfer of disease could not be accomplished with serum or lymph node cells (White 1976).

In a more recent study, Dean and Hiramoto (1984) produced inflammation in submaxillary, parotid, lacrimal and harderian glands of Wistar rats by injecting homogenized syngeneic submaxillary and sublingual glands in complete Freund's adjuvant (Fig. 1). Sera from experimental rats and from controls injected with adjuvant alone were tested by indirect immunofluorescence on a series of organs including rat salivary glands. Fluorescence was noted in cytoplasm of salivary duct cells, but this reactivity did not correlate with the presence of sialoadenitis.

Hayashi and associates (1985) emphasized the role of T lymphocytes in adjuvant-induced sialoadenitis in mice. Sialoadenitis was induced in CRJ mice thymectomized three days after birth and immunized with syngeneic submaxillary salivary

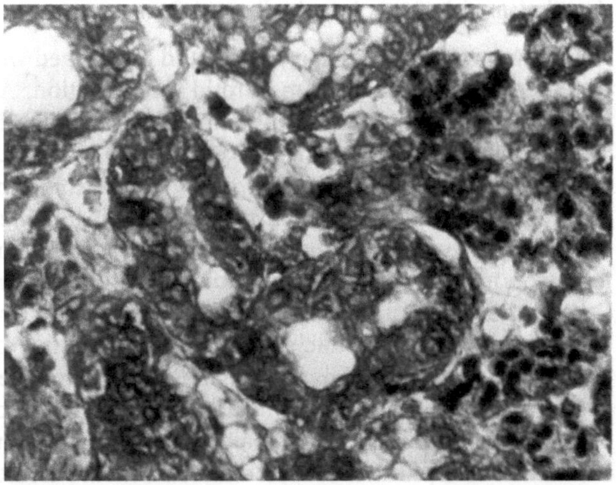

Fig. 1. Submandibular gland of a rat 14 days after injections of submandibular salivary gland plus complete Freund's adjuvant and Bortadella pertussis vaccine. The acini and granular tubules are disrupted and replaced by duct-like structures and mononuclear cell infiltrate (phosphotungstic acidhematoxylin, X 400). Photograph generously supplied by D. H. Dean, D. D. S., M. S.

glands emulsified in complete Freund's adjuvant. Inflammatory lesions, localized specifically to the submaxillary and parotid glands, were composed predominantly of small and medium lymphocytes which expressed Thy 1.2 and Lyt 2 cell surface antigens. In later stages of disease, scattered IgG-bearing cells appeared in the periphery of inflammatory lesions. Based upon these findings, the authors postulated that a population of Lyt 2^+ (suppressor/cytotoxic) cells mediated inflammation in salivary glands.

Takeda and Ishikawa (1983) studied the SL/Ni mouse strain, which spontaneously develops systemic lupus erythematosus-like illness with vasculitis, glomerulonephritis, and lymphoid infiltration in the salivary glands (Takeda et al. 1981). These autoimmune animals were unusually susceptible to induction of sialoadenitis. SL/Ni mice immunized with syngeneic salivary gland tissue in complete Freund's adjuvant developed extensive lymphoid infiltration of the submaxillary salivary glands, with proliferation of duct epithelial cells (Takeda and Ishikawa 1983).

Adjuvant models failed to reproduce the histological characteristics of Sjögren's syndrome, but they may afford the opportunity to examine factors which induce or protect from sialoadenitis. Work with related models (Ben-Nun and Cohen 1982; Holoshitz et al. 1983; Maron et al. 1983; Naparstek et al. 1983) suggested that specific lines of effector T lymphocytes, generated *in vitro* and injected into rats, specifically mediated encephalomyelitis, thyroiditis or arthritis depending upon the antigen used to generate the cell line. The same cell lines prevented later induction of adjuvant disease. For example, "arthritogenic" lymphocytes isolated from Lewis rats immunized with complete Freund's adjuvant produced transient arthritis in irradiated recipients, but the same rats were protected from subsequent induction of adjuvant arthritis (Holoshitz et al. 1983).

Instillation of Antigens into the Parotid Duct

Rats immunized with foreign protein and challenged with antigen instilled directly into the parotid duct develop parotid inflammation. A number of antigens have been used to produce gland inflammation, including human plasma (Sela et al. 1972), bovine serum albumin (Boss et al. 1977; Sela et al. 1973; Sela et al. 1975) and bovine gamma globulin (Sela et al. 1975). In some instances, sialoadenitis was induced by instilling xenogeneic protein directly into the parotid duct without prior systemic sensitization (Ulmansky et al. 1972). The pathologic findings in chronic lesions induced by multiple injections of antigen resembled Sjögren's syndrome. Parotid tissue contained atrophy of the glandular parenchyma, intralobular duct ectasia and dense mononuclear infiltration consisting of lymphocytes, histiocytes and plasma cells. No epimyoepithelial islands were noted (Boss et al. 1977).

Subsequent experiments did not determine clearly if local inflammation or a true autoimmune response was the major cause of parotid inflammation in this model. Instillation of nephrotoxic rabbit antiserum to rat basement membrane into the cannulated parotid duct produced acute necrotizing sialoadenitis and vasculitis. It was postulated that *in situ* reaction between the exogenous antibodies and tissue antigens produced parotid inflammation (Rosenmann et al. 1974). Finding immunoglobulin deposits in parotid glands of rats with sialoadenitis induced by intraductal antigen supported the theory that antibody played a role in the pathogenesis of inflammation. Attempts to produce acute sialoadenitis with preformed immune complexes placed in the parotid duct, however, produced acute acinar necrosis which did not resemble Sjögren's syndrome (Dishon et al. 1973).

Antisera to Salivary Glands or Saliva

Haferkamp (1962) gave rats intravenous injections of globulin fractions of rabbit antisera to rat lacrimal and salivary glands. Deposits of immunoglobulins were identified in acinar tissue and secretory ducts of parotid glands in recipients. If these animals received subsequent injections of antigen or foreign protein, widespread destructive changes appeared in lacrimal glands and parotid and submaxillary salivary glands.

Ichikawa et al. (1982) immunized Japanese white rabbits with Sephadex-G200-separated fractions of rat submaxillary glands. Sera from the immunized rabbits, which reacted with cell membranes, nuclear membranes and duct material in rat submaxillary glands by indirect immunofluorescent testing, was injected intraperitoneally into normal rats. Seven days later, submaxillary glands, livers and kidneys from the recipients contained scattered periductal infiltrations of mononuclear cells, polymorphonuclear cells and eosinophils. Granular deposits of rabbit gamma globulin were found by immunoflourescence in cytoplasm of infiltrating inflammatory cells and in the walls of small vessels surrounding salivary gland acini. Because the inflammatory changes and immunoglobulin deposits were nonspecific, it was suggested that lesions were caused by circulating immune complexes formed by non-organ specific antibodies contaminating the antiserum.

Weill and Goldberg (1976) found that CVA mice injected with heterologous antisera against fractionated mouse saliva developed ultrastructural cytolysis in submaxillary acinar cells, with disappearance of rough endoplasmic reticulum and dissociation of Golgi apparatus. Examination of salivary tissue by light and transmission electron microscopy showed no evidence of inflammation. No abnormalities were detected in control mice injected with normal rabbit sera or crude rabbit anti-mouse immune globulin.

Graft-versus-host Disease

In chronic graft-versus-host disease, immune complex deposits and salivary gland inflammation are induced in strains of mice which are not predisposed genetically to develop autoimmunity. Nonirradiated B10 X DBA/2 F_1 mice injected with DBA/2 spleen cells developed B cell activation, with excessive production of IgG and multiple antibodies directed preferentially against self antigens (Pals et al. 1984; Van Rappard-Van der Veen et al. 1984). Disease in these mice resembled systemic lupus erythematosus, with antibodies to DNA, lymphoid hyperplasia, periarteritis and glomerulonephritis (Gleichmann et al. 1982). Periductal lymphoid infiltrates developed in salivary glands and liver, and perivascular lymphoid infiltrates were found in salivary glands, liver, kidney and lung (Pals et al. 1984). The finding of salivary gland inflammation in murine graft-versus-host disease was of interest in view of the description of Sjögren's syndrome-like disease in humans undergoing chronic graft-versus-host reaction following allogeneic bone marrow transplantation (Gratwhol et al. 1977; Lawley et al. 1977; Shulman et al. 1978).

Viral Sialodacryoadenitis in the Rat

Infection with a specific corona virus (Kojima et al. 1980) causes swelling of the neck, ophthalmic lesions, and hypersecretion of porphyrin-stained tears in rats (Innes and Stanton 1961). Beginning 4-5 days after exposure to the virus, lacrimal glands of affected rats develop necrosis of ductal epithelial cells, interstitial edema and infiltrates of histiocytes, lymphocytes and polymorphonuclear leukocytes. Viral particles have been identified by electron microscopy in ductal epithelial lining cells (Jonas et al. 1969). Inflammatory lesions occur less commonly in the submaxillary and parotid salivary glands (Fig. 2). Inflammation of the glands is usually self-limited (Eisenbrandt et al. 1982; Jonas et al. 1969). In some instances, infection with sialodacryoadenitis virus may lead to residual inflammation of the lacrimal glands. Chronic disease has also been identified in the harderian glands, which are accessary lacrimal glands occupying much of the orbit deep to the eyeball in rats and mice (Bellhorn 1981; Innes and Stanton 1961). These chronic lesions resemble Sjögren's syndrome. A recent description of subclinical disease in young Sprague-Dawley rats documented chronic dacryoadenitis with multilobular atrophy of alveolar tissue 20-38 days after exposure to the virus (Fig. 3) (Eisenbrandt et al. 1982). Decreased tear formation in infected animals commonly results in keratoconjunctivitis (Lai et al. 1976).

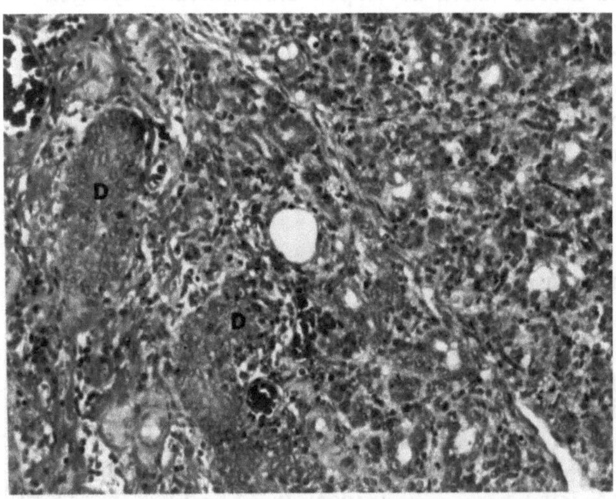

Fig. 2. Acute viral sialodacryoadenitis involving the parotid salivary gland in the rat. Degenerating acinar cells are infiltrated with lymphocytes, macrophages and plasma cells. Squamous metaplasia of duct epithelium is noted (D) (hematoxylin and eosin, X 215). Photograph supplied through the courtesy of David L. Eisenbrandt, D. V. M., Ph. D., and reprinted with permission from Lab Anim Sci 32: 655-659, 1982

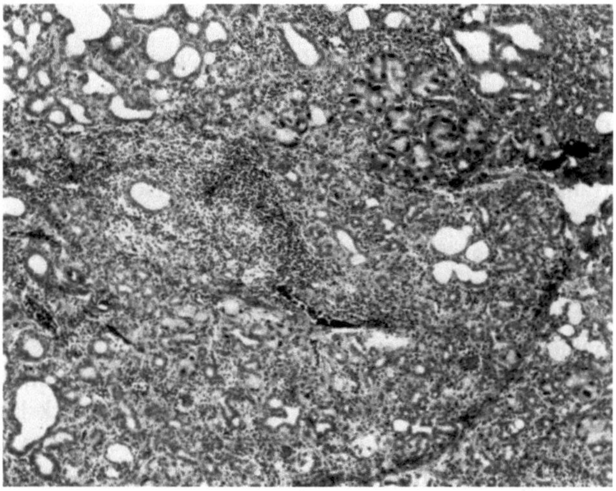

Fig. 3. Chronic lesions of viral sialodacryoadenitis. Involvement of the intraorbital lacrimal gland is characterized by infiltration of inflammatory cells as well as degenerative and atrophic changes in acinar cells (hematoxylin and eosin, X 82). Photograph supplied by David L. Eisenbrandt, D.V.M., Ph.D.

Sialoadenitis in Murine Models of Autoimmunity

Many spontaneous disorders in mice have been recognized as important models for the study of autoimmune disease. Strains of mice have been described with autoimmune hemolytic anemia (Bielschowsky et al. 1959), systemic lupus erythematosus (Howie and Helyer 1968) and rheumatoid arthritis (Hang et al. 1982; O'Sullivan et al. 1985).

Because features of Sjögren's syndrome are common in patients with systemic lupus erythematosus (Moutsopoulos et al. 1980; Ramos-Niembro and Alarcon-Segovia, 1979), mice with lupus-like diseases might be expected to have features of Sjögren's syndrome. A number of careful studies have confirmed that inflammation of lacrimal and salivary glands is common in mice with lupus, including NZB, NZB/NZW (Kessler 1968) and the MRL substrains (Hoffman et al. 1984). Severity of inflammation in autoimmune strains is summarized in Table 2. These abnormalities, however, are uncommon in normal mice (Hoffman et al. 1984).

Table 2. Sjögren's syndrome in autoimmune mice (Kessler 1968; Kessler et al. 1971; Hoffman et al. 1984)

	Conjunctivitis	Lacrimal Gland Inflammation	Salivary Gland Inflammation
NZB	Yes	Mild	Mild
NZB/NZW	Yes	Moderate	Moderate
MRL/l	Yes	Severe	Severe
MRL/n	Yes	Severe	Severe

Autoimmune Strains of Mice

Immune mediated hemolytic anemia was recognized in the New Zealand Black (NZB) mouse by Bielschowsky et al. (1959) as the first spontaneous autoimmune disease in an animal model. This strain also develops membranous glomerulonephritis (Howie and Helyer 1968) and lymphoid hyperplasia which may progress to frank lymphoid malignancy (East 1970). Howie and Helyer (1965) recognized that F_1 NZB/NZW offspring of NZB crossed with the New Zealand White (NZW) strain (Hahn and Shulman 1969; Kelley and Winkelstein 1980) developed illness resembling systemic lupus erythematosus.

MRL/l mice, which are homozygous for the lpr gene, develop accelerated autoimmune disease characterized by massive lymph node proliferation, hyperglobulinemia, antibodies to DNA and Sm, rheumatoid factor, vasculitis and glomerulonephritis. Mice of the MRL/n substrain, which lack lpr/lpr and do not develop lymphadenopathy, develop mild lupus-like disease with low levels of anti-DNA antibodies and late-onset glomerulonephritis (Andrews et al. 1978; Murphy 1981; Theofilopoulos et al. 1980; Theofilopoulos and Dixon 1985).

Abnormalities of Harderian, Lacrimal and Salivary Glands in Autoimmune Mice

Kessler (1968, 1971) was the first investigator to describe spontaneous changes of Sjögren's syndrome in NZB and NZB/NZW mice. Modified Schirmer tests in 6 NZB/NZW mice were compared to 6 control NZW mice; in NZB/NZW hybrids, mean wetting was 3.1 mm/2 minutes and in NZW mice wetting was 4.8 mm. Slit lamp biomicroscopic examinations were not successful due to the small size and extreme curvature of mouse eyes (Kessler HS, personal communication). The amylase content of saliva from NZB and NZB/NZW mice was less than half the content in NZW controls. Salivary protein was higher in NZB/NZW mice compared to NZW mice, and levels of sodium, potassium and chloride were similar in both groups of animals.

Conjunctivae from NZB/NZW mice showed increased numbers of goblet cells, epithelial cell sloughing and increased keratin granules, whereas the cornea was edematous and irregular. Round cells infiltrated the vitreous and anterior chamber. Some NZB/NZW mice had posterior synechiae of the iris.

Harderian, lacrimal and salivary glands from NZB mice and NZB/NZW mice aged 2 to 15 months were examined. Periductal and perivascular mononuclear cell infiltrates were observed in virtually every animal after 4 months of age. The cellular infiltrates consisted mainly of small lymphocytes, plasma cells and reticulum cells. Epimyoepithelial island formation was present. Figure 4 illustrates a typical lesion in the lacrimal gland of a NZB mouse. Inflammation was most severe in lacrimal glands, and infiltrates were typically smaller and fewer in number within the harderian glands. Lesions were less extensive in the salivary glands. Decreasing grades of involvement were observed in parotid, submaxillary and sublingual glands. Mononuclear infiltrates increased with age and were more pronounced in females compared to males. NZB mice had in general less extensive glandular lesions than NZB/NZW hybrids. These reports, which have been cited extensively, established NZB/NZW mice as a model of Sjögren's syndrome (Kessler 1968; Kessler et al. 1971).

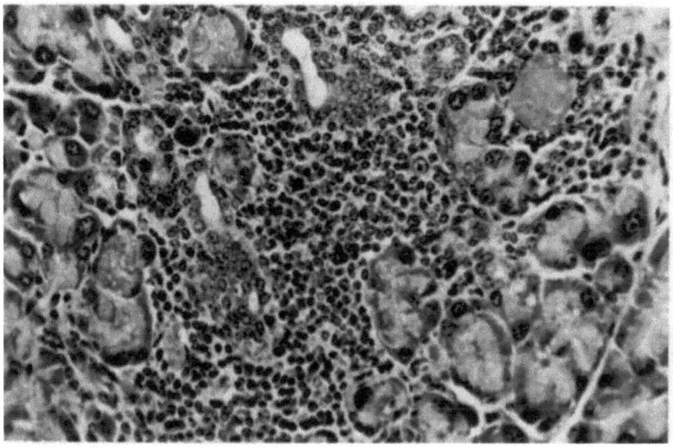

Fig. 4. A dense mononuclear cell infiltrate localized around two ducts in the lacrimal gland of an 8-month-old NZB male (hematoxylin and eosin, approximate original magnification X 250). This photograph, from the original collection of Harry S. Kessler, D. D. S., was made available through the generosity of his heirs

Greenspan et al. (1974) extended the observations of Kessler to examine populations of cells infiltrating salivary glands in NZB/NZW mice. The earliest abnormalities were observed in the submaxillary glands. Immunoglobulin-positive lymphocytes and plasma cells appeared around blood vessels related to medium sized intralobular ducts. As the infiltrates expanded, acini degenerated and the ducts became surrounded by inflammatory cells and underwent mild degenerative changes. Later in the course of disease, larger infiltrates were found; the majority of cells in these foci stained with anti-mouse thymocyte serum.

Keyes and associates (1977) were the first to note the orderly progression of cellular infiltration in NZB/NZW mice. Early lacrimal gland involvement was followed by submaxillary and parotid gland inflammation, and invading cells were centered predominantly around ducts and blood vessels. In accord with the report of Kessler (1971), structures resembling epimyoepithelial islands were found. Control CBA/Ht6 mice in this study lacked glandular inflammation.

Carlsoo and Ostberg (1978, 1979) carried out the first ultrastructural studies of NZB/NZW submaxillary and parotid glands. They reported mononuclear cells infiltrating glandular tissue adjacent to ducts and vessels, with invasion of acinar and intercalated duct cells. The infiltrates consisted primarily of lymphocytes with occasional histiocytes and plasma cells. Some acinar and duct cells were lysed, whereas others appeared damaged and contained cytoplasmic vacuoles and vesiculated endoplasmic reticulum. There was no epimyoepithelial cell proliferation, and it was concluded that the basic pathologic lesion in NZB/NZW submaxillary and parotid glands was vasculitis.

Our studies of Sjögren's syndrome in autoimmune mice employed large numbers of NZB and NZB/NZW mice and normal C57BL/6J and DBA/2 controls to extend earlier descriptions and to permit comparison between strains (Hoffman et al. 1984). We confirmed the results of Kessler (1971) showing ocular dryness in NZB/NZW mice. Tear flow was diminished significantly in autoimmune NZB/NZW mice compared to control C57BL/6J and DBA/2 mice (Hoffman et al. 1984).

Histological evidence of conjunctivitis was present in 71% of NZB and 26% of NZB/NZW mice but not in nonautoimmune control strains. Several New Zealand mice had corneal epithelial thinning with epithelial cell sloughing, but these changes were also present in nonautoimmune controls. The remainder of the eyes were unremarkable except for occasional cataracts (Hoffman et al. 1984).

In our comparative study, lacrimal glands had the most severe inflammatory changes. Submaxillary, parotid and sublinguial salivary glands were involved with diminishing severity. Inflammation was present in 85% of NZB and 57% of NZB/NZW lacrimal glands, while 32% of NZB and 40% of NZB/NZW submaxillary glands were affected. In contrast to the report of Kessler and associates (1971), we found that salivary gland inflammation in NZB mice was more severe compared to NZB/NZW mice. The NZB mice in our study were older than the mice studied by Kessler (1971), and we felt our results reflected progression of infiltrates in aging animals. We did not find epimyoepithelial islands in glands from New Zealand mice. After examining serial sections of salivary glands, we concluded that cross sections through the end of an acinar duct resembled hyperplasia of ductal cells; these structures might be mistaken for epimyoepithelial islands.

MRL mice were, to our knowledge, first mentioned as a potential model of Sjögren's syndrome by Huston and Steinberg (1979). Recently, Hang and associates (1982) reported that 60% of MRL/l mice had periductal mononuclear inflammatory cell infiltrates in salivary glands. The inflammation was felt to be nonspecific because involvement of salivary glands did not correlate with presence or absence of rheumatoid-like polyarthritis. Furthermore, similar patterns of inflammation were present in lungs and kidneys of MRL/l and MRL/n mice.

We recently reported an extensive study of features of Sjögren's syndrome in MRL/l and MRL/n mice and normal controls (Hoffman et al. 1983; Hoffman et al. 1984). Ocular pathology was common in the MRL substrains. We found band keratopathy and posterior uveitis (Hoffman et al. 1983). Conjunctivitis, involving the bulbar and palpebral conjunctiva, was associated with inflammation of adjacent sebaceous glands (Fig. 5) (Hoffman et al. 1984). Sialoadenitis in MRL mice was similar to the inflammatory changes in New Zealand mice, but the MRL substrains had more severe lesions. Detailed grading of cellular infiltrates revealed a predictable pattern of inflammation, with preferential involvement of salivary and lacrimal glands and minimal lesions in lungs and kidneys. We postulate that the infiltrates were directed specifically at gland target organs. Sialoadenitis of the lacrimal glands was found in 50% of MRL/l and 90% of MRL/n mice; 86% of MRL/l and 94% of MRL/n mice had sialoadenitis involving the submaxillary salivary glands. Infiltration of parotid and sublinguial glands occurred less frequently.

Inflammation in lacrimal and salivary glands of MRL/l and MRL/n mice was characterized by large multifocal confluent infiltrates of lymphocytes, with occasional histiocytes and plasma cells. Perivascular and periductal aggregates of cells infiltrated and led to focal destruction of secretory alveoli. Epimyoepithelial island formation was not present. Typical lesions in lacrimal glands are shown in Figs. 6 and 7. Figure 8 illustrates mononuclear infiltration of the submaxillary gland of a MRL/l female. Transmission electron microscopy identified infiltrating cells in lacrimal glands as predominantly lymphocytes (Fig. 9). Numerous lymphoblasts were present and the glandular architecture was almost completely destroyed by the

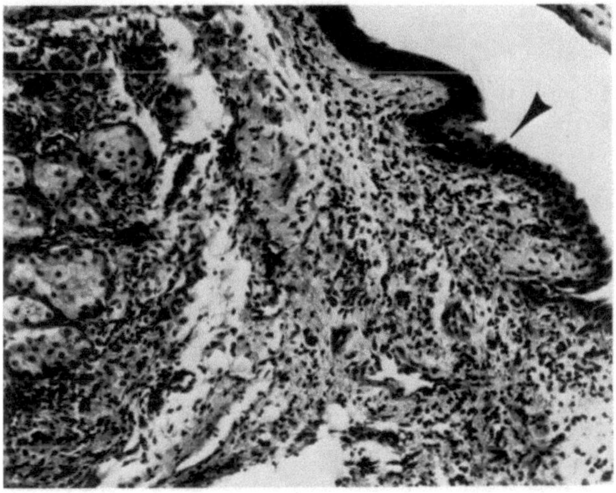

Fig. 5. Severe inflammation in a section through the superior palpebral conjunctiva of a female MRL/n mouse aged 9 months. Overlying epithelium (arrow) is hyperplastic. Conjunctival tissue contains diffuse infiltrates of mononuclear and polymorphonuclear cells. On the left, the sebaceous glands are infiltrated with inflammatory cells (hematoxylin and eosin, original magnification X 100). Reprinted with permission from Arthritis Rheum 27: 157-165, 1984

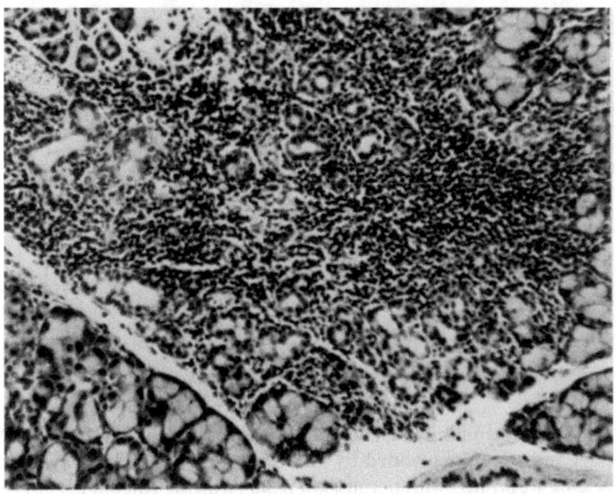

Fig. 6. A characteristic lesion in the lacrimal gland of a MRL/l male aged 4 months. Mononuclear cells infiltrate the adjacent parenchyma, resulting in focal destruction of secretory alveoli (hematoxylin and eosin, original magnification X 250). Reprinted with permission from Arthritis Rheum 27: 157-165, 1984

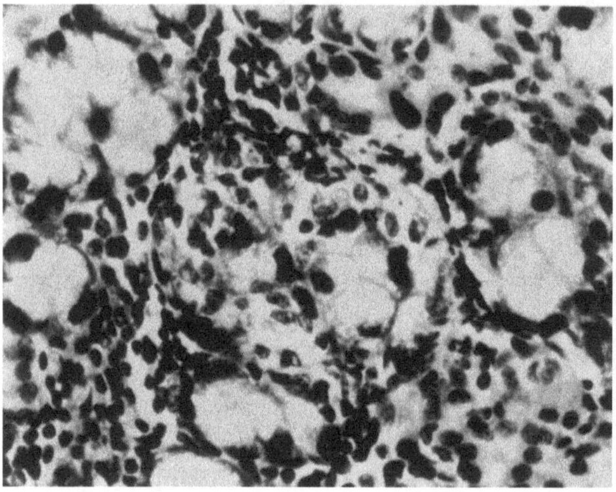

Fig. 7. Lacrimal gland tissue from a female MRL/l mouse 4 months of age, with infiltration and destruction of acini by inflammatory cells (hematoxylin and eosin, original magnification X 400)

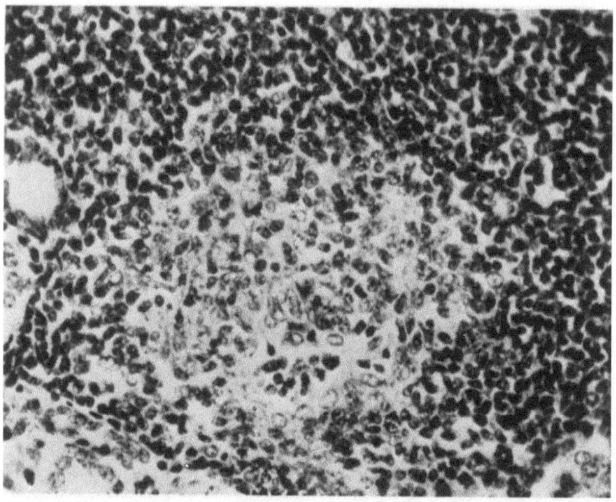

Fig. 8. Submandibular gland infiltrated with mononuclear cells, 9-month-old MRL/l female. A duct and acini are invaded by inflammatory cells (hematoxylin and eosin, original magnification X 250). Reprinted with permission from Arthritis Rheum 27: 157-165, 1984

invasive nature of these cells. No viruses or tubuloreticular structures were identified (Hoffman et al. 1984).

Antibodies to the extractable nuclear antigens SS-A and SS-B occur frequently in Sjögren's syndrome and may play a role in the pathogenesis of the disease (Whaley and Alspaugh 1985). For these reasons, sera from 10 male and 10 female NZB, NZB/NZW, MRL/l and MRL/n mice were examined for antibodies to SS-A and SS-B using the Ouchterlony technique. Immunoprecipitation was not detected with this relatively insensitive assay (Hoffman et al. 1984).

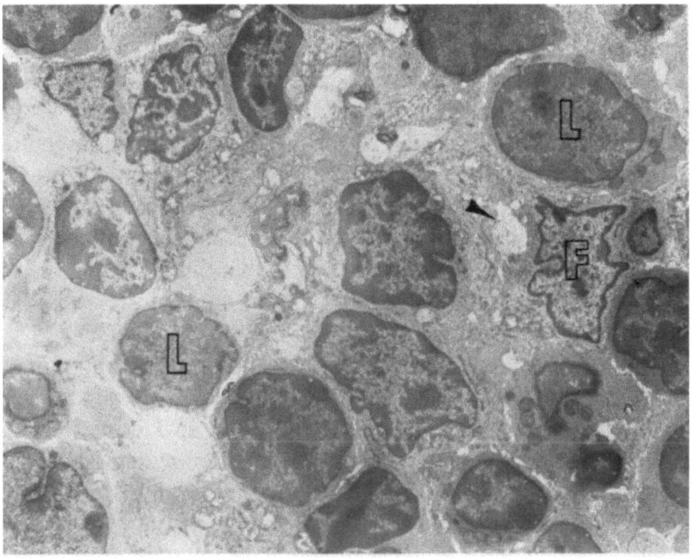

Fig. 9. Electron micrograph of lacrimal gland from a female MRL/n mouse. Architecture of the gland has been destroyed by infiltration of lymphocytes (L). Prominent endoplasmic reticulum, prominent Golgi apparatus and cytoplasmic extension identify these cells as transformed lymphocytes. A fibroblast (F) appears to be laying down collagen (arrow) (transmission electron microscopy, original magnification X 3,300). Reprinted with permission from Arthritis Rheum 27: 157-165, 1984

Autoimmune mice are promising models for studies of the pathogenesis and treatment of Sjögren's syndrome. In humans, monoclonal antibodies have been used to identify infiltrating cells in labial biopsies of patients with Sjögren's syndrome as predominantly OKT4-positive (helper-inducer) lymphocytes (Fox et al. 1982). It would be of interest to study autoimmune mice using monoclonal lymphocyte surface markers to determine if similar subsets of T lymphocytes infiltrate lacrimal and salivary glands. Murine models could also be used to evaluate therapeutic agents such as immunosuppresive drugs and monoclonal antibodies directed against lymphocyte surface antigens.

Therapy of Sialoadenitis in Autoimmune Mice

Therapy of Sjögren's syndrome with immune modulating substances has been tested in autoimmune mice. Bach and associates (1980) found diminished 99-Technetium uptake in submaxillary glands of NZB/NZW mice compared to nonautoimmune controls. The abnormal salivary scintigraphy was felt to reflect Sjögren's syndrome. Synthesized T cell-stimulating serum thymic factor ("facteur thymic serique") was administered to 6-week-old NZB/NZW females. After 20 weeks of treatment, uptake of 99-Technetium over the submaxillary glands returned to normal. Long-term therapy with the thymic factor was associated with 93% incidence of renal amyloidosis; this complication was attributed to the use of carboxymethylcellulose as a vehicle for injection. A group of NZB mice received facteur thymique serique beginning of 33 weeks of age. Ten weeks later, scintigraphic examination showed modest increases of radioisotope uptake. It was concluded that thymic factor prevented Sjögren's syndrome, but prolonged therapy was potentially hazardous.

Schot et al. (1984) described the use of a weakly androgenic steroid, nandrolone decanoate, in NZB/NZW female mice and castrated male mice. Treatment with 2.5-40 mg/kg given subcutaneously every third week for 9 months reduced significantly the number and total area of mononuclear cell infiltrates in submaxillary glands compared to untreated control mice. It was suggested that the therapeutic efficacy and weak virilizing properties of nandrolone decanoate might promote its use in treating human Sjögren's syndrome.

In summary, New Zealand mice, the prototypes of spontaneous autoimmune disease, were the first murine models of Sjögren's syndrome. They have dry eyes, conjunctivitis and mononuclear cell infiltrates in lacrimal and salivary glands. An important marker of Sjögren's syndrome, epimyoepithelial island formation, has been reported in NZB/NZW mice although examination at the ultrastructual level failed to confirm this observation. Recently, new strains of autoimmune mice have been described and studied as potential new models of Sjögren's syndrome. MRL/l and MRL/n mice, which exhibit severe inflammatory cell infiltration and destruction of lacrimal and salivary glands, afford opportunities for continued exploration of the pathogenesis and therapy of Sjögren's syndrome.

Sjögren's Syndrome in Dogs

A large number of autoimmune diseases have been reported in dogs, including Sjögren's syndrome, systemic lupus erythematosus, rheumatoid arthritis, polyarthritis, autoimmune hemolytic anemia and immune mediated thrombocytopenia (reviewed in Halliwell 1978; Halliwell 1982; Lewis 1974).

Plasmacytic Conjunctivitis

German shepherds raised in areas of high exposure to sunlight may develop plasmacytic conjunctivitis. This lesion is characterized by inflammation and thickening of the nictitating membrane which often progresses to superficial keratitis. Affected dogs usually present with epiphora or normal tear flow. Biopsy of the membrane reveals dense subconjunctival infiltration of plasma cells (Teichert 1966; Kaswan RL, personal communication).

Keratoconjunctivitis Sicca

Keratoconjunctivitis sicca is a common, potentially blinding disorder in dogs which may result from congenital deficiency in tear production (Gelatt and Gwin 1981), trauma (Brightman 1980), canine distemper (Aguirre et al. 1971; Kaswan et al. 1984) or prolonged treatment with sulphonamides (Slatter and Blogg 1978). The lacrimal gland and the seromucous gland of the nictitating membrane are the major sources of tears in the dog (Gelatt et al. 1968). Treatment of prolapse of the nictitating membrane gland by surgical removal may therefore predispose to later development of keratoconjunctivitis sicca, especially if tear production is compromised by another disorder (Gelatt and Gwin 1981).

In a recent study, 13 of 28 dogs with keratoconjunctivitis sicca had no major concurrent disease. These animals are of special interest because they may represent models of primary Sjögren's syndrome in which the gland of the nictitating membrane is readily accessible as a biopsy site (Kaswan et al. 1984) (Fig. 10). Keratoconjunctivitis sicca has also been reported in dogs with immune mediated disorders (polyarthritis, polymyositis, systemic lupus erythematosus, thyroiditis), and it may be assumed that these animals have secondary Sjögren's syndrome (Kaswan et al. 1984; Kaswan et al. 1985) (Fig. 11). Biopsies of nictitating membrane glands and main lacrimal glands in affected dogs yielded lesions typical of Sjögren's syndrome: moderate to severe infiltration with lymphocytes and plasma cells, atrophy of tubular structures, and increased intralobular fibrous connective tissue (Kaswan et al. 1984). These dogs have decreased tear flow in Schirmer's test (Kaswan et al. 1983). Antinuclear antibodies, usually a nucleolar pattern, have been found in 42 percent of dogs with keratoconjunctivitis sicca (Kaswan et al. 1985), and 34% of affected animals had rheumatoid factor detected by the Rose-Waaler test in serum diluted 1:16 or greater (Kaswan et al. 1983). Circulating antibodies to the gland of the nictitating membrane were demonstrated by indirect immunofluorescence in 9 of 31 dogs (Kaswan et al. 1985).

It is apparent that idiopathic keratoconjunctivitis sicca in dogs is often a manifestation of widespread involvement of lacrimal and salivary glands. Ten of 50 dogs with keratoconjunctivitis sicca studied by Kaswan and associates (1983) had peridontitis and apparent xerostomia. Multiple biopsies in a small number of affected

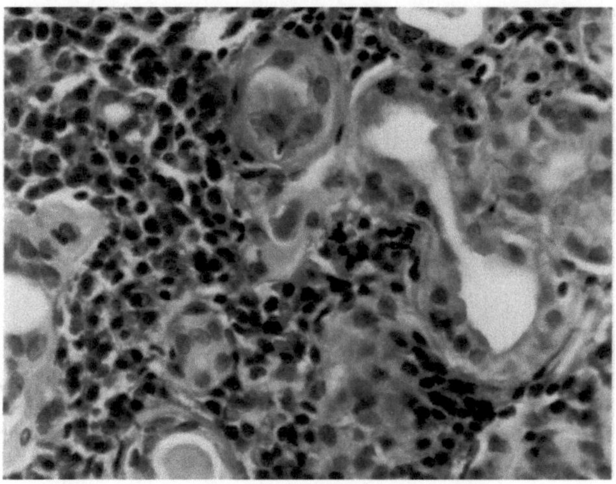

Fig. 10. Lacrimal adenitis in the nictitating membrane gland of a bulldog with idiopathic keratoconjunctivitis sicca. Functional acini are atrophied and replaced with increased amounts of fibrous connective tissue infiltrated with lymphocytes and plasma cells (hematoxylin and eosin, original magnification X 440). Photograph supplied through the courtesy of Renee L. Kaswan, D. V. M., M. S. and reprinted with permission from Am J Vet Res 45: 112–118, 1984

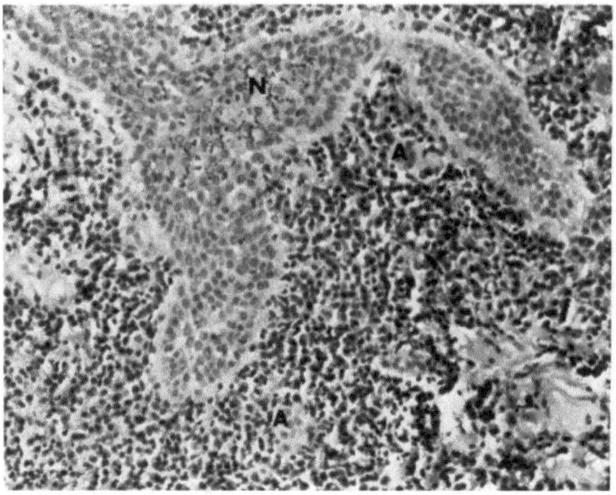

Fig. 11. Advanced inflammatory changes in the nictitating membrane gland of a dog with concurrent lymphocytic thyroiditis. Cords of hyperplastic ductal epithelial cells, which form epithelial islands, are surrounded by dense infiltration of mononuclear cells. Acini (A) are atrophied and sparse. Neutrophils (N) are in a former ductal lumen (hematoxylin and eosin, X 200). Photograph supplied by Renee L. Kaswan, D. V. M., M. S. and reprinted with permission from Am J Vet Res 45: 112-118, 1984

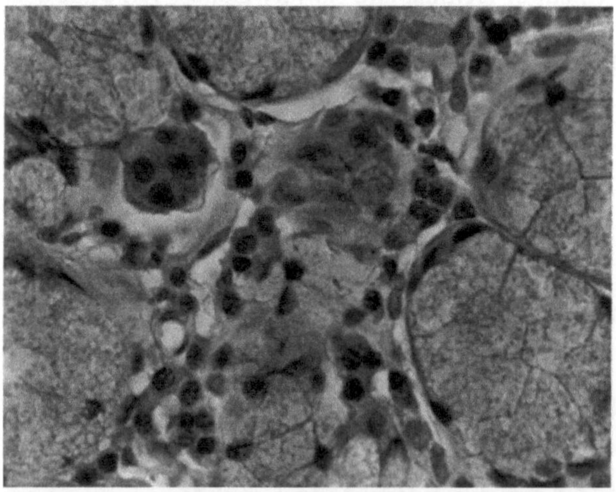

Fig. 12. Focal plasmacytic periacinar infiltrates in labial salivary gland of a dog with keratoconjunctivitis sicca. The biopsy was obtained from the ventral submucosa lateral to the lower premolar (hematoxylin and eosin, original magnification X 400). Photograph supplied by Renee L. Kaswan, D. V. M., M. S. and reprinted with permission from Am J Vet Res 46: 376-383, 1985

dogs revealed lymphocytic infiltrates in 5 of 9 labial salivary specimens (Fig. 12), 2 of 4 parotid glands, 2 of 4 mandibular salivary glands, and 2 of 3 thyroid glands (Kaswan et al. 1985).

Sjögren's Syndrome and Canine Systemic Lupus Erythematosus

Quimby et al. (1979) recognized Sjögren's syndrome in two female poodles from a colony maintained for investigations of systemic lupus erythematosus. One animal developed chronic bilateral conjunctivitis, keratitis, corneal ulceration and recurrent vaginitis at 7 years of age. Tear flow was less than 1 mm/minute (normal 15-30), and the mouth was dry. Laboratory examination revealed LE cells, antinuclear antibodies in serum diluted 1:10 and antibodies to native DNA. Indirect immunofluorescent testing with frozen sections of nictitating membrane revealed antibodies against epithelial cells. A biopsy of the nictitating membrane contained infiltrates of polymorphonuclear leukocytes, histiocytes and small lymphocytes. At necropsy, the lacrimal gland and the mandibular salivary gland had dense mononuclear cell infiltrates. A second dog from the same colony (case 4, Kaswan et al. 1984) developed conjunctivitis, severe keratoconjunctivitis and xerostomia. Schirmer tests revealed wetting of 4-10 mm/minute. This dog had positive tests for LE cells, antinuclear antibodies, anti-microsomal antibodies and antibodies to the nictitating membrane. The nictitating membrane gland was infiltrated with inflammatory cells and a thyroid biopsy contained infiltrating small lymphocytes and plasma cells that often surrounded thyroid epithelial cells.

Sjögren's Syndrome and Canine Polyarthritis

Symmetrical erosive polyarthritis in a dog was reported by Lewis and Hathaway in 1967. Subsequently, other authors described symmetrical erosive polyarthritis with radiographic, serologic and pathologic features similar to rheumatoid arthritis in humans (Newton et al. 1976; Pedersen et al. 1976; Schumacher et al. 1980). Of particular interest is a description of Sjögren's syndrome-like illness in a female poodle with chronic inflammatory polyarthritis, sialoadenitis, thyroiditis and cholangiohepatitis (Pedersen et al. 1980).

Avian Autoimmune Diseases

In 1968, Bang and Bang described lymphocyte and plasma cell invasion of harderian and lacrimal glands in domestic chickens raised under germ free conditions. The similarities to sialoadenitis in humans suggested that domestic fowls may be useful in the study of Sjögren's syndrome. More recently, a syndrome of inherited dysgammaglobulinemia with Coombs positive hemolytic anemia, cryoglobulins and rheumatoid factor has been described in chickens (Gershwin et al. 1978). Although a detailed study of harderian, lacrimal and salivary glands for features of Sjögren's syndrome was not carried out in these animals, several parenchymal organs were infiltrated diffusely with inflammatory cells (Gershwin ME, personal communication).

Attempts to Induce Sjögren's Syndrome in Primates

Although patients with Sjögren's syndrome develop autoantibodies which react equally with human or monkey parotid gland or pancreas (Ludwig et al. 1977), there is no recognized nonhuman primate model of sialoadenitis. Felsenfeld (1972) reported unsuccessful attempts to induce Sjögren's syndrome in *Macaca speciosa* using repeated injections of autologous salivary gland tissue. In monkeys, bilateral greater petrosal neurectomy with subsequent loss of parasympathetic innervation of the lacrimal glands caused selective atrophy of serous cells. Total tear secretion was diminished to 4-8% of normal values 7-15 days after surgery. Long-term effects were not evaluated (Ruskell 1969).

Conclusions

In conclusion, there are several experimentally induced and spontaneous illnesses with features of Sjögren's syndrome in animals. Experimental models of sialoadenitis have been produced with salivary gland antigens, adjuvants and allogeneic antisera. Sialodacryoadenitis in the rat is an interesting model resulting from infection with a specific corona virus. Spontaneously occurring autoimmune diseases with features of Sjögren's syndrome in mice, dogs and domestic fowl were reviewed. Among these, autoimmune NZB, NZB/NZW, MRL/l and MRL/n mice develop destructive inflammation of lacrimal and salivary glands which resemble Sjögren's syndrome in humans. Canine keratoconjunctivitis sicca and inherited dysgammaglobulinemia in chickens may also be useful models, and additional studies should be undertaken to more fully characterize lacrimal and salivary gland inflammation in these animals. A large body of information describing potential laboratory models of Sjögren's syndrome is currently available, and it is apparent that animal models will advance our understanding of the pathogenesis and treatment of this disease. This review will introduce other investigators to these models and hopefully stimulate interest in future studies of the pathogenesis and treatment of Sjögren's syndrome.

Acknowledgment

We appreciate the assistance and encouragement of the late Harry S. Kessler, D.D.S. Mrs. Ruth Kessler generously allowed access to his experimental data and his previously unpublished photomicrographs. D.H. Dean, D.D.S., M.S., contributed Figure 1, and David L. Eisenbrandt, D.V.M., Ph.D. provided photomicrographs illustrating lesions of viral sialodacryoadenitis in the rat. Renee L. Kaswan, D.V.M., M.S. reviewed the manuscript and contributed photomicrographs illustrating canine keratoconjunctivitis sicca.

References

Aguirre GD, Rubin LF, Harvey CE (1971) Keratoconjunctivitis sicca in dogs. J Am Vet Med Assoc 158: 1566-1578
Andrews BS, Eisenberg RA, Theofilopoulos AN et al (1978) Spontaneous murine lupus-like syn-

dromes. Clinical and immunopathological manifestations in several strains. J Exp Med 148: 1198–1215
Bach M-A, Droz D, Noel L-H et al (1980) Effect of long-term treatment with circulating thymic factor on murine lupus. Arthritis Rheum 23: 1351–1358
Bang BG, Bang FB (1968) Localized lymphoid tissues and plasma cells in paraocular and paranasal organ systems in chickens. Am J Pathol 53: 735–751
Bellhorn RW (1981) Laboratory animal ophthalmology. In: Gelatt KN (ed) Veterinary ophthalmology. Lea and Febiger, Philadelphia, pp 649–671
Benedict AA, Tam LQ, Chanh TC et al (1980) Inherited 7 S immunoglobulin deficiency in chickens: Late onset dysgammaglobulinemia and evaluation of the lymphocyte proliferative responses and other immunologic functions. Clin Immunol Immunopathol 17: 1–14
Ben-Nun A, Cohen IR (1982) Experimental autoimmune encephalomyelitis (EAE) mediated by T cell lines: Process of selection of lines and characterization of the cells. J Immunol 129: 303–308
Beutner EH, Djanian AY, Geckler RC, Witebsky E (1961) Serological studies of rabbit antibodies to rabbit submaxillary glands. Proc Soc Exp Biol Med 107: 486–491
Bielschowsky M, Helyer BJ, Howie JB (1959) Spontaneous haemolytic anaemia in mice of the NZB/BL strain. Proc Univ Otago Med Sch 37: 9–11
Bloch KJ, Buchanan WW, Wohl MJ, Bunim JJ (1965) Sjögren's syndrome. A clinical, pathological, and serological study of sixty-two cases. Medicine (Baltimore) 44: 187–231
Boss JH, Rosenmann E, Sela J (1977) Experimental allergic sialoadenitis X. Chronic destructive parotitis induced in immunized rats by daily intraductal challenges with antigen. J Oral Pathol 6: 96–105
Brightman AH (1980) Keratoconjunctivitis sicca. Vet Med Today 176: 710–711
Carlsoo B, Ostberg Y (1978) Ultrastructural observations on the parotitis autoimmunica in the NZB/NZW hybrid mice. Acta Otolaryngol (Stockh) 85: 298–306
Carlsoo B, Ostberg Y (1979) The autoimmune submandibular sialoadenitis of the NZB/NZW hybrid mice. A light and electron microscopical investigation. Arch Otorhinolaryngol 225: 57–65
Chan WC (1964) Experimental sialo-adenitis in guinea-pigs. J Path Bact 88: 592–595
Dean DH, Hiramoto RN (1984) Experimental auto-allergic sialoadenitis in male rats. J Oral Pathol 13: 63–68
Dishon T, Sela J, Ulmansky M et al (1973) Experimental allergic sialoadenitis VI. Prevention by antihistamine and induction by intraductal instillation of preformed immune complexes. Virchows Arch [Pathol Anat] 359: 283–288
East J (1970) Immunopathology and neoplasms in New Zealand Black (NZB) and SJL-J mice. In: Hamburger F (ed) Progress in experimental tumor research Vol 13. S Karger, Basel, pp 84–134
Eisenbrandt DL, Hubbard GB, Schmidt RE (1982) A subclinical epizootic of sialodacryoadenitis in rats. Lab Anim Sci 32: 655–659
Felsenfeld O (1972) Autoimmune diseases. In: T-W-Fiennes RN (ed) Pathology of simian primates, part I: General pathology. Karger, New York, pp 380–398
Fox RI, Carstens SA, Fong S et al (1982) Use of monoclonal antibodies to analyze peripheral blood and salivary gland lymphocyte subsets in Sjögren's syndrome. Arthritis Rheum 25: 419–426
Fox RI, Howell FV, Bone RC, Michelson P (1984) Primary Sjögren's syndrome: Clinical and immunopathologic features. Semin Arthritis Rheum 14: 77–105
Gelatt KN, Gwin RM (1981) Canine lacrimal and nasolacrimal systems. In: Gelatt KN (ed) Veterinary ophthalmology. Lea and Febiger, Philadelphia, pp 309–329
Gelatt KN, Peiffer RL, Erickson JL, Gum GG (1968) Evaluation of tear formation in the dog, using a modification of the Schirmer tear test. J Am Vet Med Assoc 166: 368–370
Gershwin ME, Erickson K, Montero J et al (1980) The immunopathology of spontaneously acquired dysgammaglobulinemia in chickens. Clin Immunol Immunopathol 17: 15–30
Gershwin ME, Montero J, Eklund J et al (1978) Spontaneous autoimmune disease with associated acquired immune deficiency in chickens. In: Rose NR, Bigazzi PE, Warner NL (eds) Genetic control of autoimmune disease. Elsevier, New York, pp 271–284
Gleichmann E, Van Elven EH, Van der Veen JPW (1982) A systemic lupus erythematosus (SLE)-like disease in mice induced by abnormal T-B cell cooperation. Preferential formation of autoantibodies characteristic of SLE. Eur J Immunol 12: 152–159
Gratwhol AA, Moutsopoulos HM, Chused TM et al (1977) Sjögren-type syndrome after allogeneic bone-marrow transplantation. Ann Intern Med 87: 703–706
Greenspan JS, Gutman GA, Weissman IL, Talal N (1974) Thymus-antigen- and immunoglobulin-

positive lymphocytes in tissue infiltrates of NZB/NZW mice. Clin Immunol Immunopathol 3: 16-31
Haferkamp O (1962) Ein tierexperimenteller Beitrag zur Immunopathologie der Speicheldrüsen. Virchow Arch Path Anat 335: 298-322
Hahn BH, Shulman LE (1969) Autoantibodies and nephritis in the white strain (NZW) of New Zealand mice. Arthritis Rheum 12: 355-364
Halliwell REW (1978) Autoimmune disease in the dog. Adv Vet Sci Comp Med 22: 221-263
Halliwell REW (1982) Autoimmune diseases in domestic animals. J Am Vet Med Assoc 181: 1088-1096
Hang L, Theofilopoulos AN, Dixon FJ (1982) A spontaneous rheumatoid arthritis-like disease in MRL/l mice. J Exp Med 155: 1690-1701
Hayashi Y, Sato M, Hirokawa K (1985) Induction of experimental allergic sialadenitis in mice. Am J Pathol 118: 476-483
Hoffman RW, Alspaugh MA, Waggie KS et al (1984) Sjögren's syndrome in MRL/l and MRL/n mice. Arthritis Rheum 27: 157-165
Hoffman RW, Yang HK, Waggie KS et al (1983) Band keratopathy in MRL/l and MRL/n mice. Arthritis Rheum 26: 645-652
Holoshitz J, Naparstek Y, Ben-Nun A, Cohen IR (1983) Lines of T lymphocytes induce or vaccinate against autoimmune arthritis. Science 219: 56-58
Howie JB, Helyer BJ (1965) Autoimmune disease in mice. Ann NY Acad Sci 124: 167-177
Howie JB, Helyer BJ (1968) The immunology and pathology of NZB mice. In: Dixon FJ, Kunkel HG (eds) Advances in immunology Vol 9. Academic Press, New York, pp 215-266
Huston DP, Steinberg AD (1979) Animal models of human systemic lupus erythematosus. Yale J Biol Med 52: 289-305
Ichikawa Y, Takaya M, Arimori S (1982) Experimental induction of sialadenitis in rats by heterologous anti-salivary gland antibodies. Tokai J Exp Clin Med 7: 53-61
Innes JRM, Stanton MF (1961) Acute disease of the submaxillary and harderian glands (sialo-dacryoadenitis) of rats with cytomegaly and no inclusion bodies. Am J Pathol 38: 455-468
Jonas AM, Craft J, Black CL et al (1969) Sialodacryoadenitis in the rat. A light and electron microscopic study. Arch Pathol (Chicago) 88: 613-622
Kaplinsky N, Revach M, Katz WA (1980) Eosinophilic fasciitis: report of a case with features of connective tissue disease. J Rheumatol 7: 536-540
Kaswan RL, Martin CL, Chapman WL (1984) Keratoconjunctivitis sicca: Histopathologic study of nictitating membrane and lacrimal glands from 28 dogs. Am J Vet Res 45: 112-118
Kaswan RL, Martin CL, Dawe DL (1983) Rheumatoid factor determination in 50 dogs with keratoconjunctivitis sicca. J Am Med Vet Assoc 183: 1073-1075
Kaswan RL, Martin CL, Dawe DL (1985) Keratoconjunctivitis sicca: immunological evaluation of 62 canine cases. Am J Vet Res 46: 376-383
Kelley VE, Winkelstein A (1980) Age- and sex-related glomerulonephritis in New Zealand White mice. Clin Immunol Immunopathol 16: 142-150
Kessler HS (1968) A laboratory model for Sjögren's syndrome. Am J Pathol 52: 671-678
Kessler HS, Cubberly M, Manski W (1971) Eye changes in autoimmune NZB and NZB × NZW mice. Arch Ophthal 85: 211-219
Keyes GG, Vickers RA, Kersey JH (1977) Immunopathology of Sjögren-like disease in NZB/NZW mice. J Oral Pathol 6: 288-295
Kojima A, Fujinama F, Doi K et al (1980) Isolation and properties of sialodacryoadenitis virus of rats. Exp Anim 29: 409-418
Kurata Y, Watanabe Y, Okada S, Fukuyama Y (1969) Immunological studies of insoluble lipoproteins II. On the salivary gland characteristic antigens. Int Arch Allerg 35: 392-401
Lai YL, Jacoby RO, Bhatt PN, Jonas AM (1976) Keratoconjunctivitis associated with sialodacryoadenitis in rats. Invest Ophthalmol 15: 538-541
Lawley TJ, Peck GL, Moutsopoulos HM et al (1977) Scleroderma, Sjögren-like syndrome, and chronic graft-versus-host disease. Ann Intern Med 87: 707-709
Lewis RM (1974) Spontaneous autoimmune diseases of domestic animals. In: Richter GW, Epstein MA (eds) International review of experimental pathology Vol 13. Academic Press, New York, pp 55-82
Lewis RM, Hathaway JE (1967) Canine systemic lupus erythematosus; presenting with symmetrical polyarthritis. J Small Anim Pract 8: 273-284

Ludwig H, Schernthaner G, Scherak O, Kolarz G (1977) Antibodies to pancreatic duct cells in Sjögren's syndrome and rheumatoid arthritis. Gut 18: 311-315

Maron R, Zerubavel R, Friedman A, Cohen IR (1983) T lymphocyte line specific for thyroglobulin produces or vaccinates against autoimmune thyroiditis in mice. J Immunol 131: 2316-2322

McAdam LP, O'Hanlan MA, Bluestone R, Pearson CM (1976) Relapsing polychondritis: prospective study of 23 patients and a review of the literature. Medicine (Baltimore) 55: 193-215

McCabe BF (1961) The evidence for an auto-immune mechanism in Mikulicz's disease. Laryngoscope 71: 396-403

Montero J, Gershwin ME, Eklund J et al (1979) Autoimmune manifestations of selective 7S immunoglobulin deficiency of chickens. Clin Immunol Immunopathol 14: 334-347

Moutsopoulos HM, Chused TM, Mann DL et al (1980) Sjögren's syndrome (sicca syndrome): current issues. Ann Intern Med 92: 212-226

Moutsopoulos HM, Klippel JH, Pavlidis N et al (1980) Correlative histologic and serologic findings of sicca syndrome in patients with systemic lupus erythematosus. Arthritis Rheum 23: 36-40

Murphy ED (1981) Lymphoproliferation (lpr) and other single-locus models for murine lupus. In: Gershwin ME, Merchant B (eds) Immunological defects in laboratory animals Vol 2. Plenum, New York, pp 143-173

Naparstek Y, Ben-Nun A, Holoshitz J et al (1983) T lymphocyte lines producing or vaccinating against autoimmune encephalomyelitis (EAE). Functional activation induces peanut agglutinin receptors and accumulation in the brain and thymus of line cells. Eur J Immunol 13: 418-423

Newton CD, Lipowtiz AJ, Halliwell RE et al (1976) Rheumatoid arthritis in dogs. J Am Vet Med Assoc 168: 113-121

O'Sullivan FX, Fassbender H-G, Gay S, Koopman WJ (1985) Etiopathogenesis of the rheumatoid arthritis-like disease in MRL/l mice. I. The histomorphologic basis of joint destruction. Arthritis Rheum 28: 529-536

Pals ST, Radaszkiewicz T, Gleichmann E (1984) Allosuppressor- and allohelper-T cells in acute and chronic graft-versus-host disease. J Immunol 132: 1669-1678

Pedersen NC, Pool RC, Castles JJ, Weisner K (1976) Noninfectious canine arthritis: rheumatoid arthritis. J Am Vet Med Assoc 169: 295-303

Quimby FW, Schwartz RS, Poskitt T, Lewis RM (1979) A disorder of dogs resembling Sjögren's syndrome. Clin Immunol Immunopathol 12: 471-476

Ramos-Niembro F, Alarcon-Segovia D (1979) Development of sicca symptoms in systemic lupus erythematosus patients with existing subclinical abnormalities of lacrimal and/or salivary glands. Arthritis Rheum 22: 935-936

Rosenmann E, Sela J, Ulmansky M et al (1974) Experimental allergic sialoadenitis II. Induction of acute sialoadenitis in rats by locally administered basement membrane antibodies. Oral Surg 37: 566-575

Ruskell GL (1969) Changes in nerve terminals and acini of the lacrimal gland and changes in secretion induced by autonomic denervation. Z Zellforsch 94: 261-281

Schot LPC, Verheul HAM, Schuurs AHWM (1984) Effect of nandrolone decanoate on Sjögren's syndrome like disorders in NZB/NZW mice. Clin Exp Immunol 57: 571-574

Schumacher HR, Newton C, Halliwell REW (1980) Synovial pathologic changes in spontaneous canine rheumatoid-like arthritis. Arthritis Rheum 23: 412-423

Sela J, Bab JA, Dishon T et al (1975) Experimental allergic sialoadenitis. VII. Reactivity of the parotid gland to antigenic challenge in passively immunized rats. J Oral Pathol 4: 11-18

Sela J, Dishon T, Rosenmann E et al (1973) Experimental allergic sialoadenitis V. Comparison of the response of the parotid gland and synovial membrane to multiple antigenic challenges. J Oral Pathol 2: 7-15

Sela J, Ulmansky M, Dishon T et al (1972) Experimental allergic sialoadenitis I. Acute sialoadenitis induced by a local immune reaction. Virchows Arch [Pathol Anat] 335: 213-219

Sharawy M, White SC (1978) Morphometric and fine structural study of experimental autoallergic sialadenitis of rat submandibular glands. Virchows Arch [Cell Pathol] 28: 255-273

Shulman HM, Sale GE, Lerner KG et al (1978) Chronic cutaneous graft-versus-host disease in man. Am J Pathol 91: 545-564

Sjögren H (1933) Zur Kenntnis der keratoconjunctivitis sicca. Acta Ophthalmol [Suppl] (Copenh) 11: 48-97

Slatter DH, Blogg JR (1978) Keratoconjunctivitis sicca in dogs associated with sulphonamide administration. Aust Vet J 54: 444-446

Takeda Y, Ishikawa G (1983) Experimental autoallergic sialadenitis in mice: Histopathological and ultrastructural studies. Virchows Arch [Pathol Anat] 400: 143–154
Takeda Y, Komori A, Ishikawa G (1981) Histopathological study of the salivary glands in SL/Ni mice. Jpn J Oral Biol 23: 427–438
Teichert VG (1966) Plasmazellulare Infiltration des dritten Augenlides beim Hund. Berl München Tieraerzl Wschr 79: 449–451
Theofilopoulos AN, Dixon FJ (1985) Murine models of systemic lupus erythematosus. In: Dixon FJ (ed) Advances in immunology Vol 37. Academic Press, New York, pp 269–390
Theofilopoulos AN, McConahey PJ, Izui S et al (1980) A comparative immunologic analysis of several murine strains with autoimmune manifestations. Clin Immunol Immunopathol 15: 258–278
Ulmansky M, Dishon T, Rosenmann E et al (1972) Experimental allergic sialoadenitis IV. Studies on the etiopathogenetic mechanisms of the acute and chronic inflammatory process. Isr J Med Sci 8: 1791–1797
Van Rappard-Van der Veen FM, Kiesel U, Poels L et al (1984) Further evidence against random polyclonal antibody formation in mice with lupus-like graft-vs-host disease. J Immunol 132: 1814–1820
Weill JC, Goldberg M (1976) Intracellular modifications induced in mouse submaxillary glands by antibodies directed against saliva. Immunology 31: 397–405
Whaley K, Alspaugh MA (1985) Sjögren's syndrome. In: Kelley WN, Harris ED, Ruddy S, Sledge CB (eds) Textbook of rheumatology, 2nd ed. Saunders, Philadelphia, pp 956–978
Whaley K, MacSween RNM (1974) Experimental induction of immune sialadenitis in guinea-pigs using different adjuvants. Clin Exp Immunol 17: 681–684
White SC, Casarett GW (1974) Induction of experimental autoallergic sialadenitis. J Immunol 112: 178–185
White SC (1976) T-cell dependence of experimental autoallergic lesions of rat submandibular glands. J Dent Res 55: B 299 (abstract)

IV. Treatment of Sjögren's Syndrome

Treatment of Sjögren's Syndrome

N. Talal and H. M. Moutsopoulos

Patients with Sjögren's syndrome should be seen regularly by a rheumatologist, an ophthalmologist, and a dentist. They need to be followed closely for significant functional deterioration, superimposed signs of disease complications or significant changes in the course of the disease. For example, regular outpatient visits with serial observations of pertinent laboratory parameters may allow for the early diagnosis of extraglandular complications or malignancy.

Sjögren's syndrome is often a neglected disease, adding greatly to the distress of the patient. The physician must remember that there is nothing minor about the symptoms of dry eyes and dry mouth. A patient of mine once wrote that "Sjögren's is misery" and so it often seems to the sufferer.

Treatment of the Glandular Disease

Ophthalmologic (Keratoconjunctivitis Sicca, KCS)

The patient may notice accumulation of thick ropy secretions along the inner canthus owing to a decreased tear film and an abnormal mucus component. Related complaints include erythema, photosensitivity, eye fatigue, decreased visual acuity, and the sensation of a "film" across the field of vision. Desiccation can cause small superficial erosions of the corneal epithelium. Slit lamp examination may reveal filamentary keratitis (filaments of corneal epithelium and debris) in severe cases. Conjunctivitis caused by Staphyloccus aureus is a complication.

The low level of humidity in air-conditioned environments may make these symptoms worse. Similar problems arise in windy or dry climates. Cigarette smoking and drugs with anticholinergic side effects may also increase symptoms. The most frequently implicated drugs are phenothiazines, tricyclic anti-depressants, antispasmodics, anti-Parkinsonian and decongestant medications. Many of these are available over-the-counter.

The mainstay of treatment for dry eyes is lubrication through the use of artificial tear drops which can be used as often as necessary (generally every 1-3 hours). A variety of such drops are readily available without prescription, differing primarily in viscosity and preservative. The thicker, more viscous drops require less frequent application, although they can cause blurring and leave a residue on the lashes. Many patients will prefer the thinner drops which require more frequent applications. Patients generally test several different preparations to determine which one is best for them. An apparent failure to respond to artificial tears may actually reflect eye irritation resulting from the topical application of preservatives such as benzalkonium chloride, chlorbutanol or thimerosal. Also available are lubricating ointments which may produce significant blurring and are best used at night to provide protection over a longer period.

More recently, a slow release tear has been marketed under the trade name *Lacrisert (Merck, Sharp and Dohme)*. It is a polymer of hydroxypropyl cellulose and comes as a cylinder which is inserted every 6-12 hours below the inferior tarsal margin. It absorbs the tears, slowly dissolves, and releases polymer. It is particularly useful in those patients who otherwise would use tear substitutes as frequently as every fifteen minutes.

Other steps can be taken to preserve tears if tear substitutes are insufficient to control symptoms. Water tight swimmer's goggles can be very helpful in creating a moist chamber effect by preventing evaporation. They also protect against wind and dust particles. The same effect can be achieved with ordinary food plastic wrap taped over the eyes. Commercial "bubble" bandages are also available.

Soft contact lenses may also help to protect the cornea, especially when filaments are a problem. However, the lenses themselves require wetting and the patients must be followed very carefully because there is an increased risk of infection. Such lenses are invaluable in the management of corneal ulcers which can arise as a complication of KCS.

Punctal occlusion is another method of conserving the few tears that patients produce. This procedure should be considered only in severe cases when there seems little likelihood of spontaneous increase in tear flow. Stents have been devised as a nonsurgical means of occlusion; this is a good way to predict the success of surgical occlusion.

Autonomic stimulation of tear flow has been relatively neglected as a form of therapy because the eye drops have generally worked well. Sympthomimetics and parasympathomimetics, especially the muscarinics, serve to stimulate tear flow. Pilocarpine taken orally has been reported as successful, as has bromhexine and psysalaemin.

In patients with a relative excess of mucin production and formation of filaments, a mucolytic agent such as acetylcysteine has been found to be useful. However other investigators have failed to confirm this.

Topical steroid use for the corneal ulcers of Sjögren's syndrome was associated with a worsening clinical course and is not recommended.

Two new approaches to topical therapy have recently been suggested. One is the use of dilute sodium hyaluronate. This compound has recently been approved for intraocular surgery, and the authors advocate making a ten per cent diluted solution for topical use. Another group of investigators have developed a procedure for taking the patient's own serum and using this as an artificial tear (Fox et al. 1984). Both of these possibilities are somewhat tedious and need further study before final recommendations can be made.

Salivary

Xerostomia is often the initial symptom of Sjögren's syndrome. However, it is a common and subjective clinical complaint with a large variety of etiologies including emotional factors, sialodochitis, chronic sialadenitis, various drugs already listed, irradiation and dehydration. It is best considered a relatively nonspecific finding requiring further evaluation by careful history, physical examination and often labial salivary gland biopsy to confirm the presence of significant lymphocytic infiltrates attaining a focus score compatible with autoimmune exocrinopathy (i.e., Sjögren's syndrome).

Complaints resulting from dryness of the mouth are varied. The "cracker sign" describes the difficulties encountered in trying to eat dry foods without sufficient lubrication. A positive "cracker sign" is almost diagnostic of true Sjögren's syndrome. Many subjects require frequent ingestion of liquids. They may resort to carrying water bottles or candy in purse or pocket. Additional features include oral soreness, adherence of food to buccal surfaces, fissuring of the tongue, and dysphagia. Angular cheilitis associated with superimposed candidiasis may occur. Patients may lose the ability to discriminate foods on the basis of taste and smell. Dental caries are accelerated. The parotid gland enlarges in many patients secondary to cellular infiltration and ductal obstruction. Usually asymptomatic and self-limited, the enlargement can be recurrent and associated with pain or erythema. Local heat and analgesics are often helpful. Because of the potential risk of malignancy, ionizing irradiation to the parotid glands is not recommended.

Treatment of xerostomia associated with Sjögren's syndrome is difficult. No single highly effective method is currently available, and most efforts are aimed only at palliation. Before any treatment program is started, it is important to identify contributing factors such as mouth breathing, heavy smoking and drugs with anticholinergic side effects which further decrease salivary flow. Stimulation of salivary flow by sucrose-free, highly flavored lozenges or chewing gums, use of lemon-flavored drinks, and dietary counseling to avoid particularly dry foods may also be of assistance. Most patients discover that it is helpful to carry water, sugarless lemon drops or chewing gums. These must be sugar-free because of the risk of rampant dental caries. Fluids ad libitum should be utilized for all meals and snacks, which should also begin and finish with highly flavored substances which tend to stimulate salivary flow. The consumption of large amounts of water during the day, while symptomatically helpful, may produce nocturia that interrupts sleep patterns and leads to fatigue.

Artificial saliva substitutes offer some additional palliation. Mucin-containing saliva substitutes seem to be more effective than substitutes based on carboxymethyl cellulose or polyethylenoxide. Mucins tend to protect against desiccation, provide for lubrication and cleaning and appear to have some antimicrobial effect. Saliva substitutes should, however, be utilized sparingly with only the minimum volume necessary for oral lubrication. This usually consists of no more than 2.0 ml before and after meals, at bedtime and following oral hygiene. The material can also be applied to any removable intraoral appliance to facilitate more sustained release.

Topical or oral treatment with stannous fluoride enhances dental mineralization retards damage to tooth surfaces. In cases of rapidly progressive dental disease, the fluoride can be directly applied to the teeth from plastic trays that are used at night. This latter method may be inconvenient but provides better exposure of gingival margins to the fluoride.

Increased salivary flow rates may be induced by potassium iodide or parasympathomimetic agents such as pilocarpine or neostigmine, systemically or as a mouthwash. Varying degrees of success have been noted. A new battery-powered electronic device for stimulating salivary flow has recently been developed and is currently under study. Bromhexine, a synthetic alkaloid originally used as a mucolytic agent in cough syrups, has been tried with limited success (Frost-Larsen et al. 1978; Nahir et al. 1981).

Increased moisture to the upper airways by use of normal saline sprays and humidifiers at night may reduce respiratory symptoms and alleviate mouth breathing. In some cases, nasal irrigation with normal saline proves helpful.

Vaginal dryness is treated with lubricants such as K-Y jelly, and dry skin with moisturizing lotions.

Treatment of Extranglandular Disease

Systemic corticosteroids and immunosuppressive drugs are only used to treat potentially life threatening disease, often involving the lung or kidney. They are not recommended for the treatment of dry eyes and dry mouth. No controlled studies have been performed because relatively few patients require systemic treatment.

A diffuse interstitial pneumonitis resulting from lymphocytic infiltration and fibrosis may cause severe exertional dyspnea. Obstructive disease (in the absence of smoking) may result from lymphocytic infiltration surrounding small airways. Pulmonary function tests should be performed and monitored twice per year to determine the extent of functional impairment. Lung biopsy should be performed before treatment is started. There is a better chance for therapeutic success if a highly cellular infiltrate is found. Conversely, one may decide against treatment if only scar tissue is present on lung biopsy.

Treatment is usually initiated with corticosteroids in the range of 0.5–1 mg/kg daily. As the patient improves, the dose can be tapered to a maintenance level 50% of the starting dose. If there is no apparent response within 3–6 months, steroids should be discontinued and a trial of cyclophosphamide considered. A range of 100 mg/day is a good starting dose. Cyclophosphamide has succeeded when other immunosuppressive drugs have been tried first and failed. Although the risk of lymphoma is an important theoretical consideration, in our experience it has not appeared in Sjögren's syndrome patients treated with cyclophosphamide.

The most common renal abnormalities in Sjögren's syndrome involve the tubules, particularly overt or latent renal tubular acidosis. Potassium and bicarbonate are generally sufficient to control the hyperchloremic acidosis. Steroids were successful in one patient (El-Mallakh et al. 1985) but we prefer cyclophosphamide (100 mg/day) based on personal experience. Peripheral and cranial neuropathy has been associated with vasculitis involving the vasa nervorum. Although there is little data concerning the treatment of this complication, bolus cyclophosphamide in a dose of 0.5 to 0.75 gm/meter^2 may be of benefit.

The incidence of lymphoma is increased 44-fold in Sjögren's syndrome. Pseudomalignant or malignant lymphoproliferation may be present initially or may develop later in the illness. Most lymphomas belong to the B cell lineage, although the histologic appearance is variable. A diminution of previously elevated immunoglobulins and loss of autoantibodies may precede a malignant transformation. Pseudolymphoma is an intermediate stage in this transition from benign to malignant lymphoproliferation.

The distinction between lymphoma and pseudolymphoma may be difficult even in the hands of highly experienced and expert pathologists. Some patients with pseudolymphoma may not require treatment if there is no functional compromise. If there is, treatment of pseudolymphoma with corticosteroids or cyclophosphamide is often successful. Treatment of lymphoma and decisions regarding chemotherapy and/or radiation therapy should be guided by experienced oncologists. In general, these lesions are highly refractory to treatment.

Use of Nonsteroidal Agents and Other Medications in Sjögren's Syndrome

Treatment of secondary Sjögren's syndrome is usually directed at the associated disease. The treatment of rheumatoid arthritis or systemic lupus erythematosus is not altered because of the concommitant presence of Sjögren's syndrome. The sicca complex is generally milder and managed as already discussed. Arthralgias or myalgias are managed with salicylates or nonsteroidal anti-inflammatory drugs.

References

El-Mallakh R, Bryan RK, Masi AT, Kelly CE, Rakowski KJ (1985) Long-term low-dose glucocorticoid therapy associated with remission of overt renal tubular acidosis in Sjögren's syndrome. Am J of Med 79: 509-514

Fox RI, Chan R, Michelson JB, Belmont JB, Michelson PE (1984) Beneficial effect of artificial tears made with autologous serum in patients with keratoconjunctivitis sicca. Arth and Rheum 27 (4): 459-461

Frost-Larsen K, Isager H, Manthorpe R (1978) Sjögren's syndrome treated with bromhexine: a randomized clinical study. Br Med J I: 579-1581

Nahir AM, Scharf Y, Ben-Aryeh H, Szargel R, Gutman D, Zonis S, Scharf J (1981) Effect of prolonged bromhexine therapy on Sjögren's syndrome. Israel J Med Sc 17 (6): 403-406

Subject Index

MIX
Papier aus verantwortungsvollen Quellen
Paper from responsible sources
FSC® C105338
FSC
www.fsc.org

If you have any concerns about our products,
you can contact us on
ProductSafety@springernature.com

In case Publisher is established outside the EU,
the EU authorized representative is:
Springer Nature Customer Service Center GmbH
Europaplatz 3, 69115 Heidelberg, Germany

Printed by Libri Plureos GmbH
in Hamburg, Germany